NUTRITION AND AIDS

NUTRITION AND AIDS

KHOMDON SINGH LISAM
SUCHITRA LISAM

KALPAZ

Nutrition and AIDS

ISBN: 978-81-7835-733-1

Published in 2009 in India by
Kalpaz Publications
C-30, Satyawati Nagar,
Delhi-110052
E-mail: kalpaz@hotmail.com
Phone : 9212729499

Lasser Type Setting by: Rudra Computer Graphics, Delhi
Printed at : Singhal Print Media, Delhi

Dedication

This book entitled "Nutrition and AIDS" is dedicated to the people living with HIV-AIDS in India.

Contents

Foreword

Today, there are more than 40 million people living with HIV/AIDS in the world. More than 95% of all the HIV infected people now live in the developing countries. UNAIDS has reported that there are 2.5 million HIV infections in India by December, 2007. HIV/AIDS has affected not only the vulnerable population but also their spouses, children and other family members and communities. It reduces household's capacities to produce and purchase food, depletes their assets and exhaust social safety nets. Nutritional deficiencies may appear in any stage of HIV infection. The importance of nutrition in the overall management of HIV/AIDS can not be over –emphasised. Timely improvement in nutritional status can help strengthen the immune system, thereby reducing the incidence of infections, preventing loss of body weight and lean body mass, and delaying disease progression. Good nutrition can help boost immune function, maximize the effectiveness of antiretroviral therapy, reduce the risk of chronic illnesses and contribute to a better quality of life. Good Nutrition is not a cure for HIV. Nutrition and HIV are closely linked. Good nutrition means eating such variety of foods each day that will give adequate proteins, fats, carbohydrates, vitamins, minerals to keep our body strong. Good nutrition can prevent many of the complications of HIV/AIDS and can improve adherence to antiretroviral drugs.

Dr. Khomdon Singh Lisam has been involved in the HIV/AIDS control programme in India since 1990. He worked as the Project Director of the Manipur State AIDS Control Society during 1995-2003. He also worked in Thailand and Myanmar in 2003 as a member of the UNODC, Yangon. He worked as a Consultant (IDUs and

Training) under the NACO and Clinton Foundation in 2005-2006. He was invited as a resource person in many countries including South Africa, Bangladesh, Nepal, Thailand and Myanmar. He has done extensive research work in HIV/AIDS in 1992 in the University of Leeds, UK and has also studied many HIV/AIDS and Drug abuse prevention projects in many countries including USA, U.K. Spain, Italy, France, Nepal, Bangladesh, Myanmar, Thailand, South Africa, Uganda and also in almost all the states in India. He was instrumental in the development of Manipur State AIDS Policy in October, 1996, which is the first and only State Policy on HIV/AIDS in India till date. He was the person who introduced the first Harm Reduction project in India called the "Rapid Intervention and Care(RIAC)" project in November, 1998. Today, this project is the first and biggest Harm Reduction project in the Government sector in the whole of South and South East Asia. After implementation of this project, the HIV seroprevalence rate among the IDUs in Manipur has shown a decline from 80.7% in 1997 to 19.8% in 2006.

Dr. Suchitra Lisam is presently working as a Senior Manager of Knowledge Management and HIV/AIDS in the International Federation of Red Cross and Red Crescents, New Delhi. She is looking after the HIV/AIDS projects in Afghanistan, Nepal, Bangladesh, Sri Lanka under the International Federation of Red Cross and Red Crescents.

I am confident that this book will be immensely useful to the people living with HIV/AIDS and organizations working in the field of HIV/AIDS and nutrition. I congratulate Dr. Khomdon Singh Lisam and Dr. Suchitra Lisam for bringing out such a useful book.

L.P. Gonmei
Commissioner (Health and Family Welfare)
Government of Manipur

Foreword

I am a young man with all the energy, hopes and aspirations in life. I have a lovely wife and one daughter who is 9 (nine) year old. I am co-infected with HIV and HCV but fortunately my wife and my child is found to be negative and I am open to public for the last 11 years. I have never experienced any kind of human rights violations from any quarter, personally in my life, except to some of my near and dear colleagues of MNP+. But I am living under constant fear of death, not from HIV but HCV. Many of my friends have already died of AIDS and HCV. And I think I will also die within 2 years if I am not treated of HCV. But advantage of antiretroviral treatment has changed my thinking, to some extent; I've no doubt that I may live a longer and healthier life thanks to antiretroviral therapy. This means I'm starting to expect things from life-not least enjoyment and fulfillment. I'm no longer prepared to accept the day -to-day drudge that accompanied my pre-treatment days with HIV

I understand that good nutrition is extremely important for a person with HIV. I have to concentrate on eating a wide variety of foods each day. There is no one type of food that has everything our bodies needs. I have to choose from the variety of foods according to my nutritional needs. Earlier, I never realized the impact of HIV on nutrition and vice versa. The doctors treating me hardly emphasized the importance of nutrition and diet in the overall medical treatment for HIV/AIDS. The importance of a good nutrition increases many fold when you are taking antiretroviral treatment. This fact was not given due priority by the medical specialist and counselors.

I had a lot of difficulty as the President of the Manipur Network of Positive People in finding resource material /books on nutrition, in local context, for people living with HIV/AIDS. It is very unfortunate that NACO and the Government of India is not giving due importance to the nutritional component of HIV/AIDS management under the NACO programme. The help and assistance from the international donor agencies is not addressing the real problem.

I have read the book entitled "Nutritional and HIV/AIDS" written by Dr. Khomdon Singh Lisam and Dr. Suchitra Lisam. Dr. Khomdon Singh Lisam needs no introduction as he is one of pioneer in India in the field of HIV/AIDS. Dr. Khomdon Singh Lisam has written many books on HIV/AIDS earlier. This is his fourth book on HIV/AIDS. Dr. Suchitra Lisam is working as a senior Manager of HIV/AIDS in the International Federation of Red Cross and Red Crescents, New Delhi. Her contribution in the field of HIV/AIDS is also commendable. The book covers all the important topics on the nutrition and HIV/AIDS. I found the book quite interesting, exhaustive, easily understandable, readable and useful for people living with HIV/AIDS.

I strongly recommend this book as a reference resource book for people with HIV/AIDS and even for common people interested in nutrition.

L. Deepak Singh
President
Manipur Network of Positive People
(MNP+)

Preface

Being diagnosed with HIV will be one of the most significant events in your life. It's very difficult to predict exactly what emotions and feelings you'll experience in the first few hours and days after finding out you have HIV. However, commonly reported reactions include feeling numb, frightened, upset, tearful, desperate or angry.

Finding out that you are HIV-positive puts you in a position where you can start to take steps to look after your health. Although there's no cure for HIV and it can still be fatal, there are treatments which mean that people with HIV can live much longer and healthier lives. The sooner your HIV infection is diagnosed, the sooner you can receive appropriate medical care.

The fact that you have HIV might be the only information you can absorb on the day of your diagnosis. You should have had post-test counselling after you received your test result, and you may have been able to ask a few questions at this stage. There are no right or wrong questions to ask, and don't worry if you didn't understand everything you were told. There'll be opportunities to get more information later. It's perfectly okay to want the most basic information, such as, 'What's the difference between HIV and AIDS?' Or, 'How long before HIV makes me ill?' Or, 'How long can I survive ? "The first chapter of this book, 'Basic Facts about HIV/ AIDS", should answer your questions.

You may also come across lots of medical terms you don't understand. Always ask your doctor, a nurse or a pharmacist to explain anything you don't understand, and ask for written information if you still have questions or uncertainties. If you want more detailed information on a particular topic, the chances are that there'll be a chapter in this book focusing on the subject you're interested in. You are going to need specialist medical care for your HIV. Most people in India are tested for HIV at VCTC/ITCT (although some people are diagnosed through other medical services). The doctor, nurse or counsellor who gave you your test result should have made a follow-up appointment for you to see a specialist HIV doctor. If this wasn't arranged, you need to make sure that you are registered with a specialist doctor who is expert and knowledgeable about HIV/AIDS as soon as possible.

If you are well at the time of your HIV diagnosis, you'll probably need to go to the clinic for a check-up every three months or so. At your appointment with your doctor you'll have an opportunity to discuss your health and ask questions, and you will have some blood tests such as CD4 count to monitor your health. Immediately after your diagnosis can be a difficult time to make major decisions. These decisions might include who to tell about your HIV diagnosis or when to start anti-HIV treatment. Take time to think about who you are going to tell that you are HIV-positive. Think about why you want to tell them and how you are going to tell them. Can you anticipate their best or worst reactions? Begin by telling the people closest to you, who will be the most supportive.

It's highly unlikely that you are asked to start taking anti-HIV treatment the day you found out that you were HIV-positive. It's more likely that your health will be monitored, so both you and your doctor can understand how your body is coping with HIV. If your immune system has already been weakened by HIV, then the decision to start taking anti-HIV drugs to prevent you getting the infections and illnesses to which HIV can make you vulnerable will be a more pressing one. But anti-HIV treatment is something that you will need to consider sooner or later.

Food is important for everyone. When we eat well we feel well. Nutrition plays an important role in helping the immune system of our bodies work well. When we feed our bodies well, most of us feel better and have a more positive attitude about life. Eating tasty meals with people who care about us can be wonderful "medicine" for our emotional health. Food provides the energy and nutrients that our bodies need to stay alive, move and work; build new cells and tissues for growth, maintenance and repair; resist and fight infections. When the body does not get enough food, it becomes weak and cannot develop or function properly. Healthy and balanced nutrition means eating the right type of foods in the right quantities to keep healthy, keep fit and enjoy ourselves. Good nutrition means eating such variety of foods each day that will give you adequate proteins, fats, carbohydrates, vitamins, minerals to keep your body strong. Good nutrition can help boost immune function, maximize the effectiveness of antiretroviral therapy, reduce the risk of chronic illnesses such as diabetes and cardiovascular disease, and contribute to a better quality of life.

There are many ways in which HIV/AIDS can affect the body's nutritional status . HIV increases the body's metabolic demands which, in turn, increase the amount of calories and protein needed to maintain body weight and muscle mass. HIV infects intestinal epithelial cells which can compromise your body's ability to absorb nutrients from food and medications. HIV/AIDS, opportunistic infections and some medications can decrease, or even eliminate your appetite, increasing the risk for weight loss and wasting. Some antiretroviral therapies can increase your cardiovascular risk factors by altering your cholesterol, triglyceride and glucose levels. Good nutrition helps keep your immune system strong, enabling you to fight the disease better . A healthy diet improves quality of life. Weight loss, wasting, and malnutrition continue to be common problems in HIV, despite more effective antiretroviral medications, and can contribute to HIV disease progression. Good nutrition helps the body process the many medications taken by people with HIV. Diet (and exercise) may help with symptoms such as diarrhoea, nausea, and fatigue, and with fat redistribution and metabolic abnormalities such as high blood sugar, cholesterol, and triglycerides. Good Nutrition is not a cure for HIV. But nutrition is one key element in the medical management of HIV.

In India, nutrition is yet to be included as an important component of the National AIDS Control Programme. There is not much resource materials available on nutrition and HIV/AIDS in India. The purpose of this book is to fill up the existing gap and to provide basic information on nutrition in relation to HIV/AIDS. It is hoped that the book will be useful as a resource material /

reference book for people with HIV/AIDS, for the State AIDS Control Societies and for NGOs and other agencies working in the field of HIV/AIDS and nutrition.

Dr. Suchitra Lisam
Dr. Khomdon Singh Lisam

Acknowledgements

The authors gratefully acknowledge the help, support and encouragement received from the following persons in bringing out this publication.

- Mr. L.P. Gonmei, Commissioner (Health and Family Welfare), Government of Manipur.
- Dr. B. S. Banerjee', Project Director, Delhi State AIDS Control Society.
- Kh. Pramodkumar Singh, Project Director, Manipur State AIDS Control Society.
- J.C. Dewri, Former Project Director, Assam State AIDS Control Society.
- Dr. Kumuni Kathipri, Director, Family Welfare, Nagaland.
- Dr. K. Ropari, Project Director, Mizoram State AIDS Control Society.
- Dr. A.K. Gupta, Additional Project Director, Delhi State AIDS Control Society.
- Mr. L. Rabindra Singh, District and Sessions Judge, Manipur (Retired).
- Sh. Naresh Kumar Sharma, Classic Offset Printers & Packagers, Delhi.
- Shri Ashok Mangla, Faridabad, Haryana.
- Kh. Kuleswar Singh, Proprietor, Video Film Production Centre, Singjamei Keithel.
- L. Deepak Singh, President, Manipur Network of Positive People.
- Mr. Rajesh Nair, Former, NGO Consultant, National AIDS Control Organization (NACO).

- Dr. Hemchandra Barman, Deputy Director, Assam State AIDS Control Society.
- Dr. Maisnam Damayanti Devi, Deputy Director of Health Services, Manipur.
- Mr. Umananda Lisam, Southern Palace Compound, Imphal.
- Mrs. Sapam Sandhyarani Devi, Southern Palace Compound, Palace Road, Imphal.
- Mr. Dayanand Lisam, Southern Palace Compound, Palace Road, Imphal Imphal.
- Korou Lisam, Southern Palace Compound, Palace Road, Imphal Imphal.
- Hyeithoi Lisam, Southern Palace Compound, Palace Road, Imphal Imphal.
- Seilendro Thokchom, Office Asstt, AIDS Consortium, Delhi.

Dr. Khomdon Singh Lisam
Dr. Suchitra Lisam

1

Basic Facts about HIV/AIDS

What is AIDS?

AIDS stands for Acquired Immuno Deficiency Syndrome. Acquired means that AID is not inborn, not inherited (many other immuno-deficiency diseases are inherited) but acquired from outside the human body; Immuno- deficiency means that the body's defence system has been weakened or damaged rendering the person unable to defend himself against diseases. Syndrome means a collection of signs and symptoms resulting from a single cause that together manifest a definite clinical picture.

The term, AIDS ; Acquired Immuno-Deficiency Syndrome (AIDS) was coined in 1982.

The first report on what is now known as AIDS appeared on the 5th June, 1981 in the Morbidity and Mortality Weekly Report Centre, published by the Centre for Disease Control (CDC), Atlanta , USA. Eight previously healthy young homosexual men had been treated for biopsy-confirmed Pneumocystis Carinii Pneumonia (PCP) at three different hospitals in Los Angeles between October 1980 and May, 1981

AIDS is a long, often painful and fatal disease that develops in people up to a decade or more after they have been infected by the Human Immuno-deficiency virus (HIV). AIDS is the late stage of HIV infection . It has got no cure, no effective treatment, no vaccine for its prevention till date. The only vaccine available against AIDS to day is education.

What is HIV ?

HIV stands for Human Immuno deficiency Virus, the virus that causes AIDS. Since HIV is the causative organism for AIDS, sometimes it is called AIDS virus. The virus was isolated in 1983 by Dr. Luc Montagnier and his team at the Pasteur Institute of Paris, France from the patients with AIDS, presenting themselves with persistent lymph-adenopathy and hence called it Lymphadenopathy Associated Virus (LAV).

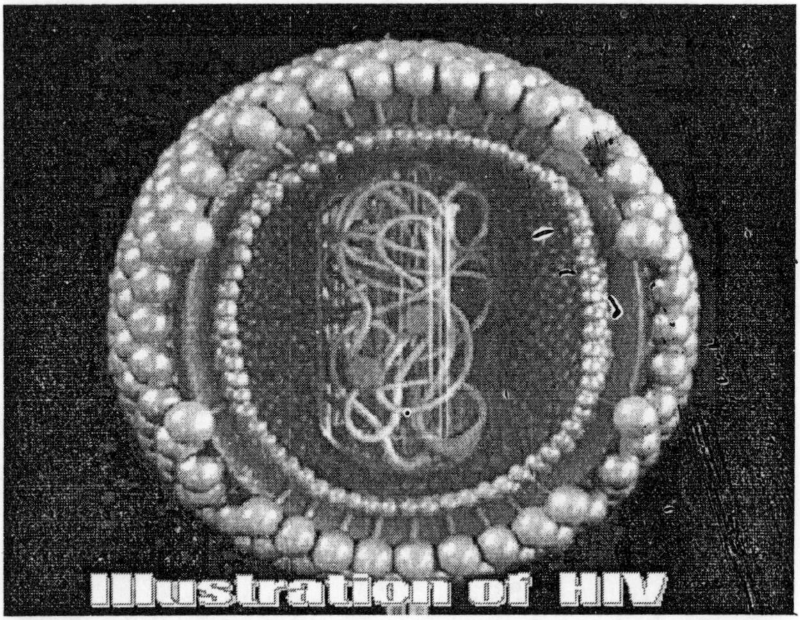

How HIV enters the body ?

The HIV invades selectively the blood cells which bear the necessary viral receptor on their surfaces. This site is called the CD-4 antigen. Chief amongst these cells are White Blood Cells, the CD-4 or T-Helper cells. HIV invades cells which carry CD-4 antigen on their surface. The virus first fuses with the CD-4 receptor site. It is then pulled inside the cell. The outside of the virus particle is stripped off and the virus RNA without its attached enzyme "reverse transcriptase" is released into the cell. Once free, the RNA makes a copy of itself in DNA. The virus then breaks the DNA in the cell's own chromosomes and then builds itself into the break. Once a person is infected with the virus, it becomes a part of the make-up of the cells of that person. It is for this reason that someone infected with the virus will stay infected for life. When the cell's own DNA become active, the viral DNA carried within it is also activated. As the cell's DNA is replicated the viral DNA is also replicated to produce more of viral proteins. These then leave the infected cell, stealing part of the cell wall to produce more virus particles and infect other cells and other people. Eventually, the infected cell dies as a result of viral load. This process can go on ultimately leading to destruction of more and more of CD4 (T-4) cells causing immuno deficiency, which renders the person unable to fight infections and tumours. This may lead to the reversal of the CD4 -CD8 (T-4/T-8) ratio. The micro organisms which cannot produce infection or disease in a person with a normally functioning immune

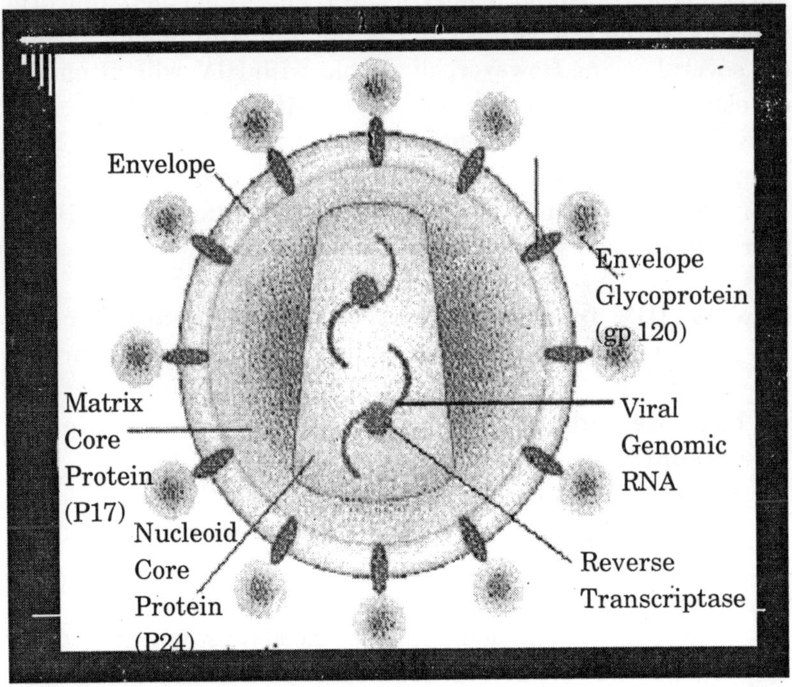

system now take full opportunity of the weakened immune system and start producing infections (opportunistic infections) in the person, such as tuberculosis, oral candidiasis, Herpes Zoster, Pneumocystis Carinii Pneumonia (PCP), Cyto-Megalo-Virus (CMV), Crypto-sporidiosis etc. and cancers like Kaposi's Sarcoma.

Body Fluids responsible for transmission of HIV infection.

The body fluids that have been proven to spread HIV are :-

- blood
- semen (semen contains a high concentration of HIV) including pre-ejaculatory fluid.
- vaginal fluid
- breast milk
- other body fluids containing blood

Difference between HIV infection and AIDS

HIV is the name of the virus that causes AIDS whereas AIDS is the name of the disease develop after 5-10 years of HIV infection. AIDS is the late stage of HIV infection. All people carrying HIV do not have AIDS. However, all people with HIV infection can transmit the infection to their sex partners and drug injecting partners. A person with HIV infection can remain healthy for several years. However, all people with HIV will ultimately develop AIDS. All people who have AIDS have HIV in their body. The only way of identifying AIDS is by testing the blood for presence of HIV.

HIV is a human virus. A person already infected with HIV is therefore the sole source of this infection.

How is HIV transmitted from one person to another ?

HIV is transmitted from one person to another through three routes :-

- **Unprotected sexual Intercourse with an infected person:**
  - heterosexual, homosexual, bisexual sex through exchange of body fluids (unprotected sex or sex without condom vaginal and anal).
- **Blood to blood or body fluids :**
  - through transfusion of infected blood (unscreened blood) or injection of infectedblood products or tattooing with contaminated instruments .
  - through sharing of contaminated syringes, needles or injection works like cooker, cotton. water as in case of transmission among Injecting Drug Users (IDUs), or use of contaminated instruments as in case of tattooing or

equipment such as sharps, other instruments and equipment used for invasive procedures or needle stick injury in health care workers caring for infected people.
- through use of infected donated organ transplant and semen (artificial insemination)

- **From infected mother to child :**
  - during pregnancy (trans-placental). - during child birth- through exposure of the child with the mother's vaginal secretions as well as with her blood during breast-feeding.

Epidemiological evidence is also firm that HIV is not spread by:

- close contact, interpersonal contact of a non sexual nature with an infected person such as shaking hands, touching, hugging, kissing.
- sharing of food, utensils, crockery, cutlery; sharing of washing and toilet facilities, bathrooms, swimming pools, telephones etc.
- living together in the same room or being part of the family.
- Working in the same workplace or schools.
- Donating blood.
- From sneezing or coughing or breathing of the infected person.
- through water, saliva, air or insect bites such as mosquitoes, fleas, bedbugs etc.
- Saliva, tears, sweat, sputum, nasal secretions, urine, stool are body substances that are not known to have transmitted HIV in any setting.

Who are at risk of acquiring HIV infection ?

Nearly all people are in one of the following population groups are risk of HIV infection.

- Injecting Drug Users who share needles and syringes or share works such as cookers, water, spoon, cotton etc. with a HIV infected person.
- Sexually active homosexual or bisexual men.
- Commercial sex workers or people who have multiple sex partners.
- Recipients of infected blood or blood products or organ transplants from an infected person.
- Male or female sex partners of individuals in any of the above groups.

- People who have sex without condom with Injecting Drug Users, Homosexuals, bisexual men or member of any high risk group mentioned above.
- Babies who has been born to a woman who contracted HIV infection before or during pregnancy.
- Babies who has been breast fed by an infected woman.
- Young men and women who indulged in sex with strangers
- Adolescents and young people
- Girls and young women
- Social, sexual, ethnic, and religious minorities
- Street children and children who work

What happened when HIV enters the body ?

The HIV may enter the body through any of the routes described earlier. The person himself may not be aware that the virus has entered his body and he may remain unaware for years together. However, he may spread the virus to others through sex or sharing of needles and syringes or through blood donation. As the virus enters the body, it gets attached to the CD4 lymphocyte and the number of virus increased. There are about 2-4 billion CD4 lymphocytes in the body. The virus multiplies rapidly and produces a high concentration of virus in the blood (viraemia). This condition is manifested as fever, headache, diarrhoea, rashes in about 20% to 30% of the cases. These symptoms appear like a common cold or flu. The symptoms pass off after a few days and the person becomes normal again. If blood sample is taken during this time – during the first 8-12 weeks for testing HIV antibodies like ELISA or Western Blot or Simple or Rapid test, the result will be negative. Because, the body has not yet produced sufficient antibodies to make the test positive. The person is already infected but the HIV antibody test is negative. This period is called " Window Period". Sometimes, the window period may be as long as six months. The negative test result is a false negative. During this time, the person may knowingly or unknowingly transmit the virus to his spouse or partners. The virus can be detected even during this window period if we do the PCR test (Polymerase Chain Reaction) by demonstrating the p24 antigen of the virus or by virus culture.

What is Immune System ?

We are surrounded by billions of germs including bacteria and viruses. Millions of germs may be entering our body when we breath, drink water or any liquid or take food or kiss somebody or have sex with somebody. The immune system protects us against billions of bacteria, viruses, and other parasites. When we hang out with our friends, watch TV, or go to school, inside our bodies, our immune system is constantly on the alert, attacking at the first sign of an invasion by harmful organisms.

To many of these germs, a human being is like a walking smorgasbord, offering nearly limitless resources that they can use for energy and reproduction. Luckily for us, getting into the human body is not an easy task. From the point of view of these tiny organisms, a human is a bit like a fortress. The skin is thick and very hard to penetrate. In addition, the skin also produces a variety of substances that are harmful to invaders. Openings such as the eyes, nose, and mouth are protected by fluids or sticky mucus that capture harmful attackers. The respiratory tract also has mechanical defenses in the form of *cilia,* tiny hairs that remove particles. Intruders that get as far as the stomach are up against a sea of stomach acid that kills most of them.

But in spite of our fantastic defenses, hostile invaders still manage to get through. Some enter along with our food, while others may sneak in via the nose. And, as we all know, many things can break through our skin. In everyday life we often receive cuts or scrapes, and every time this happens we face the risk of a full-scale invasion from bacteria or viruses. What is the secret, then, that keeps us healthy most of the time?

When we receive a cut, and when invaders enter the body, cells are destroyed. The dying cells trigger an automatic response called inflammation, which includes dilated blood vessels and increased blood flow. An inflammation is the body's equivalent to a burglar alarm. Once it goes off, it draws defensive cells to the damaged area in great numbers. Increased blood flow helps defensive cells reach the place where they're needed. It also accounts for the redness and swelling that occur.

The defensive cells are more commonly known as immune cells. They are part of a highly effective defense force called the immune system. The cells of the immune system work together with different proteins to seek out and destroy anything foreign or dangerous that enters our body. It takes some time for the immune cells to be activated - but once they're operating at full strength, there are very few hostile organisms that stand a chance.

Immune cells are white blood cells produced in huge quantities in the bone marrow. There are a wide variety of immune cells, each with its own strengths and weaknesses. Some seek out and devour invading organisms, while others destroy infected or mutated body cells. Yet another type has the ability to release special proteins called antibodies that mark intruders for destruction by other cells. But the really cool thing about the immune system is that it has the ability to "remember" enemies that it has fought in the past. If the immune system detects a "registered" invader, it will strike much more quickly and more fiercely against it. As a result, an invader that tries to attack the body a second time will most likely be wiped out before there are any symptoms of disease. When this happens, we say that the body has become immune.

Bacteria and Viruses: Our Main Enemies

Most bacteria are free living, while others live in or on other organisms, including humans. Many bacteria that have human hosts produce toxins (poisons) that damage the body. Not all bacteria are harmful, though. Some are neutral and many are even desirable as they fulfill important functions in the body. Bacteria are complete organisms that reproduce by cell division. Viruses, on the other hand, cannot reproduce on their own. They need a host cell. They hijack body cells of humans or other species, and trick them into producing new viruses that can then invade other cells. Frequently, the host cell is destroyed during the process.

An antigen is a foreign substance entering the human body that triggers a reaction from the immune system. Antigens are often found on the surfaces of bacteria and viruses. A pathogen is a microscopic organism that causes sickness. Hostile bacteria and viruses are examples of pathogens.

The immune system is very complex. It's made up of several types of cells and proteins that have different jobs to do in fighting foreign invaders.

Phagocytes

This is a group of immune cells specialized in finding and "eating" bacteria, viruses, and dead or injured body cells. There are three main types, the granulocyte, the macrophage, and the dendritic cell.

The **granulocytes** often take the first stand during an infection. They attack any invaders in large numbers, and "eat" until they die. The pus in an infected wound consists chiefly of dead granulocytes. A small part of the granulocyte community is specialized in attacking larger parasites such as worms.

The **macrophages** ("big eaters") are slower to respond to invaders than the granulocytes, but they are larger, live longer, and have far greater capacities. Macrophages also play a key part in alerting the rest of the immune system of invaders. Macrophages start out as white blood cells called monocytes. Monocytes that leave the blood stream turn into macrophages.

The **dendritic** cells are "eater" cells and devour intruders, like the granulocytes and the macrophages. And like the macrophages, the dendritic cells help with the activation of the rest of the immune system. They are also capable of filtering body fluids to clear them of foreign organisms and particles

Lymphocytes - T cells and B cells

White blood cells called lymphocytes originate in the bone marrow but migrate to parts of the lymphatic system such as the lymph nodes, spleen, and thymus. There are two main types of lymphatic cells, T cells and B cells.

T cells come in two different types, helper T cells and killer T cells. They are named T cells after the thymus, an organ situated under the breastbone. T cells are produced in the bone marrow and later move to the thymus where they mature.

Helper T cells are the major driving force and the main regulators of the immune defense. Their primary task is to activate B cells and killer T cells. However, the helper T cells themselves must be activated. This happens when a macrophage or dendritic cell, which has eaten an invader, travels to the nearest lymph node to present information about the captured pathogen. The phagocyte displays an antigen fragment from the invader on its own surface, a process called antigen presentation. When the receptor of a helper

T cell recognizes the antigen, the T cell is activated. Once activated, helper T cells start to divide and to produce proteins that activate B and T cells as well as other immune cells.

The killer T cell is specialized in attacking cells of the body infected by viruses and sometimes also by bacteria. It can also attack cancer cells. The killer T cell has receptors that are used to search each cell that it meets. If a cell is infected, it is swiftly killed. Infected cells are recognized because tiny traces of the intruder, antigen, can be found on their surface.

The B lymphocyte cell searches for antigen matching its receptors. If it finds such antigen it connects to it, and inside the B cell a triggering signal is set off. The B cell now needs proteins produced by helper T cells to become fully activated. When this happens, the B cell starts to divide to produce clones of itself. During this process, two new cell types are created, plasma cells and B memory cells.

The plasma cell is specialized in producing a specific protein, called an antibody, that will respond to the same antigen that matched the B cell receptor. Antibodies are released from the plasma cell so that they can seek out intruders and help destroy them. Plasma cells produce antibodies at an amazing rate and can release tens of thousands of antibodies per second.

When the Y-shaped antibody finds a matching antigen, it attaches to it. The attached antibodies serve as an appetizing coating for eater cells such as the macrophage. Antibodies also neutralize toxins and incapacitate viruses, preventing them from infecting new cells. Each branch of the Y-shaped antibody can bind to a different antigen, so while one branch binds to an antigen on one cell, the other branch could bind to another cell - in this way pathogens are gathered into larger groups that are easier for phagocyte cells to devour. Bacteria and other pathogens covered with antibodies are also more likely to be attacked by the proteins from the complement system.

The Memory Cells are the second cell type produced by the division of B cells. These cells have a prolonged life span and can thereby "remember" specific intruders. T cells can also produce memory cells with an even longer life span than B memory cells. The second time an intruder tries to invade the body, B and T memory cells help the immune system to activate much faster.

The invaders are wiped out before the infected human feels any symptoms. The body has achieved immunity against the invader.

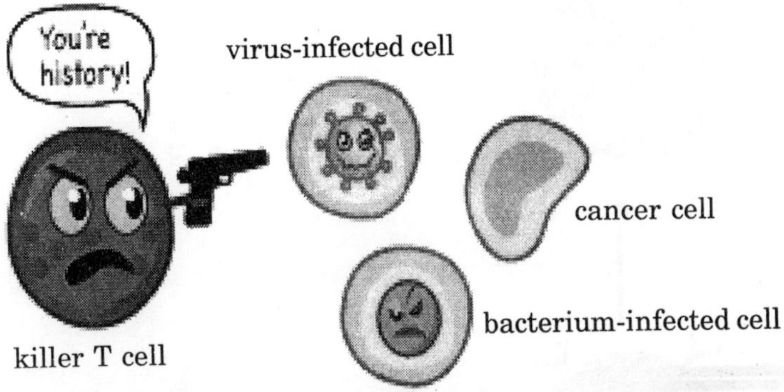

The killer T cells terminate cencer cells and cells intected by a virus or bacterirum.

Immune deficiency is, therefore, the breakdown or an inability of certain parts of the immune system to function, which renders a person susceptible to certain diseases.

What is Window Period

The time interval between the exposure and infection with HIV and the antibodies in the blood of the person becomes detectable. This time interval is called "window period". It may range from 6 weeks to 12 weeks. So the ELISA test or ERS should be performed only after 6-12 weeks after the exposure. If negative, the test should be repeated after 12 weeks or six months again.

How can HIV infection be detected ?

Infection with HIV can be detected with the help of a blood test known as : "Antibody test". HIV antibody test is a test to determine whether an individual has antibodies to HIV, the virus that causes AIDS. Presence of HIV antibody indicates that the person has been exposed to HIV and he is infected. The ELISA test is an antibody test and has become commercially available in 1985. ELISA, Rapid and Simple (ERS) tests are all HIV antibody tests. Western Blot is also an antibody test.

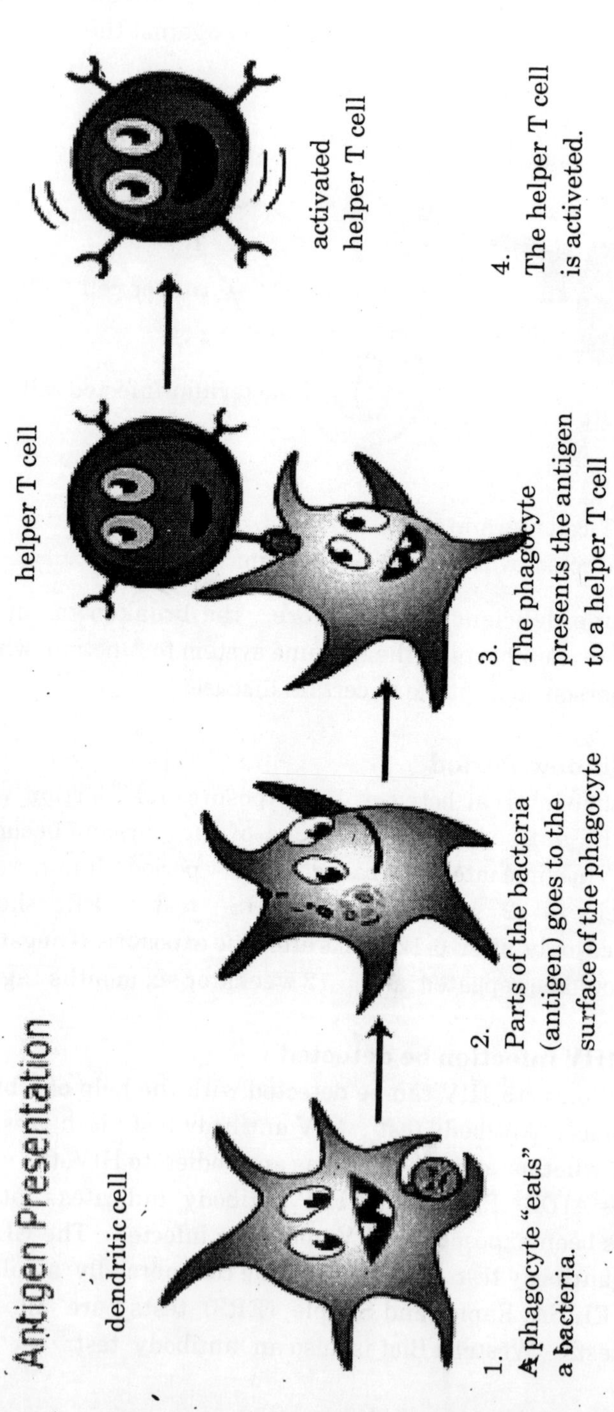
Antigen Presentation
dendritic cell
helper T cell
activated helper T cell
1. A phagocyte "eats" a bacteria.
2. Parts of the bacteria (antigen) goes to the surface of the phagocyte
3. The phagocyte presents the antigen to a helper T cell
4. The helper T cell is activeted.

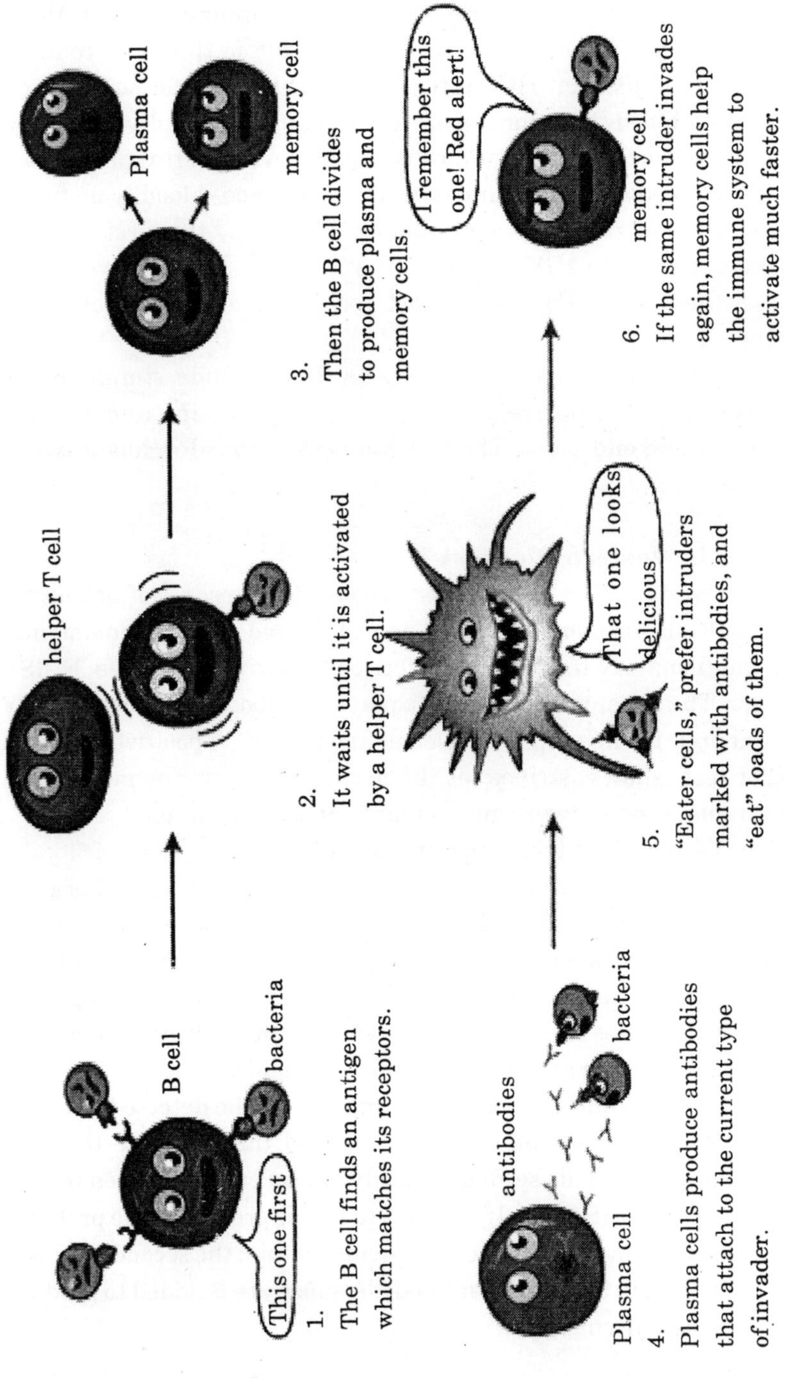
B cell
bacteria
This one first
1.
The B cell finds an antigen which matches its receptors.
helper T cell
2.
It waits until it is activated by a helper T cell.
Plasma cell
memory cell
3.
Then the B cell divides to produce plasma and memory cells.
Plasma cell
antibodies
bacteria
4.
Plasma cells produce antibodies that attach to the current type of invader.
That one looks delicious
5.
"Eater cells," prefer intruders marked with antibodies, and "eat" loads of them.
I remember this one! Red alert!
memory cell
6.
If the same intruder invades again, memory cells help the immune system to activate much faster.

What is ELISA Test ?

ELISA stands for Enzyme Linked Immuno Sorbent Assay. This is a kind of HIV antibody test. This is the most common method of test for HIV antibodies. This is used for screening of donated blood and for laboratory diagnosis of individuals who have been exposed to unprotected sex with a stranger or have shared needles and syringes or have received blood transfusion and also for sentinel surveillance. This was the first clinical screening test for HIV infection . The test will show positive results after the Window Period. The test becomes commercially available since 1985.

The advantages of the ELISA Test include simplicity in performance, relatively in-expensive equipment and kit and measurable end point. The test can be performed in about two to three hours.

What is Western Blot test ?

Western Blot Test is a test to detect the presence of antibodies to multiple antigens of HIV. The test is used as a supplemental or confirmatory test for HIV infection following a positive ELISA test. The Western Blot test displays antibodies to specific HIV viral proteins in a separate, well defined band. A positive Western Blot test shows stripes at the locations for two or more viral proteins. A negative result is blank at these locations.

The Western Blot test is performed as follows:

1. The virus is broken up and separated using special laboratory techniques. The individual viral proteins are separated into strips with each strip containing the major viral proteins.
2. The patient's serum is mixed with the strip overnight. If antibodies are present in the serum, the antibody will bind to the specific protein that is directed again.
3. The protein-antibody combination must be detected as in the ELISA. A second antibody is added that binds to the HIV antibody. This second antibody has an enzyme linked to it as in the ELISA test. If antibody to HIV is present in the protein's serum and is bound to the specific protein; the second antibody will bind to the HIV antibody. A substrate is added to produce a colour change.

What are the Simple, Rapid Tests ?

Simple rapid test format started appearing in the late 1980s. Since then, these tests have improved in accuracy, almost roughly equivalent in specificity and sensitivity to ELISA tests. Currently available format includes the following:

- Particle agglutination, where a positive result is rapidly detected by the agglutination of very fine particles such as latex particles after is mixed with the specimen Serodia-HIV).
- Autologous These tests are simple and rapid test methods, which do not require red cell agglutination, where an anti-lunar red cell monoclonal antibody HIV peptic conjugate is mixed with a test specimen of blood; the monoclonal antibody is present; the red cells are aggregation.
- Particle adherence tests, where pattern of settling (over a period of 60 to 90 minutes) of small particle bearing HIV antigens is influenced by the presence of HIV antibodies.
- Membrane immuno concentration or immunodot test which filter the specimen through the membrane into a porous absorbent matrix, followed by addition of a signal reagent to identify the presence of HIV antibody; a dot or line usually forms on the membrane signaling appositive reaction, and
- Dipstick assays where a solid- phase plastic stem is incubated briefly with specimen and washed and HIV antibodies are then detected with a signal reagents such as colloidal gold-protein A.

What do you mean by "HIV" negative ?

The test will be negative if you are not HIV infected. The test will be positive if you are HIV infected ? HIV negative means the person is not infected with HIV as determined by a negative test result for antibody to HIV or for presence of the virus .

What do you mean by HIV positive ?

HIV positive means the person is infected with HIV as determined by a positive test result for antibody to HIV or for presence of the virus. Such an individual is also called as HIV seropositive. The person does not suffer from AIDS. He or she may be perfectly healthy and can work as a normal person. He or she may be a boxer, an Olympic gold medalist or formula-1 champion or a beautiful film star. It is not possible to identify a HIV positive person just by looking at his /her eye or his/ her face. Being handsome or beautiful or clean or dressed properly does not mean that a person can not have HIV.

A HIV positive person will eventually develop AIDS- may be after five years or ten years or even longer depending upon his or her life style.

What are HIV testing and counselling?

To find out if a person is infected with the human immunodeficiency virus (HIV), it is essential to do an HIV antibody test. This uses a small amount of blood taken from the person who wants to know if he or she is HIV positive. If the first HIV test is positive, another test is usually done, to check that the first result was correct.

Deciding to ask for an HIV test depends on the affected person realising that there is some risk of being HIV positive and feeling a need to find out.

A person might be able to find information for themselves about HIV infection and about testing, but very often they might need to get more information and be reassured that it is accurate.

Fear of stigma, discrimination and violence remain one of the biggest barriers to HIV testing and counselling; they often prevent people from going to get an HIV test, or returning to find out the result.

Voluntary and confidential counselling for HIV testing (VCT) is an important method for ensuring that a person gets support before and after an HIV test, is given the right information, and is helped to deal with the consequences of the HIV test result. Wherever it is given, it should respect the person's need for privacy and confidentiality.

Pre-test counselling can be given at a special VCT Centre, but it can also be given in a health facility, over the telephone or in places where people who are at risk of being positive are likely to gather.

Post-test counselling should be provided at the same time as the result of the test is given to the person. If the person is positive, they should be helped to deal with shock, fear or self-stigma and to work out how they are going to proceed. If the result is negative, the person needs support for avoiding HIV infection and related risks in future.

What is the time interval between entry of the virus and development of AIDS?

The time interval between the entry of the virus and development of AIDs is called the "incubation period". The mean incubation period from the time of infection to the development of AIDS may be as long as ten years or even longer. The shortest incubation period of two years or less is very highly unusual. Based in four different studies as reported by John, G and Bcartlett in 1992 in USA; the incubation is as follows :-

1	Year	=	0	percent
2	Years	=	0	percent
3	Years	=	3	percent
4	Years	=	6	percent
5	Years	=	12	percent
6	Years	=	20	percent
7	Years	=	27	percent
8	Years	=	36	percent
9	Years	=	45	percent
10	Years	=	53	percent

The reasons for the great variation are unknown. One report suggest that the incubation period may be 15 years in 75% of cases, 20 years in 90% cases.

Since 1992, scientists have estimated that about half the people with HIV develop AIDS within 10 years after becoming infected. This time varies greatly from person to person and can depend on many factors, including a person's health status, nuttrional status, and their health-related behaviours. Today there are medical treatments that can slow down the rate at which HIV weakens the immune system. There are other treatments that can prevent or cure some of the illnesses associated with AIDS, though the treatments do not cure AIDS itself. As with other diseases, early detection offers more options for treatment and management.

How children become infected with HIV

Infants can acquire HIV from their infected mothers during pregnancy, at the time of labour and delivery, or after birth through breastfeeding. They can also become infected with HIV-contaminated blood or from medical equipment or sometimes through child abuse. In some populations in sub-Saharan Africa, 30 percent or more of pregnant women are infected with HIV. 24 percent 45 percent of HIV-infected mothers will pass on the virus to their infants.

What is the clinical classification of HIV disease ?

The clinical stages of the HIV disease as per World Health Organization (WHO) may be described in five stages :-

Stage-I : Acute (primary) Infection (Seroconversion Illness)

This stage starts from 8-12 weeks after entry of the virus. During this stage, the CD4 cells instruct the body's immune system to produce antibodies against the virus resulting to hypersensitivity reaction. The signs and symptoms may range from malaise to fever, skin rash, muscle pain, joint pains. Enlarged lymph nodes in the neck and axillae resembling infectious mononucleosis. Encephalitis and aseptic meningitis can occur.

These symptoms last only for 10-12 days and are usually self limiting. Only 50% of the infected individuals may experience these symptoms. HIV antibody test in this stage are often negative and therefore, diagnosis depends on PCR test.

Stage-II Early (Asymptomatic) Disease (CD4 count more than 500/mm3.

After the episode of Seroconversion illness, the person becomes completely well without any sign or symptom. although HIV can be isolated from his blood and genital fluids. He may not be aware of the infection although he himself is infected and fully infectious to others. He can spread the infection to other though sex, blood or body fluids. This stage may last for 8-10 years or even longer. During the symptomatic period, one can keep track of the progress of the infection by physical examination and with two laboratory tests. One test is CD4 Cell count in the blood. The normal CD4 cell count is 700-1300 per cu. ml of blood. In a person with HIV infection, CD4 count decrease on average by 85-100 cells cu. ml per year. Most people do not develop symptoms until this CD4 (T-4) count is below 300 and the average CD4 (T-4) cell count for a person with an AIDS defining diagnosis is 50-100, but definitely below 200.

A second method of keeping track of infection is through blood count. The blood counts must be lowered severely before symptoms occur. Thus, there may be leucopenia, thrombocytopenia, altered serum transaminase level and polyclonal activation of immune cells.

Experts say that there is a definite advantage in starting antiretroviral treatment during this period and that will delay the progression of the disease.

Stage-III Intermediate HIV Infection (CD4 count 200-500 / mm)

During this stage, CD4 count shows a declining trend. As the CD4 count falls, complications begin to occur or worsen in severity. The person may develop herpes zoster or herpes simplex, mild oropharyngeal candidiasis or vaginal candidiasis, oral hairy leukoplakia. Mycobaterium Tuberculosis is seen commonly with a CD4 count of around 250 cubic /mm If left untreated, the patient will develop AIDS defining conditions or dying within the next 18-28 months in 30% to 50% of the cases.

With antiretroviral treatment, this risk may be reduced by two or three folds.

Stage-IV Late Stage HIV Disease (CD4 count 50-200/mm)

All patients in this stage are now defined to be having AIDS. The most common opportunistic infections at this stage include cerebral toxoplasmosis, cryptococcal meningitis, PCP, cytomegalovirus retinitis (CMV).

Stage-V Advanced HIV Disease (CD4 count below 50 /cubic mm) Combination antiretroviral therapy can halt the rapid progress of the disease to a certain extent. Nutrition is very important for maintaining the immune function and delay development of wasting syndrome.

At this stage, the patient, even with antiretroviral treatment, has a likelihood of dying within two years due to any of the opportunistic infections. The common opportunistic infections are Mycobacterium Avium Complex (MAC), systematic histoplasmosis, cryptococcal meningitis, progressive multifoccal leukoencephalopathy, CMV retinitis, CMV colitis, CMV encephalitis. Many patients with CD4 count of less than 50 per cubic mm present with direct neurological effects of HIV known as AIDS Dementia Complex (ADC). Many patients in this stage develop weight loss, wasting of muscles, various types of mal absorptions, various features of Addition's disease etc. (HIV wasting syndrome)

What are the "Opportunistic infection" (O.I)

Opportunistic infections are those infections which a person with a normally functioning immune system without HIV infection is easily able to fight off. With the progression of HIV infection, more and more CD4 cells are destroyed as a result of viral load. This process can go on ultimately leading to destruction of more and more of CD4 (T-4) cells causing immuno deficiency, which renders the person unable to fight infections and tumours. Now the micro organisms which cannot produce infection or disease in a person with a normally functioning immune system now take full opportunity of the weakened immune system and start producing infections (opportunistic infections) in the person, such as tuberculosis, oral candidiasis, Herpes Zoster, Pneumocystis Carinii Pneumonia (PCP), Cyto-Megalo-Virus (CMV), Crypto-sporidiosis etc. and cancers like Kaposi's Sarcoma.

Un-fortunately drugs which work very well in someone with a normal immune system work with less well in someone person with a weakened immune system. It often happens that a person with AIDS will succumb to an opportunistic infection and die. That is why people usually said – "AIDS itself do not kill – it kills by proxy".

The commonly found opportunistic infections include:-

- Tuberculosis
- Oral and/or Oesophageal candidiasis
- Cryptosporidiosis, caused by a protozoan causing a profuse and persistent diarrhoea.
- Herpes Simplex, causing long lasting sores which do not heal.
- Cryptococcal meningitis, an inflammation of the brain caused by a yeast-type fungus.
- Cytomegalovirus (CMV), causing damage to the brain and eyes, including progressive blindness as well as gastro-intestinal and lung disease.
- Toxoplasmosis, caused by a protozoan acquired from eating row meat or from cat-faeces causing extensive lesions in the brain.
- Pneumocystis Carinii Pneumonia (PCP), a protozoal lung infection causing fever, shortness of breath and dry cough.

If I am HIV positive, what am I supposed to do ?

Knowing that you are HIV positive, it can be a terrible blow, but you need not be very much upset. You should not have a feeling of despair. There are many diseases in the world for which there is no cure. First of all, it is important to understand your test results. Being HIV positive does not mean that you have AIDS. Being HIV positive does not mean the end of your life. It may take another 7-10 years or even longer to develop AIDS. It may be even longer up to 15 years or even more. A positive result means that antibodies for HIV have been detected in your blood and that you are capable of transmitting the virus to others (infecting). It also means that now more than ever, is the time to look after yourself and practice a healthy lifestyles. Start by getting the right advice from people who are qualified to help you to manage your health.

Seek counselling from a Voluntary Counselling and Testing Centre (VCTC) and see a doctor you trust who is knowledgeable and experienced in caring for HIV positive individuals.

The doctor will clinically assess your overall health, monitor your CD4 levels by conducting a blood test. CD4 is the level of white blood cells in your immune system undamaged by HIV virus. An HIV –negative person should have between 700 to 1300 CD4 cells per cubic mm of blood while an HIV positive person may have less levels due to the virus destroying the CD4.

The lower the levels of CD4 are, the weaker the immune system and the person will become physically weaker and more prone to opportunistic infections.

Even if there is no cure for HIV but an anti retroviral drug available in India will be able to stop the virus from increasing.

Anti retroviral drugs are given free of cost under the NACO programme. Howerver only the first line of treatment is available under the free ART treatment programme. It is a combination of three drugs . That is why-this treatment is known as Triple Combination Therapy or Cocktail Therapy or Highly Active Antiretroviral Therapy (HARRT). Remember your commitment to treatment, adherence compliance to treatment schedules and ability to get triple combination therapy is very important.

There are two issues you need to consider before you start treatment: (a) cost / financial liability (b) compliance

(a) Cost/ financial liability :–

Triple combination therapy is expensive. Nowadays , these drugs are given free of cost to the people living with HIV with CD4 count below 200, to women who have participated at the Mother to Child HIV Transmission Project (PPTCT/MTCT) and to children below 15 years of age.

(b) Adherence : -

It is important that you take your treatment without fail, daily at the agreed time for the rest of your life. Poor Adherence will result in resistance in the drug. You may have to change your treatment due to resistance. Therefore, you may have fewer choices left for you in the future. Always keep your appointment with your doctor who will monitor your health. Do not stop or change the schedules of your medicines without talking to your doctor first. Be committed and take active interest in your treatment and health.

What are the symptoms to be watched after becoming HIV positive ?

People who are HIV infected do have a higher chance of getting other infections and diseases. The symptoms to be watched for after becoming HIV positive are as follows :_

- Fever
- Cough
- Loss of appetite
- Difficulty in swallowing
- Breathing problems
- Persistent headache
- Malnutrition/ Weight Loss
- Mouth problems such as white spots, sores, change in taste or loose teeth.
- Diarrhoea
- Any skin rash or itching
- Reduced vision, moving spots or lines in your vision.

What care should I take to have a healthy and useful life even if I am IV positive ?

The golden rules to be followed for keeping healthy and useful life are as follows:

- Good Nutrition: this is extremely important. Eat a well balanced diet and maintain your usual weight. This will make you strong, keep your energy up and help your body protect itself.
- Quit Smoking: if you smoke, make a conscious attempt to stop smoking. This will certainly be of help in the long term.
- Exercise: Along with good nutrition, exercise helps you maintain your muscle mass, relax and sleep better, besides giving you a sense of well-being. Choose a form of exercise that you enjoy. Walking, jogging, swimming and cycling are good examples. Exercise regularly to stay strong and fit.
- Relax: Get enough sleep and rest.
- Hygiene: maintain good personal hygiene, to prevent other infections from setting in.
- Handle pets carefully: some infections can be acquired from pets such as cats and dogs. If you have a pet at home, ask your doctor what precautions to take. Avoid stray animals.

- Take life easy: reduce stress levels and take time to relax. Many people find that prayer or meditation, along with rest and exercise, help them cope better with the stress of having HIV/AIDS.
- Avoid Alcohol and drugs: if you drink alcohol, try and stop or at least reduce it to a minimum. Regular use of alcohol or drugs like marijuana (charas, ganja, opium, heroin etc) can weaken your resistance to infection, which can be dangerous if you already have HIV/AIDS. If you are a drug user, try to stop using drugs . It may be evry difficult for you. You can start practicing Harm Reduction with the ultimate goal of achieving abstinence.
- Safe sex: persistent use of condom should be made as a part of life to avoid transmission of HIV to spouse/partner. HIV infected person should always reveal his /her status to spouse/ partner. You should be responsible for saving the lives of your loved ones.

How long a person with HIV infection survive ?

How long a person with HIV infection survive depends upon the life style, access to health care services, the amount of care and social support and the kind of nutritious diets he or she is getting. If the person with HIV infection change his or her behaviour from high risk behaviour like injecting drug use or commercial sex to healthy and safe behaviour, then he or she may survive quite a long time. He may survive even up to 15 years or twenty years or even more.

The survival of patients with AIDS from the time of diagnosis has been reported from several research studies. Old age was associated with shorter survival. Women's survival was shorter than men's and whites lived longer then blacks. In most studies of survival, the initial presenting AIDS diagnosis was the most powerful predictor of survival, Kaposi's Sarcoma was associated with the longest survival whereas PCP with one year survival is 30-45 percent.

Interestingly, Injecting Drug Users had a more favourable survival time than other groups. However Injecting Drug Users associated with fungal and bacterial infections; Crypto-coccal meningitis and disseminated disease and Mycobacterium Avium intracellular infection result in shorter survival period.

Now, with the availability of antiretroviral drugs, the prospect of a long life is increasing .In fact. HIV/AIDS is now considered to be a chronic disease. But he or she must try to delay the onset of AIDS – the signs and symptoms. He or she can take proper precautions or start medications to delay the onset of AIDS. Once AIDS develops, the survival period may not be very long.

There are drugs which can prolong the life of the people living with HIV/AIDS and also improve the quality of life . These are called " Antiretroviral drugs" (ARV) . The Government of India has already to announced to provide antiretroviral drugs free to all patients below 200 CD4 count , those women who have participated at the at the project for prevention of mother to child HIV transmission (MTCT or PPTCT) and also children below 15 years of age. The treatment or therapy with the antiretroviral drugs is called ART . (Antiretroviral Therapy)

The antiretroviral drugs act on the HIV at different stages of its lifecycle. The current goal of anti-retroviral therapy in patients with HIV disease is to suppress viral replication as much as possible and for as long as possible. It is now recognized that this can only be achieved by using a combination of several anti-retroviral drugs (three or more) at the same time.

What are the Antiretroviral drugs ?

The newest class of anti-retroviral drugs are :-

1. Inhibitors of viral attachment – Recombinant soluble CD4 or immunoglobins
2. Non-nucleoside reverse transcriptase inhibitors (NNRTI):-
   - 2.1. Nevirapine (Viramune)
   - 2.2. Delavirdine mesylate (Rescriptor)
   - 2.3. Efavirenz (Sustiva)
3. Nucleoside analogues (NRTI) :-
   - 3.1. Zidovudine (AZT, ZDV, Azidothymidine, retrovir)
   - 3.2. Didanosine (ddI, Dideoxynosine, Videx)
   - 3.3. Zalcitabine (ddC, Dideoxycytidine, HIVID)
   - 3.4. Stavudine (D4T, ZERIT)

3.5. Lamivudine (3TC, EPIVIR)

3.6 Abacabir (ddA)

4. Protease inhibitors :-

4.1. Saquinavir mesylate

4.2. Indinavir

4.3. Ritonavir

4.4. Nelfinavir mesylate

4.5 Amprenavir

5. Integrase Inhibitors – Phase- Trial not complete as yet

6. Agents that block virus assembly and budding - interferon

Fusion inhibitors are a new type of ARV that prevent HIV from binding to the surface of the T-cell and infecting the T-cell. HIV-positive people who have become resistant to NNRTIs, NRTIs, and PIs will likely benefit from fusion inhibitors, which are a different type of ARV not yet available in resource limited settings and, therefore, not discussed in this chapter.

Each type of ARV is active at different stages of the virus in the replication cycle. Combining two or more ARVs enhances drug efficacy, which is referred to as combination therapy or highly active antiretroviral therapy (HAART). For example, the action of the ARV zidovidune is enhanced if used in combination with lamivudine or didanosine. It is likely that a person receiving ART will take a combination of ARVs to best prevent replication of them HIV virus.

WHO recommends four first-line HAART regimens for adults and adolescents in resource limited settings listed in the box on the following page.

First-Line ARV Regimens Recommended by WHO for Resource Limited Settings (WHO- 2003)

1. stavudine + lamivudine + nevirapine
2. zidovudine + lamivudine + nevirapine
3. stavudine + lamivudine + efavirenz
4. zidovudine + lamivudine + efavirenz

ART is not required at all stages of HIV. Generally, ART is used when the virus has begun to significantly damage the immune system. WHO recommends a person begin ART when that person meets any of the following three conditions

- WHO stage 4 of HIV regardless of CD4 count
- WHO stage 3 of HIV with a CD4 count below 350/mm3
- WHO stages 1 or 2 of HIV with CD4 count below 200/mm3
- Or if CD4 testing is unavailable, WHO recommends a person begin ART
- when that person meets any of the following three conditions:
- WHO stage 4 of HIV regardless of total lymphocyte count
- WHO stage 3 disease regardless of total lymphocyte count
- WHO Stage 2 disease with a total lymphocyte below 1200/ mm3

Because many ARVs may negatively interact with certain foods and nutrients, dietary management of ARV-food interactions can help improve the efficacy of ARVs while also minimizing their negative nutritional impact and enhancing adherence to drug regimens.

Antiretroviral drugs should be started

- if the CD4 count is less than 200 even if the patient has no symptoms.
- the CD count is above 200 but the patient starting signs and symproms.
- the lymphocyte count is less than 1200 per cubic mm of blood.

Today, that thinking has changed. If the goal is to reduce the viral load as low as possible, then anyone with a detectable viral load should be considered a candidate for antiviral therapy. Most experts are now advocating treatment for anyone with detectable viral load.

The minimal goal of antiviral therapy is to suppress HIV replication as much as possible for as long as possible. Simply put, the purpose of any antiviral therapy is to get the viral load as low as possible and keep it down. The ultimate goal is to achieve aviraemia i.e. undetectable levels of HIV in the blood.

Antiretroviral drugs are not drugs without any side effects. Further adherence to treatment and compliance is very important. It is a life –long treatment and the patient should not miss any of the regimens for effective results.

What may be the possible side effects of Antiretroviral drugs?

The possible side effects for AZT (Zidovudine) are bone marrow suppression and anaemia, for Didanosine, pancreatitis (inflammation of pancreas), peripheral neuropathy for Stavudine, peripheral neuropathy, pancreatitis, for Lamivudine, headache, general weakness, nausea, diarrhoea and for Zalcitabine, peripheral neuropathy stomatitis (inflammation of lips). In some cases, the side effected may be very severe warranting stoppage of the drugs.

How is HIV testing and counselling related to ARV treatment?

- No-one can start ARV treatment unless they have already had an HIV test to confirm if they are HIV-positive. ARV treatment is a life-long commitment and must be used correctly, so it is important to be sure that the person is HIV positive and is able and willing to deal with long-term treatment.
- ARV treatment is not a cure for HIV. The virus remains in the body. It causes less damage to the immune system, but the person will still be HIV-positive. So it is not necessary to repeat the HIV antibody test after confirming that a person is HIV positive, because ARV treatment does not change a person's HIV-positive status.
- ARV treatment works best if a person is not too sick when they start treatment (although even people who are very sick when they start can recover very well with ART treatment)
- When ARV treatment is accessible, people are much more likely to want an HIV test because they realise that a positive test result will enable them to get treatment when they need it.
- When ARV treatment is not accessible, for example if a person cannot afford it or cannot get it from a clinic near enough to home or work, people often avoid getting an HIV test because they think there is nothing they can do to stop AIDS and early death.
- Access to ARV treatment is a powerful incentive for people to ask for HIV testing and counselling. However, people also

need to learn about the living positively in order to support the immune system and reduce the risks of opportunistic infections. This applies to all HIV positive people, whether or not they are able to have ARV treatment.

- It is very important that people should check their HIV status while they are well and before any possible symptoms of HIV appear. Knowing your status allows a person to take important steps to protect their own and other people's health.
- These steps include:
  - Asking for a CD4 test from time to time to find out if the immune system is damaged and if it is time to start ARV treatment.
  - Using prevention when engaging in sexual activity.
  - Getting prompt help for any other health problems.
  - Disclosing one's HIV status to people one can trust, and getting ongoing support for positive living, prevention and good adherence to ARV treatment when it becomes necessary.

Why do people with HIV develop TB ?

The hallmark of HIV infection is a progressive depletion and dysfunction of CD4 cells coupled with defects in macrophages and monocyte function. Because CD4 cells and macrophages have a central role in anti-mycobacterial defences, dysfunction of these cells places the person with HIV/AIDS at high risk of developing primary or reactivation of TB. Epidemiological evidences indicate that HIV infection increases the risk of reinfection of latent tuberculosis infection.

56% of AIDS patients in India, 80% in Myanmar, 75% in Nepal and 48 % in Thailand develop tuberculosis as an opportunistic infection. The parallel epidemic of TB is likely to lead to further spread of TB among the general, non-HIV infected population. The emergence of multi drug resistant TB is another concern for worry. The target is to cure 85% of detected smear positive cases by 2000 and to detect 75% of the existing cases.

What are typical signs and symptoms of TB ?

The typical signs and symptoms of TB are as follows :-

- cough for more than three weeks with or without low grade fever, night sweats
- loss of appetite
- loss of weight
- chest pain
- haemoptysis (blood in the sputum)

All patients with positive tuberculin test should be evaluated to rule out active TB.

Diagnosis of Pulmonary TB depends on three specimens of sputum.

1. Sputum specimen on the first visit, sputum container given to the patient.
2. early morning collection of sputum by the patient on the next day.
3. spot specimen on the second visit.

What is the recommended treatment for adults ?

Treatment regimen comprises of two phases – (1) intensive phase and (2) continuation phase. The intensive phase includes daily supervised treatment with four drugs for two months – Isoniazide, Rifampicin , Pyrazinamide and Ethambutol. Ethambutol and Streptomycin can be interchanged where either one of the two drugs is not available. The continuation phase means daily supervised treatment with Isoniazide and Rifampicin for four months.

Isoniazide 300 mg daily + Rifampicin 450 mg daily (600 mg for persons weighing more than 60 Kg) + Pyrazinamide -20-30 mg per kg body weight is the usual regimen Pyrazinamide is administered during the first 2 months of therapy and then discontinued. If Isoniazide resistance is suspected, ethambutol- 25 mg per kg body weight should be included in the initial treatment regimen. Treatment with Isoniazide and Rifampicin should be continued for 9 months or 6 months after documented culture conversion whichever is longer. Drug susceptibility test should be performed routinely and treatment regimen revised if there is resistance to any drug being used.

What is the impact of TB on HIV?

The impact of TB on HIV are :-

- Shortens survival of the patient
- Accelerates progression of HIV infection
- Cause of death in one-third of HIV cases worldwide
- TB can occur at any point in the course of progression of HIV infection

What is the impact of HIV on TB?

In some countries HIV epidemic has tripled TB cases due to HIV. Most powerful risk factor for progression from TB infection to disease 50% lifetime risk for people with HIV vs 10% for normal people without HIV.

- Increased number of TB cases
- Reactivation of TB
- Susceptibility to new TB infections
- Most common serious opportunistic infection in HIV positives and is the first manifestation of AIDS in >50% cases in developing countries. HIV fuels the spread of MDR TB. In India, about 50-60% of HIV positive patients will develop TB in their lifetime.

How to treat pregnant women with TB and HIV?

HIV infected pregnant women with TB should be immediately treated without delay. Benefits of treatment with Pyrazinamide outweight potential pyrazinamide –related risks to the foetus. Aminoglycosides (Streptomycin, Kanamycin, Amikacin) and Capreomycin are all contraindicated for all pregnant women because of potential adverse effects on the foetus. Appropriate antiretroviral therapy should be offered to HIV infected pregnant women.

Can TB drugs be taken along with antiretroviral drugs?

Rifabutin can be used with protease inhibitors and NNRIS. Isoniazide, Ethambutol, Pyrazinamide and Streptomycin. contraceptives, dapsone, ketoconazole, fluconazole, narcotics (methadowe), anti coagulants, corticosteroids, cardial clycosides, hypoglysemics, diazepam, beta blockers, anti-convulsants, theophyllin have drug reactions with rifampicin or rifabutin. Dose adjustments or alternative therapies are required.Protease inhibitors/ NNRTI to be given after 2 weeks of therapy.

How can HIV be transmitted from mother to child?(MTCT)

HIV can be transmitted from a mother to her infant during pregnancy, during labour and delivery, and through breastfeeding

HIV transmission during pregnancy

There is a 5 percent-10 percent risk of transmission of HIV during pregnancy. A child is considered to have been infected in utero if the HIV-1 genome is detected within 48 hours of delivery by a polymerase chain reaction test (DNA-PCR) or viral culture. (UNICEF/UNAIDS/WHO 1998a). Transmission during pregnancy occurs when the placental protection of the fetus is compromised, allowing for viral transmission. The following factors are associated with transmission during pregnancy:

- A viral, bacterial, or parasitic placental infection in the mother during pregnancy
- HIV infection of the mother during pregnancy
- Severe immune deficiency associated with advanced AIDS in the mother (WHO1999)
- Malnutrition (Semba 1997)

HIV transmission during labour and delivery

There is a 10 percent-20 percent risk of transmission of HIV during labour and delivery. WHO/UNAIDS/UNICEF (1998) consider transmission to have occurred intrapartum if the results of the diagnostic tests were negative during the first 48 hours after delivery but became positive in subsequent samples taken within 7-90 days of delivery. During labor and delivery transmission most often occurs when babies suck, imbibe, or aspirate maternal blood or cervical secretions containing HIV. Higher risks of HIV transmission during labour and delivery are associated with duration of membrane rupture, acute chorioamnionitis resulting from untreated sexually transmitted infections (STIs) or other infections, and invasive delivery techniques that increase the baby's contact with the mother's blood (WHO 1999).

HIV transmission during breast feeding

There is a 10 percent-20 percent risk of transmission of HIV through breastfeeding. The time that HIV transmission occurs following birth is difficult to determine precisely. The presence of maternal antibodies, combined with a period of time during which the infection is undetectable, makes it difficult to determine whether infection occurred during delivery or through breastfeeding. Late post-natal transmission (after 3-6 months) can be estimated with the PCR test. A meta-analysis of five studies concluded that the best available estimate of the risk of breastmilk transmission is 14 percent (Dunn et al 1992). The risk of HIV transmission through breastfeeding can be calculated for a particular population with the following formula: percentage of HIV-infected mothers at time of delivery multiplied by 14 percent.

Up to 70 percent of breastmilk samples from HIV-infected mothers have been shown to contain cell-associated and cell-free HIV. Transmission is not necessarily a result of the presence of HIV in breastmilk, however, but of a complex interaction between the anti-infective agents—macrophages, lymphocytes, and immunoglobulin— in breastmilk and HIV.

What may be the possible mechanisms for transmission of HIV through breastmilk ?

One theory to explain the transmission of HIV through breastmilk is that M-cells—specialized epithelial cells that comprise only one percent of all epithelial mucosal cells found in the Peyer's patches of intestinal mucosa—engulf the virus and allow it to pass through to the macrophages on the other side. The M-cells could facilitate passage through the single layer of cells in the gut that are connected with mostly impermeable junctions (Featherstone 1997). Another study showed the HIV-infected cells in the intestinal lumen stimulated enterocytes to engulf HIV particles (Bomsel 1997). Research conducted in Rwanda with 215 HIV-1-infected women examined how three factors (HIV-1-infected cells, deficiencies in anti-infective substances in breastmilk,m or both) influenced transmission at 15 days, 6 months, and 18 months post-partum (Van de Perre et al 1993). Immunoglobulin (Ig) G was the most frequently identified HIV-specific antibody in breastmilk, followed by immunoglobulin (Ig) M. The strongest predictor of transmission was HIV-1 infected cells in breastmilk and combined with a defective IgM response.

What are the risks of HIV transmission through breast feeding ?

The risk factors of HIV transmission through breast feeding are as follows :-

Maternal viral load

Maternal viral load is higher in mothers with recent HIV infection or advanced disease. The risk of MTCT during breastfeeding nearly doubles if the mother becomes infected while breastfeeding. An analysis of four studies in which mothers became infected post-natally found a 29 percent risk of transmission through breastfeeding (Dunn et al 1992), the increased risk provides a strong argument for voluntary counseling and testing (VCT) and prevention measures during pregnancy and delivery.

***Strong evidence*

Maternal immune status

Maternal immune status also appears to increase the risk of transmission. Immunedeficiencies in the mother, including a low CD4 or high CD8 cell count, increase the risk. A study in Kenya (Nduati et al 1995) found a strong correlation between low CD4 counts and detection of HIV DNA in breastmilk.

***Strong evidence*

Breast health

Breast health related to mastitis, cracked and bloody nipples, and other indications of breast inflammation may affect transmission of HIV. The risk is also higher in an infant with oral lesions such as thrush (Ekpini et al 1997; Semba et al 1999).

***Strong evidence*

Mastitis may be caused by infectious agents, poor positioning and attachment, or weak suckling. Deficiencies in the antioxidants vitamin E and selenium also may increase the risk of mastitis.

Mastitis causes junctions in the mammary epithelium to become "leaky," allowing blood plasma constituents (HIV) to enter breastmilk. Cytokines and other immune reactions resulting from mastitis can damage the intestines of young babies.

Pattern or mode of breastfeeding

The pattern or mode of breastfeeding also affects transmission. Babies who are exclusively breastfed may have a lower risk of becoming infected than those who consume other liquids, milks, or solid foods in addition to breastmilk during the first months of life (Coutsoudis et al 1999, 2001; Smith and Kuhn 2000). The research conducted in South Africa (Coutsoudis et al 1999, 2001) showed that mothers who exclusively breastfed their infants for 3 months were less likely to transmit the virus than mothers who introduced other foods or fluids before 3 months. At 3 months, infants who were exclusively breastfed had significantly lower transmission rates (19.4 percent) than mixed-fed infants (26.1 percent) and the same transmission rate as formula-fed infants (19.4 percent). **Limited evidene*

Mucosal integrity

Studies show that the disruption of the epithelial integrity of the mucous membranes of the intestine or mouth of the infant increases the risk of transmission (Ekpini et. al 1997). Mixed feeding, allergic reactions to complementary foods, and infectious iliness can damage the intestine and increase risk of transmission (Bobat et al 1997; Ryder et al 1991; Tess et al. 1998b). Oral thrush in an infant may also be associated with MTCT.

Breastfeeding duration

The first positive PCR cannot differentiate whether transmission occurred during late pregnancy, labor and delivery, or the early post-natal period. Studies suggest that the risk of transmission declines with the age of the infant. It is difficult, however,to ascribe increased risk only to breastfeeding duration and the age factor, as feeding patterns change over time. Breastmilk intake is gradually decreased, which reduces exposure to the virus but also causes the infant to become increasingly vulnerable to other infections. ***Strong evidence*

Maternal nutritional status

Malnutrition during pregnancy *may* increase the risk of MTCT (Semba 1997). Vitamin A deficiency may impair T and B cell function, resulting in an increased maternal viral load and reduced antibody concentrations. Vitamin A deficiency could also result from advanced HIV disease. Both malnutrition and vitamin A deficiency contribute to MTCT. A study of 1,075 HIV-infected pregnant women in Tanzania showed that taking multivitamins, not vitamin A supplements, improved birth outcomes (reduced risk of low birth weight, severe pre-term birth, and small size for gestational age) (Fawzi et al 1998). Taking multivitamins, not vitamin A, significantly increased CD4, CD8, and CD3 counts.

What are the criteria to be considered for taking a decision on breast feeding ?

IF a mother knows she is HIV infected, and

IF safer feeding options other than exclusive breastfeeding are appropriate,

IF breastmilk substitutes are affordable and can be fed safely with clean water,

IF adequate health care is available and affordable,

Then the infant's chances of survival are greater if fed with breastmilk substitutes Or if a mother chooses to breastfeed, she should do so exclusively until the infant is about six months old, when she/he is ready to take complementary foods.

HOWEVER,

IF infant mortality is high as a result of infectious diseases, or

IF hygiene, sanitation, and access to clean water are poor, or

IF safer feeding options other than exclusive breastfeeding are inappropriate,

IF the cost of breastmilk substitutes is prohibitively high, or

IF access to adequate health care is limited,

THEN breastfeeding may be the safest feeding option, even when the mother is HIV positive.

"When replacement feeding is acceptable, feasible, affordable, sustainable, and safe, avoidance of all breastfeeding by HIVinfected mothers is recommended. Otherwise, exclusive breastfeeding is recommended during the first months of life. To minimize HIV transmission risk, breastfeeding should be discontinued as soon as feasible, taking into account local circumstances, the individual woman's situation and the risks of replacement feeding (including infections other than HIV and malnutrition)." (Source: WHO. 2001)

How can we reduce the risk of HIV transmission from mother to child ?

The three most common drug regimen used for prevention of HIV transmission from mother to child are as follows :-

- Administration of Nevirapine (NVP) to the mother during labour and to infant within 72 hours of birth. This course is preferred because of the low cost and ease of administration (single dose for mother and newborn). NVP is a non-nucleoside reverse transcriptase inhibitor. Viramune is the commercial name. A clinical trial in Uganda (Guay et al 1999) showed that giving a single dose of Nevirapine to mothers during labour and another to her infant after delivery reduced transmission in breastfed infants by 42 percent through 6 weeks and by 35 percent through 12 months.
- Administration of Zidovudine (ZDV) to women from 36 weeks gestation through labour and delivery, with additional prophylactic ZDV to the mother after birth in some regimens. ZVD is a nucleoside analogue. Retrovir is the commercial name.
- Administration of ZVD and Lamivudine (3TC) to mother and baby during the antenatal, intrapartum, and post-partum periods. 3TC is also a nucleoside analogue. Epivir is the commercial name.

2

What is Good Nutrition ?

"He that takes medicine and neglects diet, wastes the skill of the physician."

What is Good Nutrition?

Food is important for everyone. Familiar foods make us feel safe and secure. Food reminds us of our childhood, home country and culture. We celebrate events by eating special foods in the company of people who are important to us. When we eat well we feel well. Nutrition plays an important role in helping the immune system of our bodies work well. When we feed our bodies well, most of us feel better and have a more positive attitude about life. Eating tasty meals with people who care about us can be wonderful "medicine" for our emotional health.

Food provides the energy and nutrients that our bodies need to:

- stay alive, move and work;
- build new cells and tissues for growth, maintenance and repair;
- resist and fight infections.

When the body does not get enough food, it becomes weak and cannot develop or function properly. Healthy and balanced nutrition means eating the right type of foods in the right quantities to keep healthy, keep fit and enjoy ourselves.

Good nutrition means eating such variety of foods each day that will give you adequate proteins, fats, carbohydrates, vitamins, minerals to keep your body strong. Good nutrition means eating foods that give you enough calories to have a healthy body weight.

It also means getting enough protein to keep your body built up and repair any damage it may have. Good nutrition can help boost immune function, maximize the effectiveness of antiretroviral therapy, reduce the risk of chronic illnesses such as diabetes and cardiovascular disease, and contribute to a better quality of life.

- Perhaps you are infected with HIV but have no signs and symptoms of the disease. Good nutrition is extremely important if you are HIV positive. In this case, concentrate on eating a wide variety of healthy foods each day. There is no one type of food that has everything our bodies need. You have to choose from the variety of foods according to your nutritional needs.
- Perhaps your HIV infection is causing minor health problems. Eating may be uncomfortable or your appetite may be poor right now, but it is so important to eat well! Sometimes you'll find that by avoiding certain foods and eating others or changing the **time** that you eat or the **amount** that you eat can make you feel a lot better.
- Perhaps your HIV infection is causing serious health problems, and you may even need assistance in shopping, cooking or eating. Keep in close contact with your doctor and use the suggestions in this book to help you carry out his advice concerning food and eating.

Why Is Nutrition Important ?

Nutrition means your intake: the amount and quality of foods you eat, the liquids you drink, and the dietary supplements you take. Nutrition also means how your foods, liquids, and supplements get digested into the nutrients that then move from your digestive system into your bloodstream to be carried to different parts of your body and used in metabolism, the functions and processes, which support life. Think of nutrition as links in a chain. The first link is what you choose to eat and drink. Second is how well it can be digested. Third is how effectively your body can utilize these nutrients. You need all three links. The one that you have most control over is intake. If any link in the chain is broken, malnutrition can result. Poor food intake hurts the first link, vomiting and diarrhoea hurt the second, and fevers, abnormal metabolism, and infections hurt the third.

HIV infects the cells that line the gastrointestinal tract and can make eating, digestion, absorption, and elimination painful, difficult, and less effective. When severe, malnutrition can cause illness and death, even with higher CD-4 cell levels.

Good nutrition means getting enough of proteins, carbohydrates, and fats which will give you calories. These are called macronutrients. They help you maintain your body weight. In addition to proteins, carbohydrates, and fats , our bodies also require vitamins and minerals. These are called micronutrients. Good nutrition can be a problem for many people with HIV. When your body fights any infection, it uses more energy and you need to eat more than normal. But when you feel sick, you eat less than normal.

Some medications can upset your stomach, and some opportunistic infections can affect the mouth or throat. This makes it difficult to eat. Also, some medications and infections cause diarrhoea. If you have diarrhoea, your body actually uses less of what you eat. When you lose weight, you might be losing fat, or you might be losing lean body weight like muscle. If you lose too much lean weight, your body chemistry changes. Wasting can kill you. If you lose more than 5% of your body weight, it could be a sign of wasting. In this case, you must talk to your doctor.

How does what we eat affect our immune system?

Nutrition Experts all over the world have proclaimed emphatically that the most important factor to a healthy immune system is nutrition. There are specific nutrients that are key components of immune function. "A deficiency of virtually any single nutrient can significantly impair immunity". Throughout the world, nutrient deficiency is by far the most common cause of poor immune function. Scientists now recognize the crucial role that nutrition plays in supporting immune function.

Research studies indicate that increasing the intake of certain vitamins, minerals and essential fatty acids can boost the immune system and help the body to fight against AIDS, thus prolonging life and improving the quality of life . Patients must also keep in mind that most of the anti-AIDS drugs deplete one or more vitamins and/or minerals in the body.

Supplements to increase immunity

The association between vitamins, minerals and AIDS is complicated and taking vast doses of certain of these micronutrients may even hamper the immune system. So let's take a brief look at some of the micronutrients and how much you should be taking:

Vitamin A: known as the anti-infective vitamin. Helps maintain skin/mucous membranes (one of your defenses). stimulate immune response and increase the number of helper T-cells

Vitamin C: helps in phagocytosis (process of phagocytes chowing down on the bacteria and viruses) as well as detoxifying the body from pollution.

Vitamin E and Selenium: deficiencies can trigger benign (harmless) viruses to become virulent (harmful) leading to infections. It restores cell-mediated immunity and increases T-cell number and activity

Vitamin B6: This vitamin nourishes the thymus. B6 also is necessary for maintaining mental equilibrium and nervous system (combats stress!). There is some evidence that oral contraceptives, antibiotics, alcohol and high fat diet interfere with metabolism of B6 and so higher doces of B6 are needed in the diet.

Iron: has been shown to improve antibody response to the herpes simplex antigen.

Zinc: this mineral is also essential for the thymus, maintains mental equilibrium.

Why is good nutrition important for people with HIV?

There are many ways in which HIV/AIDS can affect the body's nutritional status.

- HIV increases the body's metabolic demands which, in turn, increase the amount of calories and protein needed to maintain body weight and muscle mass.
- HIV infects intestinal epithelial cells which can compromise your body's ability to absorb nutrients from food and medications.
- HIV/AIDS, opportunistic infections and some medications can decrease, or even eliminate your appetite, increasing the risk for weight loss and wasting.
- Some antiretroviral therapies can increase your cardiovascular risk factors by altering your cholesterol, triglyceride and glucose levels.

- Good nutrition helps keep your immune system strong, enabling you to fight the disease better. A healthy diet improves quality of life.
- Weight loss, wasting, and malnutrition continue to be common problems in HIV, despite more effective antiretroviral medications, and can contribute to HIV disease progression.
- Good nutrition helps the body process the many medications taken by people with HIV.
- Diet (and exercise) may help with symptoms such as diarrhoea, nausea, and fatigue, and with fat redistribution and metabolic abnormalities such as high blood sugar, cholesterol, and triglycerides.

Nutrition is one key element in the medical management of HIV. Good Nutrition is not a cure for HIV. Eat right for life. People with HIV/AIDS require more calories simply to maintain their weight, due to increased metabolism, higher energy demands, hormone and cytokine imbalances, inefficient absorption and utilization of nutrients, and/or accelerated tissue breakdown (catabolism).

The nutritional needs vary widely from person to person, and there is no one diet or supplement regimen appropriate for all people with HIV/AIDS.

While weight loss, malnutrition and increased risk for cardiovascular disease frequently accompany HIV/AIDS, there are things you can do to protect yourself. Research shows that good nutrition and exercise can boost your immune function, help fight infections, improve your tolerance and response to medications, reduce fatigue and improve your strength. Nutrition can affect a person's ability to survive with HIV/AIDS. Staying nutritionally fit is difficult for everyone, but for HIV-positive people the task is even more challenging.

When you commit to yourself to improve your health, big results can happen. This is especially true when you are living with HIV/AIDS. Make the commitment to yourself to help your body fight the virus by eating well, exercising and taking your medications as prescribed. Food, exercise and medication all work as a team to build your immune system.

3

How HIV affects Nutrition and Vice Versa

Nutrition and HIV are linked. Any immune impairment as a result of HIV/AIDS can contribute to malnutrition. Malnutrition leads to immune impairment, worsens the effects of HIV, and contributes to a more rapid progression of the disease. Thus, malnutrition both contributes to and is a result of HIV disease progression.

A person who is malnourished and then acquires HIV is more likely to progress faster to AIDS because the body is already weak and cannot fight co-infections, particularly without access to ARVs and prophylactic medications. A well-nourished person has a stronger immune system for coping with HIV and fighting illness. Timely improvement in nutritional status can help strengthen the immune system, thereby reducing the incidence of infections, preventing loss of weight and lean body mass, and delaying disease progression, so that HIV has less chance to develop in a person who is well nourished.

Some nutritional deficiencies can be reversed by timely and adequate nutritional therapy. Nutritional care and support helps people living with HIV to manage HIV-related complications, promotes good responses to medical treatment, and improves the person's quality of life by maintaining strength, comfort, level of functioning, and human dignity. Nutritional care and support is especially effective for those HIV-positive people who have not yet progressed to the stage requiring ARV treatment.

Nutrition and HIV/AIDS: Basic Facts

AIDS-wasting syndrome is defined as a 10 percent weight loss of baseline body weight plus either chronic diarrhoea . People with HIV/AIDS may experience protein –calorie malnutrition or deficiencies of specific nutrients even among individuals with relatively intact immune systems. Several factors can contribute to nutritional problems in people with HIV/AIDS.

Malabsorption: HIV or associated infections can damage the lining of the gastrointestinal tract, which can interfere with absorption of nutrients. Some HIV positive people experience specific problems, such as fat malabsorption, which can impair absorption of fat-soluble vitamins.

Opportunistic infections: Various bacterial, viral, fungal, and parasitic infections can interfere with proper nutrition. Malignancies (cancers) and mycobacterial illnesses such as tuberculosis are often characterized by wasting. Several Opportunistic Infections (O.I) cause vomiting and diarrhoea, which can lead to poor absorption or loss of nutrients. Other infections — such as thrush (oral candidiasis), gingivitis (gum inflammation), and cytomegalovirus esophagitis (throat inflammation) — can make eating painful.

Medications: Antiretrovirals, OI drugs, and other medications can contribute to nutrient deficiencies and imbalances, either due to direct drug-nutrient interactions or drug side effects. Vomiting and diarrhoea can lead to dehydration and depletion of nutrients. Loss of appetite (anorexia), fatigue, and taste alterations can make it difficult to eat enough. Antibiotics may interfere with nutrition by killing off beneficial bacteria in the gut. Food requirements — the need to take medications either on a full or an empty stomach or with specific types of food — can disrupt normal eating patterns. Further, some antiretroviral medications are associated with metabolic changes such as blood lipid and glucose abnormalities.

Inadequate intake: Sick people often experience anorexia (loss of appetite). OI symptoms and medication side effects — nausea, diarrhoea, sore mouth or throat, altered sense of taste or smell - can further reduce the desire or ability to eat. This may be compounded by lack of money, depression, or feeling too fatigued to shop and prepare food.

Nutritional deficiencies can impair immune function, potentially worsening HIV disease progression. Research has shown that depletion of vitamins A, C, and E, the B-complex vitamins, and the minerals selenium and zinc can interfere with cell-mediated immunity.Depletion of nutrients such as vitamins A and E, and minerals including magnesium, selenium, and zinc appears to be common, especially among individuals with advanced HIV disease. In particular, having HIV seems to decrease the body's store of antioxidants, as they are needed to offset increased oxidative stress.

Healthy and balanced nutrition is important for people living with HIV/AIDS

Nutritional care and support promote well-being, self-esteem and a positive attitude to life for people and their families living with HIV/AIDS.

Healthy and balanced nutrition should be one of the goals of counselling and care for people at all stages of HIV infection. An effective programme of nutritional care and support will improve the quality of life of people living with HIV/AIDS, by:

- maintaining body weight and strength;
- replacing lost vitamins and minerals;
- improving the function of the immune system and the body's ability to fight infection;
- extending the period from infection to the development of the AIDS disease;
- improving response to treatment; reducing time and money spent on health care;
- keeping HIV-infected people active, allowing them to take care of themselves, their family and children; and
- keeping HIV-infected people productive, able to work, grow food and contribute to the income of their families.

What is Healthy and balanced diet ?

A healthy diet provides adequate nutrition without a lot of empty calories. "Balanced" means eating a variety of foods from all the important food groups, since no food alone provides all the nutrients the body needs. Eat vegetables of various colors — including dark green and deep orange — since these contain different vitamins, minerals, and phytochemicals. Whole fruit is preferable to juice, which is high in sugar and calories and typically lacks fibre. Since cooking can destroy vitamins, it is usually recommended to eat vegetables raw or lightly steamed. However, this may not be the best advice for people with severely compromised immunity who are at risk of infection with microorganisms that can be killed by cooking.

In the dairy group, select low-fat or non-fat products. People who choose not to consume dairy foods should be sure to obtain enough calcium from other sources. In the protein group, eating more legumes, nuts, seeds, and fish — which contains heart-healthy omega-3 fatty acids is very useful. When eating meat or poultry, remove visible fat and skin. Boiling, baking, and grilling are healthier cooking methods than frying.

In terms of fats, avoid animal-derived fats and chemically altered hydrogenated oils, instead substituting plant-derived monounsaturated and polyunsaturated oils. This is good for people who do not need to lose (or could stand to gain) weight, since animal fats increase the risk of cardiovascular disease. Another boon for the heart: a low-sodium diet can help keep blood pressure under control.

In addition to eating a balanced diet, it is also important to consume enough fluids. Experts traditionally recommend eight 8-ounce (Litres) glasses of water per day. Herbal tea, broth, and fruit or vegetable juices can also be good fluid sources. But beverages that contain caffeine or alcohol have a diuretic effect, and can cause loss of water due to increased urination. It is especially important to drink enough fluid to prevent dehydration when suffering prolonged vomiting or diarrhoea. People with very low CD4 cell counts concerned about infections such as cryptosporidiosis due to contaminated tap water should use filtered or bottled water.

More people are also adopting vegetarian diets, which have been linked to reduced risk of cardiovascular disease and cancer. Most people can obtain adequate nutrition from a diet that contains little or no meat or other animal products. Dietary supplements are products such as vitamins, minerals, amino acids, herbs, and antioxidants; they are usually taken orally in the form of tabiets, capsules, powders, or liquids. Most healthcare providers agree that

HIV positive people can benefit from a daily multivitamin and mineral supplement. Due to the potential harmful effects of iron, many recommend an iron-free supplement for anyone other than menstruating women and people with iron deficiency.

4

Your Digestive System

Your digestive system or GI Tract

In order to know about nutrition, it is essential to know a little about your digestive system.

Your **digestive system** or gastrointestinal (GI) tract is essential for your well-being. It not only provides you with your nutrition, but is also an important part of your immune system. Your total skin area is under 2 square metres, while the total area of the mucosal linings of your digestive system is more than 400 square metres (Beagley & Elson, 1992) and the GI tract makes up the largest section. The **gastrointestinal tract (GI tract)** is the system of organs that takes in food, digests it to extract energy and nutrients, and expels the remaining waste. The major functions of the GI tract are digestion and excretion. The GI tract starts with your mouth and ends with your anus

In a normal human adult male, the GI tract is approximately 6.5 meters long (20 feet) and consists of the upper and lower GI tracts.

The **upper GI tract** consists of the mouth, pharynx, oesophagus, and stomach.

- The mouth contains the buccal mucosa, which contains the openings of the salivary glands; the tongue; and the teeth.
- Behind the mouth lies the pharynx, which leads to a hollow muscular tube, the esophagus.

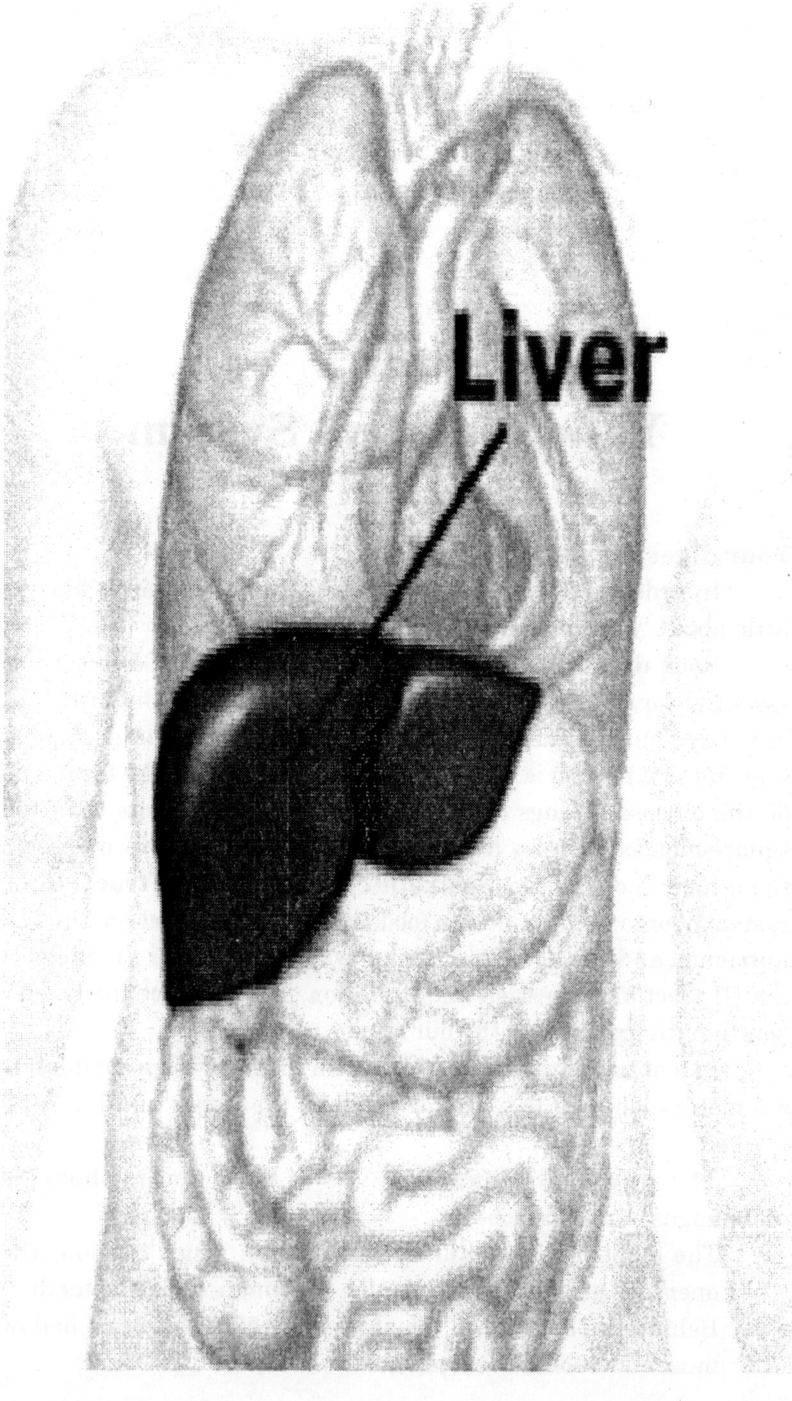
Liver

- The esophagus extends through the chest and pierces the diaphragm to reach the stomach.
- The stomach, in turn, leads to the small intestine.

  The **lower GI tract** comprises the intestines and anus.
- Bowel or intestine:
  - small intestine, which has three parts:
    - duodenum
    - jejunum
    - ileum
  - large intestine, which has three parts:
    - caecum (the vermiform appendix is attached to the caecum).
    - colon (ascending colon, transverse colon, descending colon and sigmoid flexure)
    - rectum
    - anus

Related organs

The liver secretes bile into the small intestine via the biliary system, employing the gallbladder as a reservoir. The pancreas secretes an isosmotic fluid containing bicarbonate and several enzymes, including trypsin, chymotrypsin, lipase, and pancreatic amylase, as well as nucleolytic enzymes (deoxyribonuclease and ribonuclease), into the small intestine. Both these secretory organs help in digestion.

Teeth

Teeth are structures found in the jaws of many vertebrates. The primary function of teeth is to tear and chew food, and in some animals, particularly carnivores, for fighting and/or defence. The roots of the teeth are covered by gums. Adult teeth naturally darken with age as the pulp within the tooth shrinks and dentin is deposited in its place.

While humans develop two sets of teeth throughout life (diphyodont), some animals develop only one set (monophyodont) or develop many (polyphyodont). Sharks, for example, grow a new set of teeth every two weeks. Rodent teeth grow and wear away continually through the animal's gnawing, maintaining approximately constant length.

- Humans are diphyodont, meaning that they develop two sets of teeth throughout life. The first set (the "baby," "milk," "primary" or "deciduous" set) normally starts to appear at about six months of age, although some babies are born with one or more visible teeth, known as neonatal teeth.

The second, permanent set of teeth consists of 32 teeth. Twenty-eight of them appear between the ages of about 6 and 12 years. Permanent teeth are evenly distributed across the mouth's quadrants. Each quadrant of eight teeth has a:

- central incisor (upper jaw: maxillary central incisor; lower jaw: mandibular central incisor)
- lateral incisor (upper jaw: maxillary lateral incisor; lower jaw: mandibular lateral incisor)
- cuspid (canine) (upper jaw: maxillary canine; lower jaw: mandibular canine)
- first premolar (bicuspid) (upper jaw: maxillary first premolar; lower jaw: mandibular first premolar)
- second premolar (bicuspid) (upper jaw: maxillary second premolar; lower jaw: mandibular second premolar)
- first molar (upper jaw: maxillary first molar; lower jaw: mandibular first molar)
- second molar (upper jaw: maxillary second molar; lower jaw: mandibular second molar)
- third molar (wisdom teeth) (upper jaw: maxillary third molar; lower jaw: mandibular third molar)

The permanent set may last for life if cared for properly through a regular program of dental hygiene, including regular brushing and professional cleaning by a dentist or hygienist. Teeth that are susceptible to decay may be sealed for additional protection.

Brushing teeth immediately after eating acidic foods is not recommended, because acid softens the enamel, which can then be damaged by brushing. It is better to wait at least half an hour after eating acidic foods before brushing. Rinsing the mouth and eating non-acidic foods can also speed up this process.

Tongue

The tongue is the large bundle of skeletal muscles on the floor of the mouth that manipulates food for chewing and swallowing, (deglutition). It is the primary organ of taste. Much of the surface of the tongue is covered in taste buds. The tongue with its wide variety of possible movements assists in forming the sounds of speech. It is sensitive and kept moist by saliva, richly supplied with nerves and blood vessels to help it be moved.

The dorsum (upper surface) of the tongue can be divided into two parts, an **oral part** (anterior two-thirds of the tongue) that lies mostly in the mouth and a **pharyngeal part** (posterior third of the tongue), which faces backward to the oropharynx. The two parts are separated by a V-shaped groove, which marks the **sulcus terminalis** (or **terminal sulcus**).

The oral part of the tongue is covered with small bumpy projections called papillae. There are three types of papillae: filiform (thread-shape), fungiform (mushroom-shape), and circumvallate (ringed-circle). All papillae except the filiform have taste buds on their surface. The circumvallate are the largest of the papillae. There are 8 to 14 circumvallate papillae arranged in a V-shape in front of the sulcus terminalis, creating a border between the oral and pharyngeal parts of the tongue.

There are no lingual papillae on the underside of the tongue. It is covered with a smooth mucous membrane, with a fold (the lingual frenulum) in the center.

The human tongue can detect five basic taste components, sweet, sour, salty, bitter and umami. The sense of taste is referred to as a gustatory sense. The sublingual region underneath the front of the tongue is a location where the oral mucosa is very thin, and underlied by a plexus of veins. This is an ideal location for introducing certain medications to the body.

White spots and patches or coating of the tongue are a symptom of several medical conditions:

- Antibiotics side effect
- Oral candidiasis
- Debauch
- Dehydration
- Leukoplakia
- Keratosis pharyngis
- Jaundice - causes a yellow tongue
- "Lie Bumps" - small dots usually on tip of tongue

The mouth

The human mouth is covered by an upper and lower lip. They play an important role in speech (it is part of the vocal apparatus), facial expression, kissing, drinking (especially with a straw), and smoking(which gives you cancer). Infants are born with a sucking reflex, by which they instinctively know to suck for nourishment using their lips and jaw. Lips are often adorned with lipstick or lip gloss although in most human cultures this is an affectation for females only. The philtrum is the vertical groove in the upper lip, formed where the nasomedial and maxillary processes meet during embryo development. When these processes fail to fuse fully, a hare lip and/or cleft palate can result. The nasolabial folds are the deep creases of tissue that extend from the nose to the sides of the mouth. One of the first signs of age on the human face is the increase in prominence of the nasolabial folds.

The mouth starts digestion by physically chewing the food and breaking it down with saliva.

Three possible problems in the mouth and throat are oral hairy leukophakia (OHL), aphthous ulcers, and infection by the yeast/ fungus *Candida albicans*.

Oral hairy leukoplakia is not considered as a major hazard. Some doctors use a tincture of Podophyllum on Oral hairy leukoplakia . Use of antioxidant supplements may be of benefit , although this may be of a general nature since antioxidants are generally important for immune function .

Aphthous ulcers can be painful, destroy your enjoyment of food, and should always be treated by a medical doctor. Rinsing and gargling with either a salt solution, 1-3% hydrogen peroxide can help in some cases, but should not be relied upon without also seeking expert medical advice. Corticosteroids have been prescribed for aphthous ulcers, but these should be used with caution since extensive use may make other opportunistic infections more likely

There are several ways for prevention of **thrush** in your mouth and throat. Thrush grows fastest on simple sugars, so avoid foods with high levels of these (simple sugars may be sucrose, glucose, fructose, and other names ending with 'ose'). After you've eaten, brush your teeth. Then, it's good to rinse your mouth so there will be no food particles left. Mouth wash and oral antiseptics can be used as a gargle for helping prevent yeast infection.

Pharynx

The pharynx is the part of the neck and throat situated immediately posterior to the mouth and nasal cavity, and cranial to the esophagus, larynx, and trachea.

The human pharynx is conventionally divided into three sections:

- **Nasopharynx**, lying behind the nasal cavity. Postero-superiorly this extends from the level of the junction of the hard and soft palates to the base of skull, laterally to include the fossa of Rosenmuller. The inferior wall consists of the superior surface of the soft palate.
- **Oropharynx**, which lies behind the oral cavity. The anterior wall consists of the base of the tongue and the vallecula; the lateral wall is made up of the tonsil, tonsillar fossa, and tonsillar (faucial) pillars; the superior wall consists of the inferior surface of the soft palate and the uvula.
- **Hypopharynx**, also known as the laryngopharynx, which includes the pharyngo-oesophageal junction (postcricoid area), the piriform sinus, and the posterior pharyngeal wall. Like the oropharynx above it the hypopharynx serves as a passageway for food and air and is lined with a stratified squamous epithelium. It lies directly posterior to the upright epiglottis and extends to the larynx, where the respiratory and digestive pathways diverge. At that point the laryngopharynx is continuous with the esophpagus posteriorly. The esophagus conducts food and fluids to the stomach; air enters the larynx anteriorly. During swallowing, food has the "right of way", and air passage temporarily stops.

Oesophagus

The Oesophagus or **gullet** is a muscular tube through which food passes from the mouth area to the stomach. The esophagus is continuous with the laryngeal part of the pharynx at the level of the C6 vertebra.

Food is passed through the esophagus by using the process of peristalsis. It connects the pharynx, which is the body cavity that is common to the digestive system and respiratory system behind the mouth (buccal cavity), with the stomach, where the second stage of digestion is initiated (the first stage of digestion is in the mouth, with teeth and tongue masticating food and mixing it with saliva).

The oesophagus is lined with mucous membrane, and is more deeply lined with muscle that acts with peristaltic action to move swallowed food down to the stomach.

The junction between the esophagus and the stomach (the gastroesophageal junction or GE junction) is not actually considered a valve, although it is sometimes called the cardiac valve but is actually more of a stricture.

The lining of your oesophagus can get infected with the yeast candida. This infection, called ***oesophageal candidiasis,*** makes it difficult, even painful, to swallow food, and is dangerous. If you suspect you may have this, it's important to check in right away with your doctor who can give you treatment for it. Never rely on home remedies for oesophageal candidiasis.

Since the lining of your oesophagus is part of your immune system, it may also be a place that the HIV attacks.

The important thing to remember is that the lining of your intestinal tract is a major reservoir of T-cells and therefore a site for attack by the HIV.

Stomach :

In anatomy, the **stomach** (in ancient Greek *óôüìá÷ïò*) is an organ of the gastrointestinal tract involved in the second phase of digestion, following mastication.

The stomach is generally a highly acidic environment with a pH range of 1 to 4 depending on food intake and other factors. Pepsinogen is secreted by chief cells and turns into pepsin in the presence of hydrochloric acid. The stomach's interior can secrete 2 to 3 litres of gastric fluid per day. The stomach's primary function is to break down large molecules (such as from food) into smaller ones using hydrochloric acid so that they can be absorbed from the small intestine.

Secondary functions include protein digestion using pepsin enzymes, and absorbing water, some ions, and some lipid soluble compounds such as alcohol, aspirin, and caffeine haha.

Two smooth muscle valves, or sphincters, keep the contents of the stomach contained. They are the *Cardiac or esophageal sphincter* dividing the tract above, and the *Pyloric sphincter* dividing the stomach from the small intestine.

In humans, the stomach has a volume of about 50 mL when empty. After a meal, it can expand to hold about 1 liter of food, but it can actually expand to hold as much as 4 L.

The stomach is divided into four sections, each of which has different cells and functions. The sections are:

Cardia	where the contents of the oesophagus empty into the stomach.
Fundus	formed by the upper curvature of the organ.
Body	the main central region.
Pylorus or antrum	the lower section of the organ that facilitates emptying the contents into the small intestine.

The movement and the flow of chemicals into the stomach are controlled by both the autonomic nervous system and by the various digestive system hormones:

Gastrin	The hormone gastrin causes an increase in the secretion of HCl, pepsinogen and intrinsic factor from parietal cells in the stomach. It also causes increased motility in the stomach. Gastrin is released by G-cells in the stomach to distension of the antrum, and digestive products. It is inhibited by a pH normally less than 4 (high acid), as well as the hormone somatostatin.
Cholecystokinin	Cholecystokinin (CCK) has most effect on the gall bladder, but it also decreases gastric emptying.
Secretin	In a different and rare manner, secretin, produced in the small intestine, has most effects on the pancreas, but will also diminish acid secretion in the stomach.
Gastric inhibitory peptide	Gastric inhibitory peptide (GIP) decreases both gastric acid and motility.
Enteroglucagon	enteroglucagon decreases both gastric acid and motility.

Other than gastrin, these hormones all act to turn off the stomach action. This is in response to food products in the liver and gall bladder, which have not yet been absorbed. The stomach needs only to push food into the small intestine when the intestine is not busy. While the intestine is full and still digesting food, the stomach acts as storage for food.

Some problems that can happen to the stomach when you are HIV+ may be from a decrease in the stomach acidity so that your food is more difficult to digest. Some people use either glutamic acid hydrochloride or betaine hydrochloride supplements to increase stomach acidity when they eat. Digestive enzymes such as *Daily Essential Enzymes* may help improve digestion since these don't require high acidity, and can help the breakdown of your food. If you use enzyme supplements, it's probably best if the supplement contains enzymes that digest protein, fat and carbohydrate.

Duodenum

In anatomy of the digestive system, the **duodenum** is a hollow jointed tube connecting the stomach to the jejunum. It is the first and shortest part of the small intestine. It begins with the duodenal bulb and ends at the ligament of Treitz. The name *duodenum* is from the Latin *duodenum digitorum*, twelve fingers' breadths or inches.

The duodenum is largely responsible for the breakdown of food in the small intestine. Brunner's glands are only found in the duodenum and they secrete mucus. These mucus filled glands are composed of simple cuboidal epithelial cells. The duodenum wall is composed of a very thin layer of cells that forms the muscularis mucosae.The duodenum is almost entirely retroperitoneal. The pH in the duodenum is approximately nine (slightly basic).

The duodenum is divided into four sections for the purposes of description. The first three sections form a "C" shape.

First part

The **first (superior) part** begins as a continuation of the duodenal end of the pylorus. From here it passes laterally (right), superiorly and posteriorly, for approximately 5 cm, before making a sharp curve inferiorly into the superior duodenal flexure (the end of the superior part). It is peritonised.

Second part

The **second (descending) part** of the duodenum begins at the superior duodenal flexure. It passes inferiorly to the lower border of vertebral body LIII, before making a sharp turn medially into the inferior duodenal flexure (the end of the descending part).

The pancreatic duct and common bile duct enter the descending duodenum, commonly known together as the hepatopancreatic duct (or pancreatic duct in the United States), through the major duodenal papilla. This part of the duodenum also contains the minor duodenal papilla, the entrance for the accessory pancreatic duct. The junction between the embryological foregut and midgut lies just below the major duodenal papilla.

Third part

The **third (inferior/horizontal) part** of the duodenum begins at the inferior duodenal flexure and passes transversely to the left, crossing the inferior vena cava, aorta and the vertebral column.

Fourth part

The **fourth (ascending) part** passes superiorly, either anterior to, or to the left of, the aorta, until it reaches the inferior border of the body of the pancreas. Then, it curves anteriorly and terminates at the duodenojejunal flexure where it joins the jejunum. The duodenal flexure is surrounded by a peritoneal fold containing muscle fibres: the ligament of Treitz.

Jejunum

In anatomy of the digestive system, the **jejunum** is the central of the three divisions of the small intestine and lies between the duodenum and the ileum.

In adult humans, the small intestine is usually between 2-8m (6' 7"-26' 3") long; 1-2 m of which is the jejunum.

The pH in the jejunum is usually between 7 and 8 (neutral or slightly alkaline).

The jejunum and the ileum are suspended by mesentery which gives the bowel great mobility within the abdomen.

The inner surface of the jejunum, its mucous membrane, is covered in projections called villi, which increase the surface area of tissue available to absorb nutrients from the gut contents. The villi in the jejunum are much longer than in the duodenum or ileum.

It differs from the duodenum due to lack of Brunner's glands.

It is also different from the ileum due to fewer goblet cells and generally lacks Peyer's patches.

Ileum

In anatomy of the digestive system, the **ileum** is the final section of the small intestine. It is about 2-4 m long in humans, follows the duodenum and jejunum, and is separated from the caecum by the ileocaecal valve (ICV). The pH in the ileum is usually between 7 and 8 (neutral or slightly alkaline).

Its function is to absorb the products of digestion,. The wall itself is made up of folds, each of which has many tiny finger-like projections known as villi, on its surface. In turn, the epithelial cells which line these villi possess even larger numbers of microvilli. Therefore the ileum has an extremely large surface area both for the adsorption (attachment) of enzyme molecules and for the **absorption of products of digestion.** The cells that line the ileum contain the protease and carbohydrase enzymes responsible for the final stages of protein and carbohydrate digestion. These enzymes are present in the cytoplasm of the epithelial cells. The villi contain large numbers of capillaries which take the amino acids and glucose produced by digestion to the hepatic portal vein and the liver.

Lacteals are small lymph vessels, and are present in villi. They absorb fatty acid and glycerol, the products of fat digestion. Layers of circular and longitudinal smooth muscle enable the digested food to be pushed along the ileum by waves of muscle contraction called peristalsis.

There is no line of demarcation between the jejunum and the ileum. There are, however, subtle differences between the two.

- The ileum has more fat inside the mesentery than the jejunum.
- The ileum is a paler color, and tends to be of a smaller caliber as well.
- While the length of the intestinal tract contains lymphoid tissue, only the ileum has abundant Peyer's patches. These

unencapsulated lymphoid nodules contain large amounts of lymphocytes and other cells of the immune system.

Caecum

The **cecum** or **caecum** (from the Latin *caecus* meaning blind) is a pouch connected to the ascending colon of the large intestine and the ileum. It is separated from the ileum by the ileocaecal valve (ICV) or Bauhin's valve, and is considered to be the beginning of the large intestine.

Appendix

The appendix is a branch of the caecum.

Like the human appendix, the caecum was once believed to have no function.

The term caecum comes from the Latin, meaning blind gut or divine right.

The junction between the small intestines and the colon, called the ileocecal valve, is so small in some animals that it was not considered to be a connection between the small and large intestines. During a dissection, the colon could be traced from the rectum, to the sigmoid colon, through the descending, transverse, and ascending sections. The colon seemed to dead-end into the caecum, or cul-de sac.

However, the connection between the end of the small intestines, ileum, and the start of the colon, caecum are clearly understood, but the name has not changed.

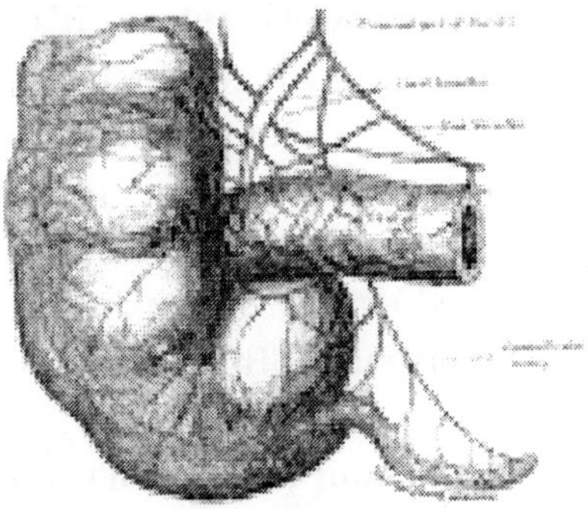

Your small intestine is also another important part of your immune system called the gut associated lymphoid tissue (GALT) -

the respiratory and urogenital tracts also have similar mucosal linings that have important immune functions The small intestine is lined with a mucosal system that provides a reservoir of T-cells called the "mucosal T-cells" (the T-cells in your blood are called the "systemic T-cells"). They are not measured by normal (blood) tests. Along the small intestine are sections called "Peyer's patches", also part of your immune system.

That the small intestinal lining is a reservoir of T-cells is only one reason why it is also a site of attack by HIV. There are several problems that can occur with your small intestine. With HIV, the 'fingers' lining the walls can get worn down to a short length because of too little nutrition. This makes it even more difficult to get your nutrition since it decreases the effective surface area for absorption of your nutrition. Several studies indicate that deterioration of the small intestine lining may be the earliest result of HIV infection, even before T-cells decline .

Vitamins B6 and B12, and the minerals magnesium and zinc are used at a faster than normal rate with HIV disease. Since these are very important for your body's ability to keep itself repaired (including replacement of the 'fingers' along the walls of your small intestine), you must make sure you keep these nutrients at a good level in your food and vitamin supplements.

You can get infection in your small intestine. When this occurs, your doctor will likely say that you have Small Bowel Disease (SBD) or Inflammatory Bowel Disease (IBD). S/he may also use names such as *ulcerative colitis* or *Crohn's disease*. Infection with parasites may also be a cause of small bowel problems. It's important to follow your doctor's instructions so it will get cured as soon as possible. S/he may give you antibiotics if s/he suspects a bacterial infection. (Normally, high stomach acidity prevents infection from entering the small intestine from the stomach; if the stomach acids are low, this protection is decreased.) In any case, a diagnosis of inflammation of the small intestine likely means that absorption of your nutrients is severely limited.

Sometimes the fat in your food doesn't finish breaking down in the small intestine, and you may even need to decrease the amount of fat in your food. Another reason to decrease dietary fat content would be diarrhoea that is difficult to get rid of.

Liver

The liver plays a major role in metabolism and has a number of functions in the body including glycogen storage, plasma protein synthesis, and drug detoxification. This organ also is the largest gland in the human body. It produces bile, which is important in digestion. It performs and regulates a wide variety of high-volume biochemical reactions requiring specialized tissues. Medical terms related to the liver often start in *hepato-* or *hepatic* from the Greek word for liver, *hepar*.

The adult human liver normally weighs between 1.3-3.0 kilograms, and it is a soft, pinkish-brown "boomerang shaped" organ. It is the second largest organ (the largest organ being the skin) and the largest gland within the human body.

It is in the on the right side of the upper abdomen body diaphragm. The liver lies on the right of the stomach and makes a kind of bed for the gallbladder (which stores bile).

The bile produced in the liver is collected in bile canaliculi, which merge to form bile ducts.

These eventually drain into the right and left hepatic ducts, which in turn merge to form the common hepatic duct. The cystic duct (from the gallbladder) joins with the common hepatic duct to form the common bile duct.

Bile can either drain directly into the duodenum via the common bile duct or be temporarily stored in the gallbladder via the cystic duct. The common bile duct and the pancreatic duct enter the duodenum together at the ampulla of Vater.

The branchings of the bile ducts resemble those of a tree, and indeed the term "biliary tree" is commonly used in this setting.

The liver is among the few internal human organs capable of natural regeneration of lost tissue; as little as 25% of remaining liver can regenerate into a whole liver again.

This is predominantly due to the hepatocytes acting as unipotential stem cells (i.e. a single hepatocyte can divide into two hepatocyte daughter cells). There is also some evidence of bipotential stem cells, called oval cells, which can differentiate into either hepatocytes or cholangiocytes (cells that line the bile ducts).

The various functions of the liver are carried out by the liver cells or hepatocytes.

- The liver produces and excretes bile required for emulsifying fats. Some of the bile drains directly into the duodenum, and some is stored in the gallbladder.
- The liver performs several roles in carbohydrate metabolism:
  - *Gluconeogenesis* (the synthesis of glucose from certain amino acids, lactate or glycerol)
  - *Glycogenolysis* (the breakdown of glycogen into glucose) (muscle tissues can also do this)
  - *Glycogenesis* (the formation of glycogen from glucose)
  - The breakdown of insulin and other hormones
  - The liver is responsible for the mainstay of protein metabolism.
- The liver also performs several roles in lipid metabolism:
  - *Cholesterol synthesis*
  - The production of triglycerides (fats).
- The liver produces coagulation factors I (fibrinogen), II (prothrombin), V, VII, IX, X and XI, as well as protein C, protein S and antithrombin.
- The liver breaks down hemoglobin, creating metabolites that are added to bile as pigment (bilirubin and biliverdin).
- The liver breaks down toxic substances and most medicinal products in a process called drug metabolism. This sometimes results in toxication, when the metabolite is more toxic than its precursor.
- The liver converts ammonia to urea.
- The liver stores a multitude of substances, including glucose in the form of glycogen, vitamin B12, iron, and copper.
- In the first trimester fetus, the liver is the main site of red blood cell production. By the 32nd week of gestation, the bone marrow has almost completely taken over that task.
- The liver is responsible for immunological effects- the reticuloendothelial system of the liver contains many immunologically active cells, acting as a 'sieve' for antigens carried to it via the portal system.

Many diseases of the liver are accompanied by jaundice caused by increased levels of bilirubin in the system. The bilirubin results from the breakup of the hemoglobin of dead red blood cells; normally, the liver removes bilirubin from the blood and excretes it through bile.

- Hepatitis, inflammation of the liver, caused mainly by various viruses(Hepatitis-A, Hepatitis-B, Hepatitis-C) but also by some poisons, autoimmunity or hereditary conditions.
- Cirrhosis is the formation of fibrous tissue in the liver, replacing dead liver cells. The death of the liver cells can for example be caused by viral hepatitis, alcoholism or contact with other liver-toxic chemicals.
- Cancer of the liver (primary hepatocellular carcinoma or cholangiocarcinoma and metastatic cancers, usually from other parts of the gastrointestinal tract).

A number of liver function tests are available to test the proper function of the liver. These test for the presence of enzymes in blood that are normally most abundant in liver tissue, metabolites or products.

Gall Blader

The **gallbladder** (or **cholecyst** sometimes **gall bladder**) is a pear-shaped organ that stores about 50 mL of bile (or "gall") until the body needs it for digestion.

The gallbladder is about 7-10cm long in humans and is dark green in appearance due to its contents (bile), not its tissue. It is connected to the liver and the duodenum by the biliary tract.

- The cystic duct leads from the gallbladder and joins with the common hepatic duct to form the common bile duct.
- The common bile duct then joins with the pancreatic duct, and enters the duodenum through the hepatopancreatic ampulla at the major duodenal papilla.

The gallbladder stores bile, which is released when food containing fat enters the digestive tract, stimulating the secretion of cholecystokinin (CCK). The bile emulsifies fats and neutralizes acids in partly digested food.

After being stored in the gallbladder, the bile becomes more concentrated than when it left the liver, increasing its potency and intensifying its effect on fats. Most digestion occurs in the duodenum.

Spleen

The **spleen** is a ductless, vertebrate gland that is closely associated with the circulatory system, where it functions in the destruction of old red blood cells in holding a reservoir of blood. It is regarded as one of the centres of activity of the reticuloendothelial system. Until recently, the purpose of the spleen was not known. It is increasingly recognized that its absence leads to a predisposition to certain infections.

The human spleen is located in the upper left part of the abdomen, behind the stomach and just below the diaphragm. In normal individuals this organ measures about 125 × 75 × 50 mm (5 × 3 × 2 inches) in size, with an average weight of 150 g.

The spleen is the largest organ derived from mesenchyme and lying in the mesentery. The spleen consists of masses of lymphoid tissue of granular appearance located around fine terminal branches of veins and arteries. These vessels are connected by modified capillaries called splenic sinuses.

Approximately 10% of people have one or more accessory spleens. They may form near the hilum of the main spleen, the junction at which the splenic vessels enter and leave the organ.

Cross sections of the spleen reveal a red soft surface which is divided into two types of pulp which correspond to the two most important functional roles of the spleen, summarized below:

Area	*Composition*	*Function*
red pulp	Composed largely of: * "sinuse" (or "sinusoids") which are filled with blood * "splenic cords" of reticular fibers * "marginal zone" bordering on white pulp	Mechanical filtration. Removes unwanted materials from the blood, including senescent red blood cells.
white pulp	Composed of nodules , called Malpighian corpuscles. These are composed of: * "lymphoid follicles" (or "follicles"), rich in B-lymphocytes * "periarteriolar lymphoid sheaths" (PALS), rich in T-lymphocytes	Helps fight infections.

Other functions of the spleen are less prominent, especialy in the healthy adult:

- Production of opsonins, properdin, and tuftsin.
- Creation of red blood cells. While the bone marrow is the primary site of hematopoeisis in the adult, up until the fifth month of gestation, the spleen has important hematopoietic functions. After birth, no significant hematopoietic function is left in the spleen except in some hematologic disorders: e.g. myelodysplastic syndrome, hemoglobinopathies.
- Storage of red blood cells and other formed elements. This is more common in the adult than the creation of new red blood cells.

Pancreas

The **pancreas** is an organ in the digestive and endocrine system that serves two major functions: exocrine (producing pancreatic juice containing digestive enzymes) and endocrine (producing several important hormones, including insulin).

In humans, the pancreas is a 15-25 cm (6-10 inch) elongated organ in the abdomen located retroperitoneal. It is located posterior to the stomach and in close association with the duodenum.

It is often described as having three regions: a head, body and tail.

- The body of the pancreas lies at the level of L2 on the spine.
- The pancreatic head abuts the second part of the duodenum.
- The tail of the pancreas extends towards the spleen.

The pancreatic duct runs the length of the pancreas and empties into the second part of the duodenum at the ampulla of Vater. The common bile duct commonly joins the pancreatic duct at or near this point.

Under a microscope, when properly stained, it is easy to distinguish two different tissue types in the pancreas. These regions correspond to the main pancreatic functions:

There are four main types of cells in the islets of Langerhans. They are relatively difficult to distinguish using standard staining techniques, but they can be classified by their secretion:

Name of cells	*Product*	*% of islet cells*	*Function*
beta cells	Insulin and Amylin	50-80%	lower blood sugar
alpha cells	Glucagon	15-20%	raise blood sugar
delta cells	Somatostatin	3-10%	inhibit endocrine pancreas
PP cells	Pancreatic polypeptide	1%	inhibit exocrine pancreas

The islets are a compact collection of endocrine cells arranged in clusters and cords and are crisscrossed by a dense network of capillaries.

There are two main classes of exocrine pancreatic secretions:

Colon

In the anatomy of the digestive system, the **colon** (> Greek κῶλον is the part of the large intestine between the cecum to the rectum. Its primary purpose is to extract water from faeces. It consists of the ascending colon, transverse colon, the descending colon, and the sigmoid colon.

Ascending colon

The ascending colon is on the right side of the abdomen. It is the part of the colon from the caecum to the hepatic flexure (the turn of the colon by the liver). It is retroperitoneal in most humans.

Transverse colon

The transverse colon is the part of the colon from the hepatic flexure (the turn of the colon by the liver) to the splenic flexure (the turn of the colon by the spleen). The transverse colon hangs off the stomach, attached to it by a wide band of tissue called the greater omentum. On the posterior side, the transverse colon is connected to the posterior abdominal wall by a mesentery known as the transverse mesocolon.

The transverse colon is encased in peritoneum, and is therefore mobile (unlike the parts of the colon immediately before and after it). More cancers form as the large intestine goes along and the contents become more solid (water is removed) in order to form

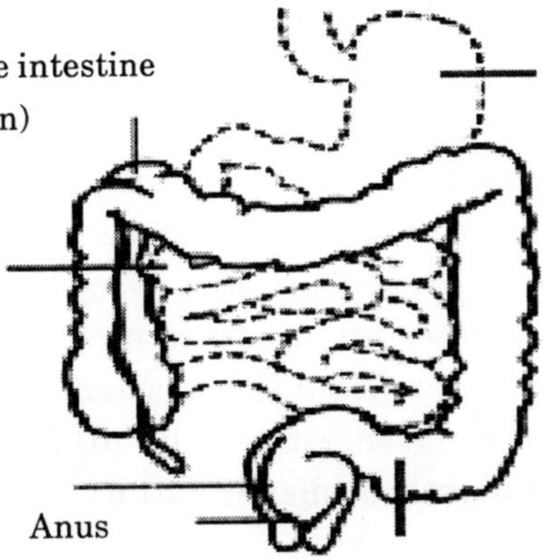

feces. It is primarily supplied by the middle colic artery, a branch of superior mesenteric artery.

Descending colon

The descending colon is the part of the colon from the splenic flexure to the beginning of the sigmoid colon. It is retroperitoneal in two-thirds of humans. In the other third, it has a (usually short) mesentery.

Sigmoid colon

The **sigmoid colon** is the part of the large intestine after the descending colon and before the rectum. The name *sigmoid* means S-shaped (see sigmoid). The walls of the sigmoid colon are muscular, and contract to increase the pressure inside the **colon,** causing the stool to move into the rectum.

Due to the intermittent high pressure within it, the colon can develop pockets called *diverticuli* in its walls. The presence of diverticuli, whether harmful or not, is called *diverticulosis*. An infection of the diverticuli is called *diverticulitis*.

The large intestine comes after the small intestine in the digestive tract and measures approximately 1.5 meters in length. By the time the chyme has reached this tube, almost all nutrients and 90% of the water have been absorbed by the body. At this point some electrolytes like sodium, magnesium, and chloride are left as well as indigestible carbohydrates known as dietary fibre. As the chyme moves through the large intestine, most of the remaining water is removed, while the chyme is mixed with mucus and bacteria known as gut flora, and becomes faeces. The bacteria break down some of the fibre for their own nourishment and create acetate, propionate, and butyrate as waste products, which in turn are used by the cell lining of the colon for nourishment. This is an example of a symbiotic relationship and provides about 100 Calories a day to the body. The large intestine produces no digestive enzymes — chemical digestion is completed in the small intestine before the chyme reaches the large intestine. The pH in the colon varies between 5.5 and 7 (slightly acidic to neutral).

Rectum

The **rectum** (from the Latin *rectum intestinum*, meaning *straight intestine*) is the final straight portion of the large intestine terminating in the anus.

For the diagnosis of certain ailments, a rectal exam may be done.

Suppositories may be inserted into the rectum as a route of administration for medicine.

Body temperature can also be taken in the rectum. Rectal temperature can be taken by inserting a mercury thermometer for 3 to 5 minutes, or a digital thermometer until it "beeps", not more than 25 mm (1 inch) into the rectum via the anus.

Many pediatricians recommend that parents take infants and toddler's temperature in the rectum for two reasons:

- (1) Rectal temperature is the closest to core body temperature and in children that young, accuracy is critical.
- (2) Younger children are unable to cooperate when having their temperature taken by mouth (oral) which is recommended for children, ages 6 and above and for adults.

Not all the food you eat is used by your body for nutrition. Some of it is unused, and after being solidified in the large intestine is eliminated from your body. For this function of elimination, the anal canal and rectum should be maintained as healthy as possible. Since anal sex is common in the gay lifestyle, it's also important to keep the anal canal and rectum healthy for your enjoyment within the confines of safer sex.

Your rectum may also get infections. Soreness or itching may be a sign something is wrong. It may mean simply that you have hemorrhoids (piles) , enlarged veins in the anal canal, but even so, make sure your doctor checks it out. Even hemorrhoids should be treated since the irritation from them will make other infections easier to set in.

The rectum in human defaecation

The rectum ampulla acts as a temporary storage facility for faeces. As the rectal walls expand due to the materials filling it from within, stretch receptors from the nervous system located in the rectal walls stimulate the desire to defaecate. If the urge is not acted upon, the material in the rectum is often returned to the colon where more water is absorbed. If defaecation is delayed for a prolonged period, constipation and hardened feces results. When the rectum is full the increase in intrarectal pressure forces the walls of the anal canal apart allowing the faecal matter to enter the canal. The rectum shortens as material is forced into the anal canal and peristaltic waves propel the faeces out of the rectum. The internal and external sphincter allow the faces to be passed by muscles pulling the anus up over the exiting faces.

Sexual stimuli

Due to the proximity of the anterior wall of the rectum to the vagina in females or to the prostate in males and the shared nerves thereof, rectal stimulation can result in sexual arousal.

Anus

In anatomy, the **anus** (from Latin *ânus* "ring, anus") is the external opening of the rectum. Closure is controlled by sphincter muscles. Faces are expelled from the body through the anus during the act of defecation, which is the primary function of the anus. The anus is often considered a taboo part of the body, and is known by a large number of usually vulgar slang terms.

The anus is situated between the buttocks, posterior to the perineum. It has two anal sphincters, one internal, the other external. These hold the anus closed until time to defaecate. One sphincter consists of smooth muscle and its action is involuntary;

the other consists of striated muscle and its action is voluntary. When the rectum is full, the increase in intrarectal pressure forces the walls of the anal canal apart allowing the facal matter to enter the canal. The rectum shortens as material is forced into the anal canal and peristaltic waves propel the faces out of the rectum. The internal and external sphincters of the anus allow the faeces to be passed by muscles pulling the anus up over the exiting feces.

To prevent diseases of the anus and to promote general hygiene, humans often clean the anus after emptying the bowels. A wash with a bidet or a wiping with toilet paper are often used to clear the anus of facal matter.

Role in sexuality

The anus has a relatively high concentration of nerve endings and is an erogenous zone. Anal intercourse can be pleasurable for both the insertive partner and the receptive partner. For the receptive partner, pleasure from anal intercourse is also thought to be related to the shared wall between the rectum and the vagina (for females) as well as the G-spot or Prostate (for males). For the insertive partner, the tightness of the anus is often said to be a source of pleasure in penetrative anal sex.

Anal intercourse, sometimes referred to as sodomy or buggery, is a human sexual activity, but is considered taboo in a number of moral systems, and it has been, and in some jurisdictions continues to be, a crime carrying severe punishment. Anal sexual activity need not include penetration. The anus also plays an important role in face sitting, coprophilia and anilingus. Anal stretching can stimulate the nerves around the anus and can be considered pleasurable. Care must be taken to maintain elasticity.

Hygiene is important for good anal health and anal sex. Washing with a mild soap and water will keep the anus clean. Harsh soaps or wiping vigorously with toilet paper can irritate the skin around the anus, making it itchy or sore. Pinworms are sometimes the source of anal itching.

Care should be taken not to strip the anus of natural oils that keep the skin around the opening supple and elastic. Penetration with a penis or sex toy can irritate or tear the inside of the anus. Lubrication is often recommended to ease penetration. The risk of injury to the anal sphincter should be a concern, which can lead on to lack of control of defaecation and faecal incontinence. Similarly if the anus is torn, this can occasionally cause a fistula formation which can not only cause fecal leaking, but also can be very difficult to treat.

5

Proteins, Carbohydrates and Fats

Food is essential for life, providing the fuel the body needs to function and the building blocks that make up cells, tissues, and organs. Vegetables, fish, chicken, mutton, pog, egg etc are the food we eat but the food our cells and organs receives are called nutrition in the form of proteins, carbohydrates, fats, vitamins and minerals . These are called five proximate principles of food. The energy provided by food is expressed in terms of calories. The body requires a certain number of calories simply to carry out its basic metabolic functions such as respiration and maintenance of body temperature. Additional calories are needed to support physical activity, fight infection, and rebuild damaged tissues.

If a person does not take in enough calories, fat is broken down to provide fuel. Once the fat is consumed — or if an individual's metabolism is disrupted due to illness — lean body mass (muscles and organs) is then used for fuel and raw materials. Conversely, if a person takes in more calories than needed, the extra energy will be stored as fat. The average person needs about 10-20 calories per pound (depending on physical activity level and other factors) to maintain a stable body weight; this requirement is likely to be higher for people with HIV, especially those with advanced disease.

But all food is not equal. While all contain calories, different foods vary widely in the nutrients they provide.

Food supplies energy for physical activity, and for the building blocks of our bodies. The major components of food are ***proteins, carbohydrates and fats***.

Protein

The name *protein* comes from the Greek *ðñþôá* ("prota"), meaning *"of primary importance"* and were first described and named by Jöns Jakob Berzelius in 1838. However, their central role in living organisms was not fully appreciated until 1926, when James B. Sumner showed that the enzyme urease was a protein. The first protein structures to be solved included insulin and myoglobin; the first was by Sir Frederick Sanger who won a 1958 Nobel Prize for it, and the second by Max Perutz and Sir John Cowdery Kendrew in 1958. Both proteins' three-dimensional structures were amongst the first determined by X-ray diffraction analysis; the myoglobin structure won the Nobel Prize in Chemistry for its discoverers. Berzelius proposed the name "protein" for this substance in a letter dated 10 July 1838.

Protein is vital to everyone's good health and survival. Protein is a nutrient in the foods we eat. It is also a component of muscle, organs, hormones, immune cells and more. Proteins are involved in many body functions and are necessary to build and repair body tissues and essential to fight infections. Protein can be used as a fuel source when energy demands are greater than food intake. It is important to eat enough foods containing carbohydrate and fat so that protein in the muscle and organs and from the diet are protected and reserved to perform its life sustaining functions.

Protein provides the building blocks of lean body mass. Proteins are large molecules made from about 20 different amino acids which are small molecules needed by all living things. Several of these, ***lysine, methionine*** and ***cysteine***, are easily destroyed in your food by heat and by oxidation during processing and storage. When a protein-rich food is consumed, it is broken down into amino acids, which are reassembled to create enzymes, hormones, and bodily tissues. Our body can not produce or manufacture some amino acids and therefore these are to be given as part of the food. These are called essential amino acids.

Essential Amino acids	*Nonessential Amino acids*
Isoleucine	Alanine
Leucine	Asparagine
Lysine	Aspartate
Methionine	Cysteine
Phenylalanine	Glutamate
Threonine	Glutamine
Tryptophan	Glycine
Valine	Proline
Arginine*	Serine
Histidine*	Tyrosine

Methionine and cysteine are sulphur-containing amino acids, and healthy people are able to make cysteine from methionine in their livers. This means that some methionine is used to make cysteine when cysteine is low from dietary sources or when extra demands for cysteine result from certain types of stress. Both lysine and the sulphur-containing amino acids are particularly subject to destruction during food processing such that they may become no longer available for normal body metabolism. Furthermore, both cysteine and methionine have been reported to tend to be low in HIV disease. This may be because both cysteine and methionine are readily oxidized, reversibly under lower oxidation stress, but irreversibly under more severe oxidation. The irreversibly oxidized forms are not available for normal body metabolism. Cysteine is very important for several reasons. Along with two other amino acids that are usually plentiful in our bodies, cysteine is required to make a compound called ***glutathione***, an antioxidant that the body keeps in all its cells and is especially important for the liver and lungs. For example, the air we breathe into our lungs contains free radicals (cigarette smoke is high in free radicals!). Glutathione neutralizes, or kills, these free radicals so that they don't harm us. "The more glutathione patients have in their CD4 T cells - the primary cells targeted by the HIV virus - the longer they are likely to survive, they found. People with HIV who have lower glutathione levels have a much lower probability of surviving over the course of three years than do people with normal glutathione levels.

Our bodies also contain a protein called ***metallothionein*** that regulates zinc and copper levels. Thirty percent of this protein is made of cysteine. Metallothionein is also an antioxidant that helps protect us from disease. This protein is particularly important for our bone marrow, thymus gland (where our T cells come from), kidneys, liver and intestines (Cousins, 1989). If glutathione is low because of cysteine deficiency, then metallothionein will also likely be low. Again, maintaining our levels of cysteine should help maintain this important antioxidant, as well as regulate zinc and copper.

Turnover of body protein increases in HIV infection, and this increase accelerates with disease progression (Macallan & Griffin, 1992). A decrease in any of our essential amino acids can cause problems (Millward *et al*, 1990). The sulphur-containing amino acids, however, are particularly critical to our health, and they are the most sensitive. A low cysteine level in the body is a source of wasting even in the absence of HIV disease. This results partly when the body cannibalizes lean body mass to maintain an important enzyme, high in cysteine content, required for digestion (Liener & Kakade, 1980). Low glutathione levels may make this wasting worse. Finally, another way in which wasting is encouraged is that when cysteine is low, the body tries to convert some of its methionine to cysteine, and this leaves less methionine which is required for making an important compound, carnitine, required in turn to get energy from fat. When carnitine levels get low with HIV infection (De Simone *et al*, 1992, 1993) long chain fatty acid oxidation is impaired so that the body is encouraged to burn up other compounds such as protein as an energy source, resulting in loss of lean body mass.

Then how can we help to keep our cysteine at a healthy level?

In our foods, eggs and dairy are probably the best sources of cysteine, although processing of these may destroy some of it. Dairy whey proteins have been shown to help boost deficient glutathione levels (Bounous *et al*, 1993). Vegetables and cereals are low in the sulphur-containing amino acids, and this should be of concern for vegetarians; however, the *cruciferous* vegetables may help prevent oxidation processes, and therefore protect cysteine to some degree.

The severity of HIV infection makes supplementation important to consider. It is advisable to take **N-acetyl cysteine (NAC)** which is available as a dietary supplement, and can be used by the body to make cysteine. Information from the 1992 Amsterdam International AIDS Conference indicates that 600-1200 mg/day may be enough to maintain normal glutathione levels. Many people take up to 1800 mg/day. NAC has been used previously for bronchitis and for acetaminophen poisoning with no major toxicity problems noted.

Daily Protein Intake

The Recommended Dietary Allowance (RDA), set for healthy men 25 years and older is 63 grams of protein a day. For healthy women 25 years and over, the RDA is 50 grams of protein a day. A person living with HIV may sometimes need twice as much, 10-16 ounces of protein or about 80-120 grams a day. When consuming only protein from plant sources, a little more protein is needed. For people living with HIV, foods rich in protein should be part of every meal.

Which Proteins?

Protein should be of high quality. Egg, rice, soybean, casein and whey are some sources of good proteins. Egg, casein or whey proteins are normally very high in quality. Partially hydrolyzed protein may be useful if digestion is difficult.. Some proteins are easier to digest than others. In general, milk proteins are easy to digest; however, the carbohydrate lactose may be a problem for some people. Soy-based products may be useful as a source of protein, and of calcium. Not only may soy protein be difficult to digest, but its use is frequently accompanied by allergies.

Sources of Protein

Foods rich in protein also contain fat, water vitamins and minerals. Except for dairy, animal sources of protein do not contain carbohydrates or fiber.

Sources of protein are **red meats, fish, poultry, eggs, nuts, beans, peas, grains** and other **seeds**. Red meat is the only really good source of carnitine, an important tool that your body needs in order to get its energy from fats and some amino acids. Red meat is also a good source of the antioxidant **CoEnzyme Q-10.** Meats and eggs are good sources of methionine and cysteine. Strict vegetarians need a variety of different cereals and vegetables to avoid deficiencies of lysine, methionine and cysteine. Combinations are better than any one; oats and rice and peas and beans provide reasonable quantities of protein. It's important for strict vegetarians who are HIV-positive to consider supplementation with carnitine.

Carbohydrates

Carbohydrates are large molecules that are built from individual sugars of which glucose is the most common. You need these for energy. Carbohydrates, which are converted to glucose in the body, are a primary source of energy.

Foods that are high in carbohydrates

Rice, Breads, pastas, beans, potatoes, bran and cereals are all high in carbohydrates.

Classification of carbohydrates

Dietitians and nutritionists commonly classify carbohydrates as simple (monosaccharides and disaccharides) or complex (oligosaccharides and polysaccharides). The term *complex carbohydrate* was first used in the Senate Select Committee publication *Dietary Goals for the United States* (1977), where it denoted "fruit, vegetables and whole-grains". Complex carbohydrates take more time to break down, and thus provide fuel over a longer period of time. The carbohydrates normally contains some simple sugars such as sucrose to improve taste. A major portion of the carbohydrate, however, should be provided by maltodextrins that have a low "dextrose equivalent", *i.e.*, DE, value, preferably 10 to 30. Despite the recent popularity of "low carbohydrate " diets, most nutrition experts recommend that carbohydrates — primarily complex ones — should make up at least 50% of one's total daily calorie intake. Simple carbohydrates are found in processed sugar, honey, fruit and juice, and lactose (milk sugar). Complex carbohydrates are found in grain products such as bread, pasta, and rice; legumes; and starchy foods such as corn, potatoes, winter squash, and root vegetables.

The basic carbohydrate units are called monosaccharides, such as glucose, galactose, and fructose. The general chemical formula of an unmodified monosaccharide is $(C \cdot H_2O)_n$, where n is any number of three or greater. All carbohydrates have a hydrogen to oxygen ratio of 2:1. Monosaccharides can be linked together in almost limitless ways. Two joined monosaccharides are called disaccharides, such as sucrose and lactose. Carbohydrates containing between about three to six monosaccharide units are termed oligosaccharides; anything larger than this is a polysaccharide. Polysaccharides, such as starch, glycogen, or cellulose, can reach many thousands of units in length. Many carbohydrates contain one or more modified monosaccharide units that have had one or more groups replaced or removed. For example, deoxyribose, a component of DNA, is a modified version of ribose; chitin is composed of repeating units of N-acetylglucosamine, a nitrogen-containing form of glucose.

Monosaccharides

Monosaccharides, also called *simple sugars*, are the basic units of carbohydrates. The general chemical formula of an unmodified monosaccharide is $(C \cdot H_2O)_n$, where n is any number of three or greater.

Monosaccharides are classified according to three different characteristics: the placement of its carbonyl group, the number of carbon atoms it contains, and its chiral handedness. If the carbonyl group is an aldehyde, the monosaccharide is an aldose; if the carbonyl group is a ketone, the monosaccharide is a ketose. The smallest possible monosaccharide, those with three carbon atoms, are called trioses. Those with four are called tetroses, five are called pentoses, six are hexoses, and so on.

Disaccharides

Disaccharides are the simplest polysaccharides. They are composed of two monosaccharide units bound together by a covalent glycosidic bond formed via a dehydration reaction, resulting in the loss of a hydrogen atom from one monosaccharide and a hydroxyl group from the other, so the formula of unmodified disaccharides is $C_{12}H_{22}O_{11}$. Although there are numerous kinds of disaccharides, a handful of disaccharides are particularly notable.

Sucrose is the most abundant disaccharide and the main form in which carbohydrates are transported in plants. It is composed of one glucose molecule and one fructose molecule. The systematic name for sucrose, *O*-á-D-glucopyranosyl-(1'!2)-D-fructofuranoside, indicates four things:

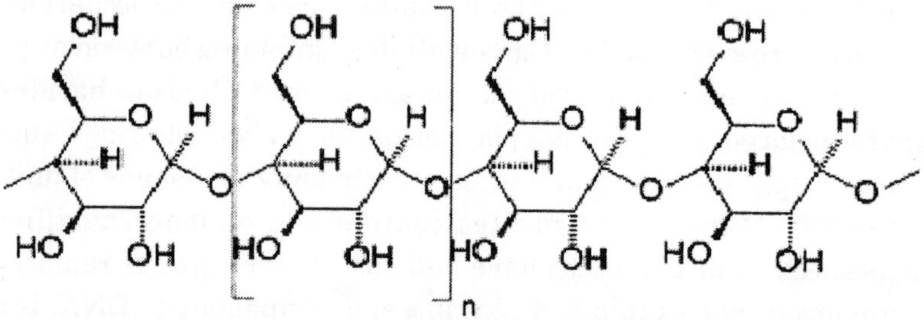

- Its monosaccharides: glucose and fructose
- Their ring types: glucose is a pyranose, and fructose is a furanose
- How they're linked together: the oxygen on the number 1 carbon (C1) of á-glucose is linked to the C2 of fructose.
- The *-oside* suffix indicates that the anomeric carbon of both monosacchaides participates in the glycosidic bond.

Lactose, a disaccharide composed of one galactose molecule and one glucose molecule, occurs naturally only in milk. The systematic name for lactose is *O*-â-D-galactopyranosyl-(1'!4)-D-glucopyranose. Other notable disaccharides include maltose (two glucoses linked á-1,4) and cellobiose (two glucoses linked â-1,4).

Oligosaccharides and polysaccharides

Oligosaccharides and polysaccharides are composed of longer chains of monosaccharide units bound together by glycosidic bonds. The distinction between the two is based upon the number of monosaccharide units present in the chain. Oligosaccharides typically contain between two and nine monosaccharide units, and polysaccharides contain greater than ten monosaccharide units. Examples of oligosaccharides include the disaccharides mentioned above, the trisaccharide raffinose and the tetrasaccharide stachyose.

Oligosaccharides are found as a common form of protein posttranslational modification. Such posttranslational modifications include the Lewis oligosaccharides responsible for blood group incompatibilities, the alpha-Gal epitope responsible for hyperacute rejection in xenotransplanation, and O-GlcNAc modifications.

Polysaccharides represent an important class of biological polymer. Examples include starch, cellulose, chitin, glycogen, callose, laminarin, xylan, and galactomannan.

Carbohydrates should provide you with a good level of soluble dietary fibre which helps control both diarrhoea and constipation. Dietary fibres are types of carbohydrates. For practical purposes, we can consider two types of fibre:

1. **Insoluble fibre** is mostly not digested. Some if it provides roughage, controls stool movement, cleanses the intestinal walls, and provides food for the gut bacteria (the "**gut flora**"). Bran types of insoluble fibre can make diarrhoea worse, so should be reduced or avoided when you have diarrhoea.
2. **Soluble fibre** is often digested, but can also help control stool movement, and it provides a source of food to keep your gut flora happy and growing. Controlling the bile acids in the intestine is an important function of soluble fibre. These acids help you to digest fats.

Good sources of insoluble fibre are grains (that still have the bran part), celery and cooked lentils. Good sources of soluble fibre are apples, bananas, broccoli, Brussels sprouts, citrus fruits, carrots, oats, blackberries, blueberries, loganberries and boysenberries. Beans, peas and flax are good sources of both soluble and insoluble fibre. The fibres in bananas, oats and flax help control both constipation and diarrhoea. Berries, and unrefined/unbleached fibre also contain important antioxidants, some even more potent than vitamin C.

Dietary fibre also provides food for your intestinal flora ('gut bugs') which discourage intestinal infection, and produce vitamins and other important compounds. Poor growth of the friendly gut bacteria encourages yeast growth.

PLWHAs need to be aware of the sugar content of foods they eat. A good practice following meals is to rinse the mouth out with water to get rid of residual materials from your food that may promote thrush. Gargling with a mixture of water with a few drops (per tablespoon of water) of antiseptic mouthwash, grapefruit seed extract; or a solution of from 1% to 3% food grade hydrogen peroxide may help discourage yeast infections. It is important not to swallow hydrogen peroxide since it can damage the oesophagus as well as the stomach.

Which Carbohydrates?

Carbohydrates require less water to digest than proteins or fats and are the most common source of energy. Proteins and fat are vital building components for body tissue and cells, and thus it could be considered advisable not to deplete such resources by necessitating their use in energy production. However, carbohydrates are not essential nutrients. It is possible for the body to obtain all its energy from protein and fats. The brain cannot burn fat and needs glucose for energy, but the body can make this glucose from protein. Carbohydrates, like proteins, contain 4 kilocalories per gram while fats contain 9 kilocalories and alcohol contains 7 kilocalories per gram.

The Food and Agriculture Organization and World Health Organization jointly recommend that national dietary guidelines set a goal of 55-75% of total energy from carbohydrates.

Many PLWHAs have experienced the importance of keeping simple sugars low in their diet. The yeast of concern here is one called Candida albicans and is the cause of thrush, oesophageal candidiasis and other infections. Generally, one recognizes the simple sugars by the ending "ose"; common simple sugars are either monosaccharides such as glucose (dextrose) and fructose, or disaccharides such as sucrose and maltose.

There are, again, special concerns regarding use of liquid food supplements by PLWHAs. The carbohydrates used in these vary from maltodextrins to simple sugars. Sipping these over a period of time exposes any residual candida in the mouth to its favourite food thus encouraging its growth.

While oral candidiasis continues to be common in HIV disease , candida infections in the oesophagus are of greater concern. It is reported that the relative hazard associated with oesophageal candidiasis was 1.5 times higher than from P.C pneumonia, and that there was poorer survival at 12 months after diagnosis than for either cryptococcal meningitis or disseminated CMV. Oesophageal candidiasis has been frequently reported among people living with HIV/AIDS.

Moreover, while some very good antifungal drugs have been developed, there is increasing evidence of resistance to those that are available (Millon et al, 1994; Vuffray et al, 1994).

Clearly, candidiasis must be considered a serious opportunistic infection, and those living with HIV/AIDS (PLWHAs) should do whatever possible to prevent its occurrence or slow its growth. Restriction of simple sugars from the diet is one thing that PLWHAs can do. Carbohydrates that are more complex are not as readily available for yeast growth, especially in the mouth and oesophagus where natural prevention is weaker than in other parts of the gastrointestinal tract. It is important to be aware that major sources of sugar include not only soft drinks.

Fats

Fat is a major source of energy in our diet and has a high concentration of calories. Fat, like protein and carbohydrate, is a major nutrient in the food we eat and is necessary to support life. Eating adequate amounts of fats and carbohydrates provides the body with its needed fuel to preserve protein for tissue growth and repair, immune function and other vital functions. Dietary fat is necessary for absorption of the fat-soluble vitamins A, D, E & K. Fat in food can give a sense of fullness, satisfaction and reduced desire to eat. Fat is flavourful. If fat absorption is a problem, too much fat may cause intestinal problems (diarrhoea, foul smelling stools and gas, abdominal pain), and eating smaller amounts may be helpful. Food eaten in amounts greater than the body's need for energy is converted and stored as fat and it doesn't matter if the food is rich in protein, fat or carbohydrate. Excess calories equals weight gain.

Fats are sources of essential fatty acids, an important dietary requirement.. Vitamins A, D, E, and K are fat-soluble, meaning they can only be digested, absorbed, and transported in conjunction with fats. Fats play a vital role in maintaining healthy skin and hair, insulating body organs against shock, maintaining body temperature, and promoting healthy cell function. They also serve as energy stores for the body. Fats are broken down in the body to release glycerol and free fatty acids. The glycerol can be converted to glucose by the liver and thus used as a source of energy. The fatty acids are a good source of energy for many tissues, especially heart and skeletal muscle. Fat also serves as a useful buffer towards a host of diseases. When a particular substance, whether chemical or biotic — reaches unsafe levels in the bloodstream, the body can effectively dilute — or at least maintain equilibrium of — the offending substances by storing it in new fat tissue. This helps to protect vital organs, until such time as the offending substances can be metabolized and/or removed from the body by such means as excretion, urination, accidental or intentional bloodletting, sebum excretion, and hair growth.

Fats provide us with energy

While fats may give high calories in foods producing energy. In producing energy for our bodies, the fatty acids are burned in cells of the body by a process called *beta* oxidation in small organelles (inside the cells) called mitochondria. This occurs in our muscles and liver. The long chain fatty acids are taken into the mitochondria by a compound called carnitine. Carnitine is normally found at high levels in the muscles of the body. This is particularly important for supply of energy to the body muscles since carnitine transports long-chain fatty acids into mitochondria, where they are oxidized to provide energy. This process also requires vitamins B_2, B_3, B_{12}, and biotin. Carnitine also helps remove short- and medium-chain fatty acids that accumulate in the mitochondria as the result of abnormal metabolism.

In HIV disease, the result is unusually high storage of fat. The inability to properly produce energy from fat is likely partly from problems in maintaining carnitine levels. There is likely increased burning up of protein to provide the energy that should have come from fat. Even if this does not occur, protein stores become difficult to maintain simply from the low levels of cysteine and methionine. Thus body lean mass is decreased and the body becomes fatty at the expense of protein. Since the immune system requires protein stores for its energy, this is devastating in a disease where the immune system is already under heavy siege.

Type of fat - The Good, The Bad, and The Healthy Diet

The *type of fat* in the diet is more important than low fat . Research has shown that eating a low-fat diet for 8 years did not prevent heart disease, breast cancer, or colon cancer, and didn't do much for weight loss, either.

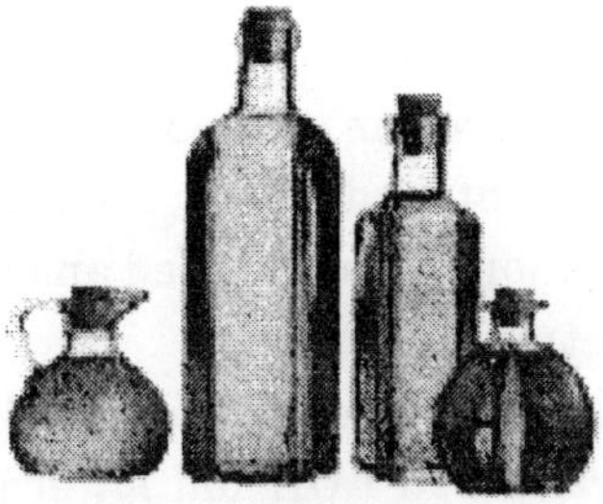

What is more important is that bad fats, meaning saturated and trans fats, increase the risk for certain diseases while good fats, meaning monounsaturated and polyunsaturated fats, lower the risk. The key is to substitute good fats for bad fats.

The Bad Fats

Some fats such as Saturated and Trans fats are bad because they tend to worsen blood cholesterol levels.

Saturated Fats

Saturated fats are mainly animal fats. They are found in meat, seafood, whole-milk dairy products (cheese, milk, and ice cream), poultry skin, and egg yolks. Some plant foods are also high in saturated fats, including coconut and coconut oil, palm oil, and palm kernel oil. Saturated fats raise total blood cholesterol levels more than dietary cholesterol because they tend to boost both good HDL and bad LDL cholesterol. The net effect is negative, meaning it's important to limit saturated fats.

High triglyceride and cholesterol levels are associated with a higher risk of heart attacks and stroke. Until recently, this was not too much of a concern for HIV+ people, because people with HIV had been observed to have low cholesterol levels. Cholesterol is necessary for your body. It is used to create cell membranes, and to make your body's hormones. Because of this, people with HIV may want to take advantage of their low cholesterol levels, and eat animal fats both as a source of cholesterol and energy. Recently, both high triglyceride and cholesterol levels have been observed in some HIV+ people on antiretroviral therapy. If your cholesterol and triglycerides are both high, you should consider limiting your saturated fat intake.

Trans Fats

Trans fatty acids are fats produced by heating liquid vegetable oils in the presence of hydrogen. This process is known as hydrogenation. The more hydrogenated an oil is, the harder it will be at room temperature.

Trans fats are even worse for cholesterol levels than saturated fats because they raise bad LDL and lower good HDL. They also fire inflammation, an overactivity of the immune system that has been implicated in heart disease, stroke, diabetes, and other chronic conditions. While you should limit your intake of saturated fats, it is important to eliminate trans fats from partially hydrogenated oils from your diet

Tips for lowering trans fat intake

- Choose liquid vegetable oils, or a choose a soft tub margarine that contains little or no trans fats.
- Reduce intake of commercially prepared baked goods, snack foods, and processed foods, including fast foods. To be on the safe side, assume that all such products contain trans fats unless they are labeled otherwise.
- When foods containing partially hydrogenated oils can't be avoided, choose products that list the partially hydrogenated oils near the end of the ingredient list.
- To avoid trans fats in restaurants, one strategy is to avoid deep-fried foods, since many restaurants continue to use partially hydrogenated oils in their fryers. You may be able to help change this cooking practice by asking your server, the chef, or manager if the establishment uses trans-free oils.

Some HIV+ people have difficulty absorbing fats. This condition is called steatorrhea. It may be due to intestinal damage caused by opportunistic infections, or by HIV itself. Steatorrhea can cause diarrhoea, bloating, or changes in the colour of your stool. If you have steatorrhea, you are probably absorbing very little of the fat you eat. Since it is still important to have some fat in your diet, you may want to drink liquid supplements or other products that contain a type of fat called MCT (medium-chain triglycerides). This type of fat is easy to absorb.

The Good Fats

Some fats like unsaturated fats- monounsaturated and polyunsaturated fats are good because they can improve blood cholesterol levels.

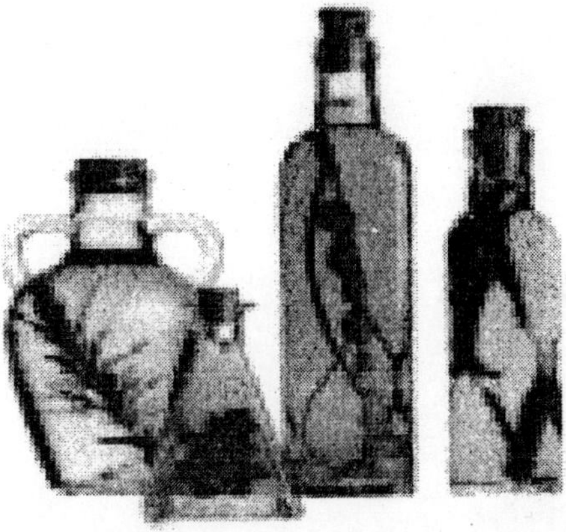

Unsaturated Fats—Polyunsaturated and Monounsaturated

Unsaturated fats are found in products derived from plant sources, such as vegetable oils, nuts, and seeds. There are two main categories: polyunsaturated fats (which are found in high concentrations in sunflower, corn, and soybean oils) and monounsaturated fats (which are found in high concentrations in canola, peanut, and olive oils). In studies in which polyunsaturated and monounsaturated fats were eaten in place of carbohydrates, these good fats decreased LDL levels and increased HDL levels.

Polyunsaturated Fats are found in some vegetable oils such as corn and peanut oil, and in most margarines. In some studies, polyunsaturated fats been shown to reduce T-cells, and with them the functioning of the immune system. While these studies were not HIV-specific, it may still be wise for HIV+ people to avoid eating

Percentage of Specific Types of Fat in Common Oils and Fats*

Oils	*Saturated*	*Mono-unsaturated*	*Poly-unsaturated*	*Trans*
Canola	7	58	29	0
Safflower	9	12	74	0
Sunflower	10	20	66	0
Corn	13	24	60	0
Olive	13	72	8	0
Soybean	16	44	37	0
Peanut	17	49	32	0
Palm	50	37	10	0
Coconut	87	6	2	0
Cooking Fats				
Shortening	22	29	29	18
Lard	39	44	11	1

(Contd.)

(Contd Table.)

Oils	*Saturated*	*Mono-unsaturated*	*Poly-unsaturated*	*Trans*
Butter	60	26	5	5
Margarine/Spreads				
70% Soybean Oil, Stick	18	2	29	23
67% Corn & Soybean Oil Spread, Tub	16	27	44	11
48% Soybean Oil Spread, Tub	17	24	49	8
60% Sunflower, Soybean, and Canola Oil Spread, Tub	18	22	54	5

*Values expressed as percent of total fat; data are from analyses at Harvard School of Public Health Lipid Laboratory and U.S.D.A. publications.

a lot of polyunsaturated fat. Polyunsaturated fats are much less likely to increase cholesterol than saturated fats.

Monounsaturated Fats are also found in vegetable oils like olive oil and canola oil. These are not suspected of being immune suppressive. Monounsaturated fats do not normally increase your cholesterol levels like saturated fats, but they are sometimes modified when heated during processing. For this reason, many people look for olive oil that is "cold pressed."

Omega-3 Fatty Acids are called essential fatty acids because they must be present in your diet. Your body can't manufacture them. They are found in the oils of most fish and seafood, as well as in flaxseed and some beans and peas. Eating foods rich in omega-3 fatty acids has been shown to reduce the risk of heart attack, and to have a positive influence on cell-mediated immunity (the part of the immune system most damaged by HIV infection).

Correct fat digestion tends to be poor with HIV. "Futile cycling" of free fatty acids is associated with a tendency for the body to become fatty at the expense of body protein (Grunfeld & Kotler, 1992; Hellerstein, 1992). Several ways to reduce this tendency may be to:-

- ensure adequate intake of vitamin C and NAC to encourage the body to make carnitine which you need to burn fat for your energy (instead of your protein stores),
- keep red meat, a good source of carnitine, in the diet,
- take supplemental carnitine, or
- replace some of your fat intake with medium chain length glycerides, usually in the form of purified MCT (medium chain triglycerides from coconut fat) or directly as coconut butter. Your body should be able to use medium chain fatty acids (from the medium chain glycerides) without carnitine.

If you have HIV infection, there is no reason to restrict fat from your diet in order to lose weight. If blood triglycerides have become higher than normal (for you), then a generally low fat diet may be advisable. Otherwise, a normal-to-low fat intake would seem to be in order (*e.g.*, about 20% of your calories), keeping in mind the above issues so that quality is emphasized. It may help to take extra vitamins C and E and beta (ß) -carotene. These antioxidants help protect you from damage by fat oxidation which tends to be high with HIV infection (Hommes *et al*, 1991).

What does this mean for those living with HIV?

In HIV disease, it is likely that hypertriglyceridemia occurs primarily, perhaps exclusively, from carnitine deficiency. Futile cycling and low cholesterol are similarly likely results. Contribution to fatigue and wasting is also highly likely.

It is likely that those who supplement with NAC have less severe carnitine deficiency since methionine should not get used up in helping maintain adequate cysteine levels. If these same people also maintain red meat in their diet, this also should help.

An additional advantage will be achieved if part of the dietary fat is fat composed of medium-chain length fatty acids, *i.e.*, medium-chain glycerides of which the most common is the product called medium-chain triglycerides (MCT). Use of these by the body is possible without carnitine. Coconut oil/fat is the source of the commercial MCT product. An alternative to using the purified MCT product is therefore to use coconut fat directly.

Carnitine tends to become low in HIV disease, although those who supplement with N-acetyl cysteine (NAC) are less likely to become as deficient as those who do not take this supplement. Medium chain length fats can provide energy without requiring carnitine for transport. Some of the fat we eat gets converted back to fat and is stored in our body. This can be used later as required. Our body fat also comes from non-fat parts of our food - from proteins and carbohydrates, so that eating a fat-free meal doesn't mean we'll not store fat in our bodies. In HIV disease there is often an increased tendency for formation of fat, likely a result of low carnitine. Thus, instead of being burned for energy, fatty acids are converted back to fat which in turn gets re-broken down to fatty acids, then re-made back to fat in a process referred to as *futile cycling*. This cycling wastes energy and contributes to weight loss that may encourage loss of protein, since protein is then forced to provide a large part of the energy required for this futile cycling. The result can be a body that has high levels of triglycerides, and, generally, a higher proportion of fat, at the expense of valuable protein.

Fats provide materials that regulate much of our bodies' chemistries, especially immunity.

Very special, and very important, compounds called *eicosanoids* are made in our bodies from the fat we eat. The process involves an initial formation of arachidonic acid and other related compounds which then are converted to the eicosanoids - the process is called the *eicosanoid cascade*. There are three subdivisions to these eicosanoids - *thromboxanes, leukotrienes* and *prostaglandins*. These are hormone-like materials that control many processes in our bodies such as blood flow, platelet aggregation, digestion mechanics, breathing functions, *etc*. Some of them work as pairs so that one will turn on a process while the other shuts the same process off. They do their work only in the cells in which they are made (Hunt and Groff, 1990).The eicosanoids interact with and help control the immune system, especially those parts involving inflammatory reponse (Kinsella *et al*, 1990; Yaqoob and Calder, 1993). Control of several cytokines such as interleukin-1 and tumour necrosis factor is by the eicosanoids. Sperm-associated immune suppression derives from this route (Stites and Terr, 1991). The balance of the various eicosanoids derives partly from compounds that change the behaviours of the enzymes involved in eicosanoid formation. For example, aspirin is well-known to inhibit the enzyme cyclo-oxygenase, thus reducing prostaglandin and thromboxane formation, hence providing an anti-inflammatory response. Another factor that influences the eicosanoid balance appears to be the type of polyunsaturated fats dominant in the diet. An excess of polyunsaturated fatty acids in the diet is highly immunosuppressive, and this is effected mainly in the cell-mediated immune response, whereas a deficiency can reduce the humoral response (Stites and Terr, 1991). Since cell-mediated and humoral immunity tend to see-saw with each other, a deficiency of polyunsaturated fatty acids enhances cell-mediated immunity (Kinsella *et al*, 1990).

While polyunsaturated fatty acids, in general, may cause certain types of immune suppression, those from corn, soy, sunflower, safflower are of greatest concern. Those from fish may have some beneficial effects. Corn oil has been observed in many studies to cause dramatic immunosuppressive effects (Kinsella et al, 1990).

Practical Considerations

Fat should be in a form that's easy to digest. Oils containing only long-chain fatty acids may be difficult for PLWHAs to properly digest, especially when the compound carnitine is deficient. It is still important, however, that adequate essential fatty acids are provided. A solution to these issues is to choose products containing a blend of polyunsaturated with monounsaturated oil and/or saturated fat, and medium chain-length glycerides. Olive and canola oils are sources of monounsaturated oils. Beef, milk and coconut fats are sources of saturated fatty acids.Cold pressed flax, evening primrose, cold water fish such as mackerel and salmon, and extra virgin olive oils are other reasonable sources of fat. Peanut oil is preferable to corn or soy. Olive and canola are both sources of monunsaturated fats and should be considered superior to corn, soy, safflower and regular sunflower. A special sunflower oil which is high in monunsaturated fats can be considered as equivalent to olive and canola oils. In general, PLWHAs should avoid products whose sole fat source is corn, soy, safflower or regular sunflower.

Fibre: Also known as "roughage," fibre is indigestible plant matter such as cellulose. Insoluble fibre plays an important role in digestion, helping food move smoothly through the colon (large intestine); this type of fibre is found in the skin and pulp of many fruits and vegetables, whole grains, popcorn, and seeds. Soluble fibre helps stabilize blood sugar and may reduce LDL cholesterol levels; this type of fibre is found in oatmeal and oat bran, legumes, nuts, and fruits such as apples, oranges, pears, and grapes.

Cholesterol in food

Although it is still important to limit the amount of cholesterol you eat, especially if you have diabetes. Cholesterol in the bloodstream is what's most important. High blood cholesterol levels greatly increase the risk for heart disease. But the average person makes about 75% of blood cholesterol in his or her liver, while only about 25% is absorbed from food. The biggest influence on blood cholesterol level is the mix of fats in the diet.

The Cholesterol—Heart Disease Connection

Cholesterol is a wax-like substance. The liver makes it and links it to carrier proteins called lipoproteins that let it dissolve in blood and be transported to all parts of the body. Why? Cholesterol plays essential roles in the formation of cell membranes, some

DIETARY FATS

Type of Fat	*Main Source*	*State at Room Temperature*	*Effect on Cholesterol Levels Compared with Carbohydrates*
Monounsaturated	Olives; olive oil, canola oil, peanut oil; cashews, almonds, peanuts, and most other nuts; avocados	Liquid	Lowers LDL; raises HDL
Polyunsaturated	Corn, soybean, safflower, and cottonseed oils; fish	Liquid	Lowers LDL; raises HDL
Saturated	Whole milk, butter, cheese, and ice cream; red meat; chocolate; coconuts, coconut milk, and coconut oil	Solid	Raises both LDL and HDL
Trans	Most margarines; vegetable shortening; partially hydrogenated vegetable oil; deep-fried chips; many fast foods; most commercial baked goods	Solid or semi-solid	Raises LDL*

*Trans fat increases LDL, decreases HDL, and increases triglycerides when compared to monounsaturated or polyunsaturated fat.

hormones, and vitamin D. Too much cholesterol in the blood can lead to problems. In the 1960s and 70s, scientists established a link between high blood cholesterol levels and heart disease. Deposits of cholesterol can build up inside arteries. These deposits, called plaque, can narrow an artery enough to slow or block blood flow. This narrowing process, called atherosclerosis, commonly occurs in arteries that nourish the heart (the coronary arteries). When one or more sections of heart muscle fail to get enough blood, and thus the oxygen and nutrients they need, the result may be the chest pain known as angina. In addition, plaque can rupture, causing blood clots that may lead to heart attack, stroke, or sudden death. Fortunately, the buildup of cholesterol can be slowed, stopped, and even reversed.

Cholesterol-carrying lipoproteins play central roles in the development of atherosclerotic plaque and cardiovascular disease. The two main types of lipoproteins basically work in opposite directions. Low-density lipoproteins (LDL) carry cholesterol from the liver to the rest of the body. When there is too much LDL cholesterol in the blood, it can be deposited on the walls of the coronary arteries. Because of this, LDL cholesterol is often referred to as the "bad" cholesterol. High-density lipoproteins (HDL) carry cholesterol from the blood back to the liver, which processes the cholesterol for elimination from the body. HDL makes it less likely that excess cholesterol in the blood will be deposited in the coronary arteries, which is why HDL cholesterol is often referred to as the "good" cholesterol.In general, the higher your LDL and the lower your HDL, the greater your risk for atherosclerosis and heart disease.

For adults age 20 years or over, the latest guidelines recommend the following optimal levels:

- Total cholesterol less than 200 milligrams per deciliter (mg/dl)
- HDL cholesterol levels greater than 40 mg/dl
- LDL cholesterol levels less than 100 mg/dl

Dietary Fat, Dietary Cholesterol, and Blood Cholesterol Levels

One of the most important determinants of blood cholesterol level is fat in the diet - not total fat, as mentioned already, but specific types of fat. Some types of fat are clearly good for cholesterol levels and others are clearly bad for them.

While it is well known that high blood cholesterol levels are associated with an increased risk for heart disease, scientific studies have shown that there is only a weak relationship between the amount of cholesterol a person consumes and their blood cholesterol levels or risk for heart disease. For some people with high cholesterol, reducing the amount of cholesterol in the diet has a small but helpful impact on blood cholesterol levels. For others, the amount of cholesterol eaten has little impact on the amount of cholesterol circulating in the blood.

Eggs

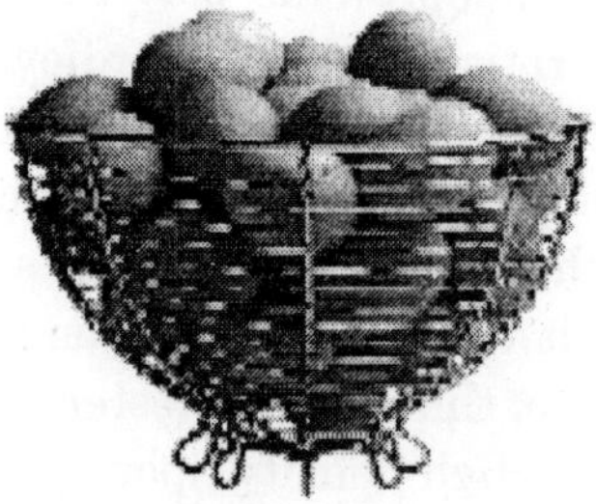

Recent research by Harvard investigators has shown that moderate egg consumption—up to one a day—does not increase heart disease risk in healthy individuals.While it's true that egg yolks have a lot of cholesterol and, therefore may slightly affect blood cholesterol levels—eggs also contain nutrients that may help lower the risk for heart disease, including protein, vitamins B12 and D, riboflavin, and folate.

So, when eaten in moderation, eggs can be part of a healthy diet. People with diabetes should probably limit themselves to no more than two or three eggs a week. Similarly, people who have difficulty controlling their blood cholesterol may also want to be cautious about eating egg yolks and choose foods made with egg whites instead.

Dietary Fats and Heart Disease:

Fish, an important source of the polyunsaturated fat known as omega-3 fatty acid, has received much attention for its potential to lower heart disease risk. There is strong evidence that fish and fish oil consumption reduces the risk of heart disease deaths and so-called "sudden deaths.

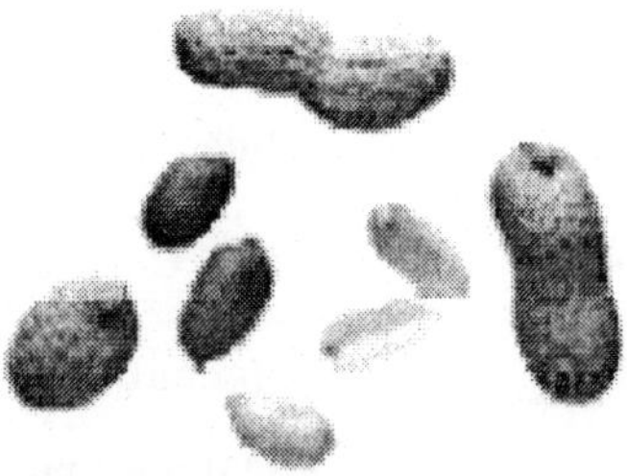

Eating fish may help prevent heart disease in several ways. It may replace red meat or other less-healthy sources of protein. More importantly, the omega-3 fats in fish appear to protect the heart against the development of erratic and potentially deadly cardiac rhythm disturbances.

If you eat a lot of fish - five or more servings a week - be sure to vary the types of fish you eat and limit consumption of the four species that are higher in mercury (swordfish, tilefish/golden bass, shark, and king mackerel).

What Do Your Cholesterol Numbers Mean?

Everyone age 20 and older should have their cholesterol measured at least once every 5 years. It is best to have a blood test called a "lipoprotein profile" to find out your cholesterol numbers. This blood test is done after a 9- to 12-hour fast and gives information about your:

- **Total cholesterol**
- **LDL (bad) cholesterol** — the main source of cholesterol buildup and blockage in the arteries
- **HDL (good) cholesterol** — helps keep cholesterol from building up in the arteries
- **Triglycerides** — another form of fat in your blood

If it is not possible to get a lipoprotein profile done, knowing your total cholesterol and HDL cholesterol can give you a general idea about your cholesterol levels. If your total cholesterol is 200 mg/dL* or more or if your HDL is less than 40 mg/dL, you will need to have a lipoprotein profile done. See how your cholesterol numbers compare to the tables below.

Total Cholesterol Level	*Category*
Less than 200 mg/dL	Desirable
200-239 mg/dL	Borderline high
240 mg/dL and above	High

LDL Cholesterol Level	*LDL Cholesterol Category*
Less than 100 mg/dL	Optimal
100-129 mg/dL	Near optimal/above optimal
130-159 mg/dL	Borderline high
160-189 mg/dL	High
190 mg/dL and above	Very high

* Cholesterol levels are measured in milligrams (mg) of cholesterol per deciliter (dL) of blood.

HDL (good) cholesterol protects against heart disease, so for HDL, higher numbers are better. A level less than 40 mg/dL is low and is considered a major risk factor because it increases your risk for developing heart disease. HDL levels of 60 mg/dL or more help to lower your risk for heart disease. Triglycerides can also raise heart disease risk. Levels that are borderline high (150-199 mg/dL) or high (200 mg/dL or more) may need treatment in some people.

What Affects Cholesterol Levels?

A variety of things can affect cholesterol levels. These are things you can do something about:

- **Diet :** Saturated fat and cholesterol in the food you eat make your blood cholesterol level go up. Saturated fat is the main culprit, but cholesterol in foods also matters. Reducing the amount of saturated fat and cholesterol in your diet helps lower your blood cholesterol level.
- **Weight :** Being overweight is a risk factor for heart disease. It also tends to increase your cholesterol. Losing weight can help lower your LDL and total cholesterol levels, as well as raise your HDL and lower your triglyceride levels.

- **Physical Activity :** Not being physically active is a risk factor for heart disease. Regular physical activity can help lower LDL (bad) cholesterol and raise HDL (good) cholesterol levels. It also helps you lose weight. You should try to be physically active for 30 minutes on most, if not all, days.
- Things you cannot do anything about also can affect cholesterol levels. These include:
- **Age and Gender :** As women and men get older, their cholesterol levels rise. Before the age of menopause, women have lower total cholesterol levels than men of the same age. After the age of menopause, women's LDL levels tend to rise.
- **Heredity :** Your genes partly determine how much cholesterol your body makes. High blood cholesterol can run in families.

- **Physical Activity:** Not being physically active is a risk factor for heart disease. Regular physical activity can help lower LDL (bad) cholesterol and raise HDL (good) cholesterol levels. It also helps you lose weight. You should try to be physically active for 30 minutes on most, if not all, days.
- Things you cannot control also can affect cholesterol levels. These include:
- **Age and Gender:** As women and men get older, their cholesterol levels rise. Before the age of menopause, women have lower total cholesterol levels than men of the same age. After the age of menopause, women's LDL levels tend to rise.
- **Heredity:** Your genes partly determine how much cholesterol your body makes. High blood cholesterol can run in families.

6

Vitamins

Vitamins are nutrients required in very small amounts for essential metabolic reactions in the body. The term **vitamin** does not include other essential nutrients such as dietary minerals, essential fatty acids, or essential amino acids. Nor does the term refer to the large number of other nutrients that promote health, but are not strictly essential.

Until the 1900s, vitamins were obtained solely through food intake. Many food sources contain different ratios of vitamins. Therefore, if the only source of vitamins is food, changes in diet will alter the types and amounts of vitamins ingested. However, as many vitamins can be stored by the body, short-term deficiencies (e.g. during a particular growing season) do not usually cause disease.

Vitamins have been produced as commodity chemicals and made widely-available as inexpensive pills for several decades allowing supplementation of the dietary intake.

Fruits and vegetables are often a good source of vitamins.

History

The value of eating certain foods to maintain health was recognized long before vitamins were identified. The ancient Egyptians knew that feeding a patient liver would help cure night blindness, now known to be caused by a vitamin A deficiency. In 1747, the Scottish surgeon James Lind discovered that citrus foods helped prevent scurvy, a particularly deadly disease in which collagen is not properly formed, and is characterized by poor wound healing, bleeding of the gums, and severe pain. In 1753, Lind published his "Treatise on the Scurvy",which recommended using lemons and limes to avoid scurvy, which was adopted by the British Royal Navy. This led to the nickname Limey for sailors of that organization. In 1897, Christiaan Eijkman discovered that eating unpolished rice instead of the polished variety helped to prevent the disease beriberi. The following year, Frederick Hopkins postulated that some foods contained "accessory factors"—in addition to proteins, carbohydrates, fats, etc.—that were necessary for the functions of the human body. Hopkins was awarded the 1929 Nobel Prize for Physiology or Medicine, with Christiaan Eijkman, for their discovery of several vitamins.Kazimierz Funk was the first to isolate the water-soluble complex of micronutrients, whose bioactivity Fletcher had identified, and Funk proposed the complex be named "Vitamine". The name soon became synonymous with Hopkins' "accessory factors", and by the time it was shown that not all vitamins were amines, the word was already ubiquitous. In 1920, Jack Cecil Drummond proposed that the final "e" be dropped, to deemphasize the "amine" reference, after the discovery that vitamin C had no amine component.

In 1931, Albert Szent-Györgyi and his research fellow Joseph Svirbely, determined that "hexuronic acid" was actually vitamin C and noted its anti-scorbutic activity, and 1937 Szent-Györgyi was awarded the Nobel Prize for his discovery. In 1943 Edward Adelbert Doisy and Henrik Dam were awarded the Nobel Prize for their discovery of vitamin K and its chemical structure.

Human vitamins

Vitamins are classified as either water soluble, meaning that they dissolve easily in water, or fat soluble which are absorbed through the intestinal tract with the help of lipids. When you eat foods that contain **fat-soluble** vitamins, the vitamins are stored in the fat tissues in your body and in your liver. They go and wait around in your body fat until your body needs them. Fat-soluble vitamins are happy to stay stored in your body for awhile - some stay for a few days, some for up to 6 months! Then, when it's time

Vitamin name	*Chemical name*	*Solubility*	*Deficiency disease*	*Recommended Dietary Allowances (male, age 19–70)*	*Upper Intake Level (UL/day)*[8]
Vitamin A	Retinoids (include: retinol, retinal, retinoic acid, 3-dehydroretinol and its derivatives)	Fat	Night-blindness, Keratomalacia[9]	**900 μg**	3,000 μg
Vitamin B_1	Thiamine	Water	Beriberi	**1.2 mg**	(N/D)[10]
Vitamin B_2	Riboflavin	Water	Ariboflavinosis	**1.3 mg**	N/D
Vitamin B_3	Niacin	Water	Pellagra	**16.0 mg**	35.0 mg

(Contd.)

(Contd. Table)

Vitamin name	*Chemical name*	*Solubility*	*Deficiency disease*	*Recommended Dietary Allowances (male, age 19–70)*	*Upper Intake Level (UL/day)*[8]
Vitamin B_5	Pantothenic acid	Water	Paresthesia	5.0 mg [11]	N/D
Vitamin B_6	Pyridoxine	Water	Anemia[12]	**1.3-1.7 mg**	100 mg
Vitamin B_7	Biotin	Water	n/a	30.0 μg	N/D
Vitamin B_9	Folic acid	Water	Deficiency during pregnancy is associated with birth defects.	**400 μg**	1,000 μg

(Contd.)

(Contd. Table)

Vitamin name	*Chemical name*	*Solubility*	*Deficiency disease*	*Recommended Dietary Allowances (male, age 19–70)*	*Upper Intake Level (UL/day)*[8]
Vitamin B_{12}	Cyanocobalamin	Water	Megaloblastic anaemia[13]	**2.4 µg**	N/D
Vitamin C	Ascorbic acid	Water	Scurvy	**90.0 mg**	2,000 mg
Vitamin D_2–D_4	Lumisterol, Ergocalciferol, Cholecalciferol, Dihydrotachysterol, 7-Dehydrocholesterol	Fat	Rickets (in adults, a.k.a. Osteomalacia)	5.0 µg-10 µg [14]	50 µg

(Contd.)

(Contd. Table)

Vitamin name	*Chemical name*	*Solubility*	*Deficiency disease*	*Recommended Dietary Allowances (male, age 19–70)*	*Upper Intake Level (UL/day)*[8]
Vitamin E	Tocopherol, Tocotrienol	Fat	deficiency is very rare, mild hemolytic anemia in newborn infants [15]	**15.0 mg**	1,000 mg
Vitamin K	Naphthoquinone	Fat	Bleeding diathesis	120 µg	N/D

for them to be used, special carriers in your body take them to where they're needed. Vitamins A, D, E, and K are all fat-soluble vitamins. **Water-soluble** vitamins are different. When you eat foods that have water-soluble vitamins, the vitamins don't get stored as much in your body. Instead, they travel through your bloodstream. And whatever your body doesn't use comes out when you urinate. So these kinds of vitamins need to be replaced often because they don't like to stick around. This crowd of vitamins includes vitamin C and the big group of B vitamins - B1 (thiamin), B2 (riboflavin), niacin, B6 (pyridoxine), folic acid, B12 (cobalamine), biotin, and pantothenic acid.

Each vitamin is typically used in multiple reactions and therefore, most have multiple functions.

Vitamins in nutrition and disease

Vitamins are essential for normal growth and development. Using the genetic blueprint inherited from its parents, a foetus begins to develop, at the moment of conception, from the nutrients it absorbs. The developing foetus requires certain vitamins and minerals to be present at certain times. These nutrients facilitate the chemical reactions that produce, among other things, skin, bone, and muscle. If there is serious deficiency in one or more of these nutrients, a child may develop a deficiency disease. Even minor deficiencies have the potential to cause permanent damage.

For the most part, vitamins are obtained through food sources. However, a few vitamins are obtained by other means: for example, microorganisms in the intestine - commonly known as "gut flora" - produce vitamin K and biotin, while one form of vitamin D is synthesized in the skin with the help of natural ultraviolet in sunlight. Some vitamins can be obtained from precursors that are obtained in the diet. Examples include vitamin A, which can be produced from beta carotene and niacin, from the amino acid tryptophan.

Once growth and development are completed, vitamins remain essential components of the healthy maintenance of the cells, tissues, and organs that make up the human body, and enable the body to efficiently use the calories provided by the food that we eat, and to help process proteins, carbohydrates, and fats.

Foods rich in vitamins

Vitamin A - liver, milk, and cheese

Beta-carotene (converted to Vitamin A) - dark green vegetables, and orange fruits such as apricots, mango and papaya.

Vitamin B_1 (Thiamine) - meat, liver, nuts, whole grains

Vitamin B_2 (Riboflavin) - dairy products, beans, leafy green vegetables

Vitamin B_6 - meats, beans, nuts, leafy green vegetables, bananas

Vitamin B_{12} - meats, fortified soy products

Biotin - egg yolks, fish, beans

Folate - meats, beans, liver, broccoli, leafy green vegetables, cantaloupe

Niacin - chicken, fish, peanuts, dried beans

Vitamin C - citrus fruits, dark green vegetables, bell peppers, tomatoes

Vitamin D- sunshine, also added to milk

Vitamin E - plant oils, leafy green vegetables, nuts

Copper - oysters, peas, beans, organ meats

Iron - meat, liver, peas, beans, whole grains, eggs

Selenium - seafood, egg yolks, whole grains

Magnesium - nuts, whole grains, dark green vegetables

Zinc - liver, sea food, whole grains

Vitamin deficiencies

Deficiencies of vitamins are classified as either primary or secondary. A primary deficiency occurs when you do not get enough of the vitamin in the food you eat. A secondary deficiency may be due to an underlying disorder that prevents or limits the absorption or use of the vitamin, due to a "lifestyle factor", such as smoking, excessive alcohol consumption, or the use of medications that interfere with the absorption or the body's use of the vitamin. Individuals who eat a varied diet are unlikely to develop a severe primary vitamin deficiency. Whereas, restrictive diets have the potential to cause prolonged vitamin deficits, which may result in often painful and potentially deadly diseases.

Because most vitamins are not stored in the body, a person must consume them regularly to avoid deficiency. Body stores for different vitamins vary widely; vitamins A, D, and B_{12} are stored in significant amounts in the body, mainly in the liver, and an adult may be deficient in vitamin A and B_{12} for long periods of time before developing a deficiency condition. Vitamin B_3, is not stored in the body in significant amounts, and stores may only last a couple of weeks.

Well-known vitamin deficiencies involve thiamine (beriberi), niacin (pellagra), vitamin C (scurvy) and vitamin D (rickets).

Supplements

Dietary supplements, often containing vitamins, are used to ensure that adequate amounts of nutrients are obtained on a daily basis, if optimal amounts of the nutrients cannot be obtained through a varied diet. Scientific evidence supporting the benefits of some dietary supplements is well established for certain health conditions, but others need further study.

Supplements are, as required by law, not intended to treat, diagnose, mitigate, prevent, or cure disease. In some cases, dietary supplements may have unwanted effects, especially if taken before surgery, with other dietary supplements or medicines, or if the person taking them has certain health conditions. Vitamin supplements may also contain levels of vitamins many times higher, and in different forms, than one may ingest through food. Before taking a supplement, it is important to check with a knowledgeable health care provider, especially when combining or substituting supplements with other foods or medicine.

The B Vitamins

There's more than one B vitamin. Here's the list: B1, B2, B6, B12, niacin, folic acid, biotin, and pantothenic acid. Whew - that's quite a group!

The B vitamins are important in metabolic activity - this means that they help make energy and set it free when your body needs it.

The following foods are rich in vitamin B?

- whole grains, such as wheat and oats
- fish and seafood
- poultry and meats

- eggs
  dairy products, like milk and yogurt
- leafy green vegetables
- beans and peas
- citrus fruits, such as oranges

Vitamin B-1 (Thiamin)

Plays a key role in the body's metabolic cycle for generating energy; helps in the digestion of carbohydrates; essential for the normal functioning of the nervous system, muscles and heart; stabilizes the appetite; promotes growth and good muscle tone.

Deficiency symptoms: May lead to the loss of appetite ; weakness and feeling tired; paralysis and nervous irritability; insomnia; loss of weight; vague aches and pains; mental depression and constipation; heart and gastrointestinal problems.

Thiamin structure

Thiamin is also known as vitamin B_1. A deficiency in thiamin intake leads to a severely reduced capacity of cells to generate energy as a result of its role in these reactions. The dietary requirement for thiamin is proportional to the caloric intake of the diet and ranges from 1.0 - 1.5 mg/day for normal adults. If the carbohydrate content of the diet is excessive then an in thiamin intake will be required.

Clinical Significances of Thiamin Deficiency

The earliest symptoms of thiamin deficiency include constipation, appetite suppression, nausea as well as mental depression, peripheral neuropathy and fatigue. Chronic thiamin deficiency leads to more severe neurological symptoms including ataxia, mental confusion and loss of eye coordination. Other clinical symptoms of prolonged thiamin deficiency are related to cardiovascular and musculature defects. The severe thiamin deficiency disease known as Beriberi, is the result of a diet that is carbohydrate rich and thiamin deficient. An additional thiamin deficiency related disease is known as Wernicke-Korsakoff syndrome. This disease is most commonly found in chronic alcoholics due to their poor dietetic lifestyles.

Vitamin B-2 (Riboflavin)

Necessary for carbohydrate, fat and protein metabolism; aids in the formation of antibodies and red blood cells; maintains cell respiration; necessary for the maintenance of good vision, skin, nails and hair; alleviates eye fatigue; promotes general health.

Deficiency symptoms: May result in itching and burning eyes; cracks and sores in the mouth and lips; bloodshot eyes; purplish tongue; dermatitis; retarded growth; digestive disturbances; trembling; sluggishness; oily skin.

Riboflavin is also known as vitamin B_2. Riboflavin is the precursor for the coenzymes, flavin mononucleotide (FMN) and flavin adenine dinucleotide (FAD).

Clinical Significances of Riboflavin Deficiency

Riboflavin deficiencies are rare nowadays due to the presence of adequate amounts of the vitamin in eggs, milk, meat and cereals. Riboflavin deficiency is often seen in chronic alcoholics due to their poor dietetic habits. Symptoms associated with riboflavin deficiency include, glossitis, seborrhea, angular stomatitis, cheilosis and photophobia. Riboflavin decomposes when exposed to visible light. This characteristic can lead to riboflavin deficiencies in newborns treated for hyperbilirubinemia by phototherapy.

Niacinamide (Niacin- vitamin B-3)

Improves circulation and reduces the cholesterol level in the blood; maintains the nervous system; helps metabolize protein, sugar and fat; reduces high blood pressure; increases energy through proper utilization of food; prevents pellagra; helps maintain a healthy skin, tongue and digestive system.

Deficiency symptoms: May result in pellagra, gastrointestinal disturbance, nervousness, headaches, fatigue, mental depression, vague aches and pains, irritability, loss of appetite, insomnia, skin disorders, muscular weakness, indigestion, bad breath, canker sores.

Niacin (nicotinic acid and nicotinamide) is also known as vitamin B_3. Both nicotinic acid and nicotinamide can serve as the dietary source of vitamin B_3. Niacin is required for the synthesis of the active forms of vitamin B_3, nicotinamide adenine dinucleotide (NAD^+) and nicotinamide adenine dinucleotide phosphate ($NADP^+$).

Both NAD^+ and $NADP^+$ function as cofactors for numerous dehydrogenase, e.g., lactate and malate dehydrogenases.

Niacin is not a true vitamin in the strictest definition since it can be derived from the amino acid tryptophan. However, the ability to utilize tryptophan for niacin synthesis is inefficient (60 mg of tryptophan are required to synthesize 1 mg of niacin). Also, synthesis of niacin from tryptophan requires vitamins B_1, B_2 and B_6 which would be limiting in themselves on a marginal diet.

The recommended daily requirement for niacin is 13 - 19 niacin equivalents (NE) per day for a normal adult. One NE is equivalent to 1 mg of free niacin).

Clinical Significances of Niacin and Nicotinic Acid

A diet deficient in niacin (as well as tryptophan) leads to glossitis of the tongue, dermatitis, weight loss, diarrhoea, depression and dementia. The severe symptoms, depression, dermatitis and diarrhoea, are associated with the condition known as **pellagra**. Several physiological conditions (e.g. Hartnup disease and malignant carcinoid syndrome) as well as certain drug therapies (e.g. isoniazid) can lead to niacin deficiency.

Nicotinic acid (but not nicotinamide) when administered in pharmacological doses of 2 - 4 g/day lowers plasma cholesterol levels and has been shown to be a useful therapeutic for hypercholesterolemia. The major action of nicotinic acid in this capacity is a reduction in fatty acid mobilization from adipose tissue. Although nicotinic acid therapy lowers blood cholesterol it also causes a depletion of glycogen stores and fat reserves in skeletal and cardiac muscle. Additionally, there is an elevation in blood glucose and uric acid production. For these reasons nicotinic acid therapy is not recommended for diabetics or persons who suffer from gout.

Pantothenic acid

Participates in the release of energy from carbohydrates, fats and protein, aids in the utilization of vitamins; improves the body's resistance to stress; helps in cell building and the development of the central nervous system; helps the adrenal glands, fights infections by building antibodies.

Deficiency symptoms: May lead to painful and burning feet, skin abnormalities, retarded growth, dizzy spells, digestive disturbances, vomiting, restlessness, stomach stress, muscle cramps.

Pantothenic acid is also known as vitamin B_5. Pantothenic acid is formed from ?-alanine and pantoic acid. Pantothenate is required for synthesis of coenzyme A, CoA and is a component of the acyl carrier protein (ACP) domain of fatty acid synthase. Pantothenate is, therefore, required for the metabolism of carbohydrate via the TCA cycle and all fats and proteins. At least 70 enzymes have been identified as requiring CoA or ACP derivatives for their function. Deficiency of pantothenic acid is extremely rare due to its widespread distribution in whole grain cereals, legumes and meat. Symptoms of pantothenate deficiency are difficult to assess since they are subtle and resemble those of other B vitamin deficiencies.

Vitamin B-6 (Pyridoxine) :

Necessary for the synthesis and breakdown of amino acids, the building blocks of protein; aids in fat and carbohydrate metabolism; aids in the formation of antibodies; maintains the central nervous system; aids in the removal of excess fluid of premenstrual women; promotes healthy skin; reduces muscle spasms, leg cramps, hand numbness, nausea and stiffness of hands; helps maintain a proper balance of sodium and phosphorous in the body.

Deficiency symptoms: May result in nervousness, insomnia, skin eruptions, loss of muscular control, anaemia, mouth disorders, muscular weakness, dermatitis, arm and leg cramps, loss of hair, slow learning, and water retention.

Pyridoxal, pyridoxamine and pyridoxine are collectively known as vitamin B_6. All three compounds are efficiently converted to the biologically active form of vitamin B_6, pyridoxal phosphate. This conversion is catalyzed by the ATP requiring enzyme, pyridoxal kinase.

Pyridoxal phosphate functions as a cofactor in enzymes involved in transamination reactions required for the synthesis and catabolism of the amino acids as well as in glycogenolysis as a cofactor for glycogen phosphorylase. The requirement for vitamin B_6 in the diet is proportional to the level of protein consumption ranging from

1.4 - 2.0 mg/day for a normal adult. During pregnancy and lactation the requirement for vitamin B_6 increases approximately 0.6 mg/day. Deficiencies of vitamin B_6 are rare and usually are related to an overall deficiency of all the B-complex vitamins. Isoniazid and penicillamine (used to treat rheumatoid arthritis and cystinurias) are two drugs that complex with pyridoxal and pyridoxal phosphate resulting in a deficiency in this vitamin.

Biotin

Helps in the utilization of protein, folic acid, Pantothenic acid, and Vitamin B-12, promotes healthy hair.

Deficiency symptoms: May lead to extreme exhaustion, drowsiness, muscle pain, loss of appetite, depression, grayish skin color.

Biotin is the cofactor required of enzymes that are involved in carboxylation reactions, e.g. acetyl-CoA carboxylase and pyruvate carboxylase. Biotin is found in numerous foods and also is synthesized by intestinal bacteria and as such deficiencies of the vitamin are rare. Deficiencies are generally seen only after long antibiotic therapies which deplete the intestinal fauna or following excessive consumption of raw eggs. The latter is due to the affinity of the egg white protein, avidin, for biotin preventing intestinal absorption of the biotin.

Vitamin B-12 (Cobalamin) :

Helps in the formation and regeneration of red blood cells, thus helping prevent anaemia; necessary for carbohydrate, fat and protein metabolism; maintains a healthy nervous system; promotes growth in children; increases energy; needed for Calcium absorption.

Deficiency symptoms: May lead to pernicious anaemia, poor appetite, growth failure in children, tiredness, brain damage, nervousness, neuritis, degeneration of spinal cord, depression, lack of balance.Cobalamin is more commonly known as vitamin B_{12}. Vitamin B_{12} is composed of a complex tetrapyrrol ring structure (corrin ring) and a cobalt ion in the center. Vitamin B_{12} is synthesized exclusively by microorganisms and is found in the liver of animals bound to protein as methycobalamin or 5'-deoxyadenosylcobalamin. The vitamin must be hydrolyzed from protein in order to be active.

Hydrolysis occurs in the stomach by gastric acids or the intestines by trypsin digestion following consumption of animal meat. The vitamin is then bound by intrinsic factor, a protein secreted by parietal cells of the stomach, and carried to the ileum where it is absorbed. Following absorption the vitamin is transported to the liver in the blood bound to transcobalamin II.

There are only two clinically significant reactions in the body that require vitamin B_{12} as a cofactor. During the catabolism of fatty acids with an odd number of carbon atoms and the amino acids valine, isoleucine and threonine the resultant propionyl-CoA is converted to succinyl-CoA for oxidation in the TCA cycle. One of the enzymes in this pathway, methylmalonyl-CoA mutase, requires vitamin B_{12} as a cofactor in the conversion of methylmalonyl-CoA to succinyl-CoA. The 5'-deoxyadenosine derivative of cobalamin is required for this reaction.

The second reaction requiring vitamin B_{12} catalyzes the conversion of homocysteine to methionine and is catalyzed by methionine synthase. This reaction results in the transfer of the methyl group from N^5-methyltetrahydrofolate to hydroxycobalamin generating tetrahydrofolate (THF) and methylcobalamin during the process of the conversion.

Clinical Significances of B_{12} Deficiency

The liver can store up to six years worth of vitamin B_{12}, hence deficiencies in this vitamin are rare. Pernicious anaemia is a megaloblastic anaemia resulting from vitamin B_{12} deficiency that develops as a result a lack of intrinsic factor in the stomach leading to malabsorption of the vitamin. The anaemia results from impaired DNA synthesis due to a block in purine and thymidine biosynthesis. The block in nucleotide biosynthesis is a consequence of the effect of vitamin B_{12} on folate metabolism. When vitamin B_{12} is deficient essentially all of the folate becomes trapped as the N^5-methylTHF derivative as a result of the loss of functional methionine synthase. This trapping prevents the synthesis of other THF derivatives required for the purine and thymidine nucleotide biosynthesis pathways.

Neurological complications also are associated with vitamin B_{12} deficiency and result from a progressive demyelination of nerve cells. The demyelination is thought to result from the increase in methylmalonyl-CoA that result from vitamin B_{12} deficiency. Methylmalonyl-CoA is a competitive inhibitor of malonyl-CoA in fatty acid biosynthesis as well as being able to substitute for malonyl-CoA in any fatty acid biosynthesis that may occur. Since the myelin sheath is in continual flux the methylmalonyl-CoA-induced inhibition of fatty acid synthesis results in the eventual destruction of the sheath. The incorporation methylmalonyl-CoA into fatty acid biosynthesis results in branched-chain fatty acids being produced that may severely alter the architecture of the normal membrane structure of nerve cells.

Folic acid

Necessary for DNA and RNA synthesis, which is essential for the growth and reproduction of all body cells; essential to the formation of red blood cells by its action on the bone marrow; aids in amino acid metabolism.

Deficiency symptoms: May result in gastrointestinal disorders, anemia, Vitamin B-12 deficiency, pre-mature gray hair.

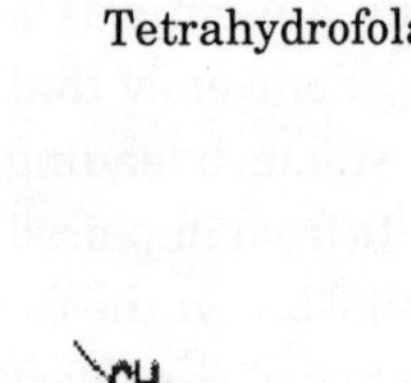

Tetrahydrofolate

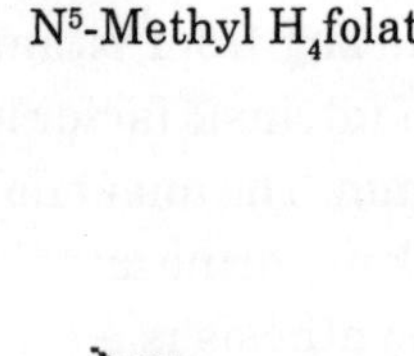

N^5-Methyl H_4folate

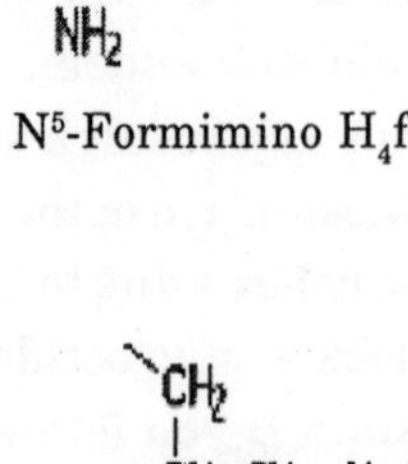

N^5-Formimino H_4folate

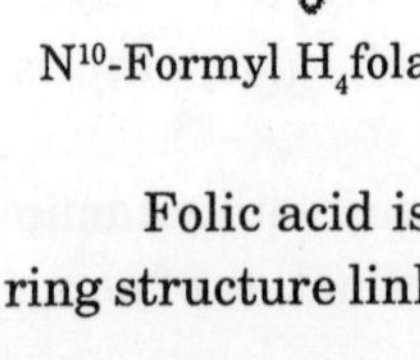

N^{10}-Formyl H_4folate

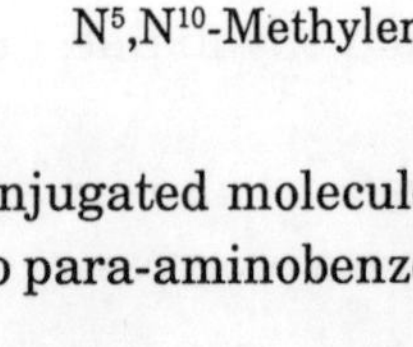

N^5,N^{10}-Methylene

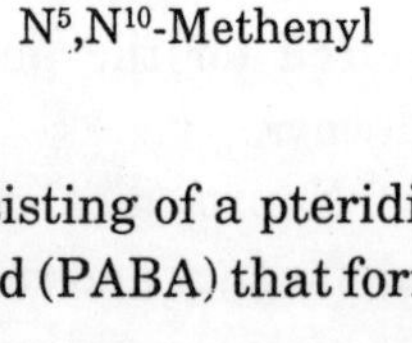

N^5,N^{10}-Methenyl

Folic acid is a conjugated molecule consisting of a pteridine ring structure linked to para-aminobenzoic acid (PABA) that forms pteroic acid. Folic acid itself is then generated through the conjugation of glutamic acid residues to pteroic acid. Folic acid is obtained primarily from yeasts and leafy vegetables as well as animal liver. Animal cannot synthesize PABA nor attach glutamate residues to pteroic acid, thus, requiring folate intake in the diet.

When stored in the liver or ingested folic acid exists in a polyglutamate form. Intestinal mucosal cells remove some of the glutamate residues through the action of the lysosomal enzyme, conjugase. The removal of glutamate residues makes folate less negatively charged (from the polyglutamic acids) and therefore more capable of passing through the basal lamenal membrane of the epithelial cells of the intestine and into the bloodstream. Folic acid is reduced within cells (principally the liver where it is stored) to tetrahydrofolate (THF also H_4folate) through the action of dihydrofolate reductase (DHFR), an NADPH-requiring enzyme.

The function of THF derivatives is to carry and transfer various forms of one carbon units during biosynthetic reactions. The one carbon units are either methyl, methylene, methenyl, formyl or formimino groups.

These one carbon transfer reactions are required in the biosynthesis of serine, methionine, glycine, choline and the purine nucleotides and dTMP.

Active center of tetrahydrofolate (THF). Note that the N^5 position is the site of attachment of methyl groups, the N^{10} the site for attachment of formyl and formimino groups and that both N^5 and N^{10} bridge the methylene and methenyl groups.

The ability to acquire choline and amino acids from the diet and to salvage the purine nucleotides makes the role of N^5,N^{10}-methylene-THF in dTMP synthesis the most metabolically significant function for this vitamin. The role of vitamin B_{12} and N^5-methyl-THF in the conversion of homocysteine to methionine also can have a significant impact on the ability of cells to regenerate needed THF.

Clinical Significance of Folate Deficiency

Folate deficiency results in complications nearly identical to those described for vitamin B_{12} deficiency. The most pronounced effect of folate deficiency on cellular processes is upon DNA synthesis. This is due to an impairment in dTMP synthesis which leads to cell cycle arrest in S-phase of rapidly proliferating cells, in particular hematopoietic cells. The result is megaloblastic anaemia as for vitamin B_{12} deficiency. The inability to synthesize DNA during erythrocyte maturation leads to abnormally large erythrocytes termed macrocytic anemia.

Folate deficiencies are rare due to the adequate presence of folate in food. Poor dietary habits as those of chronic alcoholics can lead to folate deficiency. The predominant causes of folate deficiency in non-alcoholics are impaired absorption or metabolism or an increased demand for the vitamin. The predominant condition requiring an increase in the daily intake of folate is pregnancy. This is due to an increased number of rapidly proliferating cells present in the blood. The need for folate will nearly double by the third trimester of pregnancy. Certain drugs such as anticonvulsants and oral contraceptives can impair the absorption of folate. Anticonvulsants also increase the rate of folate metabolism.

Vitamin C (Ascorbic Acid)

This vitamin is important for keeping body tissues, such as gums and muscles in good shape. C is also key if you get a cut or wound because it helps you heal. This vitamin also helps your body resist infection. This means that even though you can't always avoid getting sick, vitamin C makes it a little harder for your body to become infected with an illness.

The following foods are rich in vitamin C ?

- citrus fruits, like oranges
- cantaloupe
- strawberries
- tomatoes
- broccoli
- cabbage

Essential for healthy teeth, gums and bones; helps heal wounds, scar tissue, and fractures; prevents scurvy; builds resistance to infection; aids in the prevention and treatment of the common cold; gives strength to blood vessels; aids in the absorption of iron. It is required for the synthesis of collagen, the intercellular "cement" which holds tissues together. It is also one of the major antioxidant nutrients. It prevents the conversion of nitrates (from tobacco smoke, smog, bacon, lunch meats, and some vegetables) into cancer-causing substances. According to Dr. Lines Pauling, the foremost authority on Vitamin C, Vitamin C will decrease the risk of getting certain cancers by 75%.

DEFICIENCY SYMPTOMS: May lead to soft and bleeding gums, swollen or painful joints, slow-healing wounds and fractures, bruising, nosebleeds, tooth decay, loss of appetite, muscular weakness, skin haemorrhages, capillary weakness, anaemia, impaired digestion.

Ascorbic acid is more commonly known as vitamin C. Ascorbic acid is derived from glucose via the uronic acid pathway. The enzyme L-gulonolactone oxidase responsible for the conversion of gulonolactone to ascorbic acid is absent in primates making ascorbic acid required in the diet.

The active form of vitamin C is ascorbate acid itself. The main function of ascorbate is as a reducing agent in a number of different reactions. Vitamin C has the potential to reduce cytochromes a and c of the respiratory chain as well as molecular oxygen. The most important reaction requiring ascorbate as a cofactor is the hydroxylation of proline residues in collagen. Vitamin C is, therefore, required for the maintenance of normal connective tissue as well as for wound healing since synthesis of connective tissue is the first event in wound tissue remodeling. Vitamin C also is necessary for bone remodeling due to the presence of collagen in the organic matrix of bones.

Several other metabolic reactions require vitamin C as a cofactor. These include the catabolism of tyrosine and the synthesis of epinephrine from tyrosine and the synthesis of the bile acids. It is also believed that vitamin C is involved in the process of steroidogenesis since the adrenal cortex contains high levels of vitamin C which are depleted upon adrenocorticotropic hormone (ACTH) stimulation of the gland.

Deficiency in vitamin C leads to the disease scurvy due to the role of the vitamin in the post-translational modification of collagens. Scurvy is characterized by easily bruised skin, muscle fatigue, soft swollen gums, decreased wound healing and hemorrhaging, osteoporosis, and anemia. Vitamin C is readily absorbed and so the primary cause of vitamin C deficiency is poor diet and/or an increased requirement. The primary physiological state leading to an increased requirement for vitamin C is severe stress (or trauma). This is due to a rapid depletion in the adrenal stores of the vitamin. The reason for the decrease in adrenal vitamin C levels is unclear but may be due either to redistribution of the vitamin to areas that need it or an overall increased utilization.

Vitamin A

This vitamin plays a really big part in eyesight. It's great for night vision. Vitamin A helps you see in color, too, from the brightest yellow to the darkest purple. In addition, it helps you grow properly and helps in healthy skin.

The following foods are rich in vitamin A?

- eggs
- milk
- apricots
- nectarines
- cantaloupe
- carrots
- sweet potatoes
- spinach

Necessary for growth and repair of body tissues; helps maintain smooth, soft disease-free skin; helps protect the mucous membranes of the mouth, nose , throat and lungs, thereby reducing susceptibility to infections; protects against air pollutants; counteracts night-blindness and weak eyesight; aids in bone and teeth formation. Current medical research shows that foods rich in Beta Carotene will help reduce the risk of lung cancer and certain oral cancers. Unlike Vitamin A from fish liver oil, Beta Carotene is non-toxic.

Deficiency symptoms: May result in night blindness; increased susceptibility to infections; rough, dry, scaly skin; loss of smell and appetite; frequents fatigue; lack of tearing; defective teeth and gums' retarded growth.

Vitamin A consists of three biologically active molecules, retinol, retinal (retinaldehyde) and retinoic acid. Each of these compounds are derived from the plant precursor molecule, á-carotene (a member of a family of molecules known as carotenoids). Beta-carotene, which consists of two molecules of retinal linked at their aldehyde ends, is also referred to as the provitamin form of vitamin A.

Vision and the Role of Vitamin A

Photoreception in the eye is the function of two specialized cell types located in the retina; the rod and cone cells. Both rod and cone cells contain a photoreceptor pigment in their membranes. The photosensitive compound of most mammalian eyes is a protein called opsin to which is covalently coupled an aldehyde of vitamin A. The opsin of rod cells is called scotopsin. The photoreceptor of rod cells is specifically called rhodopsin or visual purple. This compound is a complex between scotopsin and the 11-*cis*-retinal (also called 11-*cis*-retinene) form of vitamin A. Rhodopsin is a serpentine receptor imbedded in the membrane of the rod cell. Coupling of 11-*cis*-retinal occurs at three of the transmembrane domains of rhodopsin. Intracellularly, rhodopsin is coupled to a specific G-protein called transducin.

When the rhodopsin is exposed to light it is bleached releasing the 11-*cis*-retinal from opsin. Absorption of photons by 11-*cis*-retinal triggers a series of conformational changes on the way to conversion all-*trans*-retinal. One important conformational intermediate is metarhodopsin II. The release of opsin results in a conformational change in the photoreceptor. This conformational change activates transducin, leading to an increased GTP-binding by the a-subunit of transducin. Binding of GTP releases the ?-subunit from the inhibitory?- and ?-subunits. The GTP-activated ?-subunit in turn activates an associated phosphodiesterase; an enzyme that hydrolyzes cyclic-GMP (cGMP) to GMP. Cyclic GMP is required to maintain the Na^+ channels of the rod cell in the open conformation. The drop in cGMP concentration results in complete closure of the Na^+ channels. Metarhodopsin II appears to be responsible for initiating the closure of the channels. The closing of the channels leads to hyperpolarization of the rod cell with concomitant propagation of nerve impulses to the brain.

Additional Role of Retinol

Retinol also functions in the synthesis of certain glycoproteins and mucopolysaccharides necessary for mucous production and normal growth regulation. This is accomplished by phosphorylation of retinol to retinyl phosphate which then functions similarly to dolichol phosphate.

Clinical Significances of Vitamin A Deficiency

Vitamin A is stored in the liver and deficiency of the vitamin occurs only after prolonged lack of dietary intake. The earliest symptoms of vitamin A deficiency are night blindness. Additional early symptoms include follicular hyperkeratinosis, increased susceptibility to infection and cancer and anaemia equivalent to iron deficient anaemia. Prolonged lack of vitamin A leads to deterioration of the eye tissue through progressive keratinization of the cornea, a condition known as xerophthalmia.

The increased risk of cancer in vitamin deficiency is thought to be the result of a depletion in Beta-carotene. Beta-carotene is a very effective antioxidant and is suspected to reduce the risk of cancers known to be initiated by the production of free radicals. Of particular interest is the potential benefit of increased Beta-carotene intake to reduce the risk of lung cancer in smokers. However, caution needs to be taken when increasing the intake of any of the lipid soluble vitamins. Excess accumulation of vitamin A in the liver can lead to toxicity which manifests as bone pain, hepatosplenomegaly, nausea and diarrhea.

Vitamin D

No bones about it . . . vitamin D is the vitamin you need for strong bones! It's also great for forming strong teeth. Vitamin D even lends a hand to an important mineral - it helps your body absorb the amount of calcium it needs.

The following foods are rich in vitamin D ?

- milk and other dairy products fortified with vitamin D
- fish

egg yolks

Improves absorption and utilization of Calcium and Phosphorous; required for bone and teeth formation; maintains a stable nervous system and normal heart action.

Deficiency symptoms: May lead to rickets, tooth decay, softening of bones, improper healing of fractures, lack of vigour, muscular weakness, inadequate absorption of calcium, retention of phosphorous in the kidneys.

Vitamin D is a steroid hormone that functions to regulate specific gene expression following interaction with its intracellular receptor. The biologically active form of the hormone is 1,25-dihydroxy vitamin D_3 (1,25-$(OH)_2D_3$, also termed calcitriol). Calcitriol functions primarily to regulate calcium and phosphorous homeostasis.

Active calcitriol is derived from ergosterol (produced in plants) and from 7-dehydrocholesterol (produced in the skin). Ergocalciferol (vitamin D_2) is formed by uv irradiation of ergosterol. In the skin 7-dehydrocholesterol is converted to cholecalciferol (vitamin D_3) following *uv* irradiation.

Vitamin D_2 and D_3 are processed to D_2-calcitriol and D_3-calcitriol, respectively, by the same enzymatic pathways in the body. Cholecalciferol (or egrocalciferol) are absorbed from the intestine and transported to the liver bound to a specific vitamin D-binding protein. In the liver cholecalciferol is hydroxylated at the 25 position by a specific D_3-25-hydroxylase generating 25-hydroxy-D_3 [25-$(OH)D_3$] which is the major circulating form of vitamin D. Conversion of 25-$(OH)D_3$ to its biologically active form, calcitriol, occurs through the activity of a specific D_3-1-hydroxylase present in the proximal convoluted tubules of the kidneys, and in bone and placenta. 25-$(OH)D_3$ can also be hydroxylated at the 24 position by a specific D_3-24-hydroxylase in the kidneys, intestine, placenta and cartilage.

Calcitriol functions in concert with parathyroid hormone (PTH) and calcitonin to regulate serum calcium and phosphorous levels. PTH is released in response to low serum calcium and induces the production of calcitriol. In contrast, reduced levels of PTH stimulate synthesis of the inactive 24,25-$(OH)_2D_3$. In the intestinal epithelium, calcitriol functions as a steroid hormone in inducing the expression of calbindinD_{28K}, a protein involved in intestinal calcium absorption. The increased absorption of calcium ions requires concomitant absorption of a negatively charged counter ion to maintain electrical neutrality. The predominant counter ion is Pi. When plasma calcium levels fall the major sites of action of calcitriol and PTH are bone where they stimulate bone resorption and the kidneys where they inhibit calcium excretion by stimulating reabsorption by the distal tubules. The role of calcitonin in calcium homeostasis is to decrease elevated serum calcium levels by inhibiting bone resorption.

Clinical Significance of Vitamin D Deficiency

As a result of the addition of vitamin D to milk, deficiencies in this vitamin are rare in this country. The main symptom of vitamin D deficiency in children is **rickets** and in adults is **osteomalacia**. Rickets is characterized improper mineralization during the development of the bones resulting in soft bones. Osteomalacia is characterized by demineralization of previously formed bone leading to increased softness and susceptibility to fracture.

Vitamin- E

Everybody needs E. This hard-working vitamin maintains a lot of your body's tissues, like the ones in your eyes, skin, and liver. It protects your lungs from becoming damaged by polluted air. And it is important for the formation of red blood cells.

The following foods are rich in vitamin E?

- whole grains, such as wheat and oats
- wheat germ
- leafy green vegetables
- sardines
- egg yolks
- nuts

Major anti-oxidant nutrient; retards cellular aging due to oxidation; supplies oxygen to the blood which is then carried to the heart and other organs; thus alleviating fatigue; aids in bringing nourishment to cells; strengthens the capillary walls and prevents the red blood cells from destructive poisons; prevents and dissolves blood clots; has also been used by doctors in helping prevent sterility, muscular dystrophy, calcium deposits in blood walls and heart conditions.

What is the difference between d-alpha and dl-alpha? Both work exactly the same in the body. There is some evidence that d-alpha is about 20% more powerful, but it costs about 400% more. In other words 800 I.U. of d-alpha would work as well as 1000 I.U. of dl-alpha. But, the 800 I.U. d-alpha would cost 4 times as much as 1000 I.U. of dl-alpha. The best buy by far is dl-alpha.

Deficiency symptoms: May lead to a rupture of red blood cells, loss of reproductive powers, lack of sexual vitality, abnormal fat deposits in muscles, degenerative changes in the changes in the heart and other muscles; dry skin.

Vitamin E is a mixture of several related compounds known as tocopherols. The á-tocopherol molecule is the most potent of the tocopherols. Vitamin E is absorbed from the intestines packaged in chylomicrons. It is delivered to the tissues via chylomicron transport and then to the liver through chylomicron remnant uptake. The liver can export vitamin E in VLDLs. Due to its lipophilic nature, vitamin E accumulates in cellular membranes, fat deposits and other circulating lipoproteins. The major site of vitamin E storage is in adipose tissue.

The major function of vitamin E is to act as a natural antioxidant by scavenging free radicals and molecular oxygen. In particular vitamin E is important for preventing peroxidation of polyunsaturated membrane fatty acids. The vitamins E and C are interrelated in their antioxidant capabilities. Active ?-tocopherol can be regenerated by interaction with vitamin C following scavenge of a peroxy free radical. Alternatively, ?-tocopherol can scavenge two peroxy free radicals and then be conjugated to glucuronate for excretion in the bile.

Clinical Significances of Vitamin E Deficiency

No major disease states have been found to be associated with vitamin E deficiency due to adequate levels in the average Indian diet. The major symptom of vitamin E deficiency in humans is an increase in red blood cell fragility. Since vitamin E is absorbed from the intestines in chylomicrons, any fat malabsorption diseases can lead to deficiencies in vitamin E intake. Neurological disorders have been associated with vitamin E deficiencies associated with fat malabsorptive disorders. Increased intake of vitamin E is recommended in premature infants fed formulas that are low in the vitamin as well as in persons consuming a diet high in polyunsaturated fatty acids. Polyunsaturated fatty acids tend to form free radicals upon exposure to oxygen and this may lead to an increased risk of certain cancers.

Vitamin K

Vitamin K is the clotmaster! Remember the last time you got a cut? Your blood did something special called clotting. This is when certain cells in your blood act like glue and stick together at the surface of the cut.

Which foods are rich in vitamin K?

- leafy green vegetables
- liver
- pork
- dairy products, like milk and yogurt

The K vitamins exist naturally as K_1 (phylloquinone) in green vegetables and K_2 (menaquinone) produced by intestinal bacteria and K_3 is synthetic menadione. When administered, vitamin K_3 is alkylated to one of the vitamin K_2 forms of menaquinone.

The major function of the K vitamins is in the maintenance of normal levels of the blood clotting proteins, factors II, VII, IX, X and protein C and protein S, which are synthesized in the liver as inactive precursor proteins. Conversion from inactive to active clotting factor requires a posttranslational modification of specific glutamate (E) residues. This modification is a carboxylation and the enzyme responsible requires vitamin K as a cofactor. The resultant modified E residues are ?-carboxyglutamate (gla). This process is most clearly understood for factor II, also called preprothrombin. Prothrombin is modified preprothrombin. The *gla* residues are effective calcium ion chelators. Upon chelation of calcium, prothrombin interacts with phospholipids in membranes and is proteolysed to thrombin through the action of activated factor X (Xa).

During the carboxylation reaction reduced hydroquinone form of vitamin K is converted to a 2,3-epoxide form. The regeneration of the hydroquinone form requires an uncharacterized reductase. This latter reaction is the site of action of the dicumarol based anticoagulants such as warfarin.

Clinical Significance of Vitamin K Deficiency

Naturally occurring vitamin K is absorbed from the intestines only in the presence of bile salts and other lipids through interaction with chylomicrons. Therefore, fat malabsorptive diseases can result in vitamin K deficiency. The synthetic vitamin K_3 is water soluble and absorbed irrespective of the presence of intestinal lipids and bile. Since the vitamin K_2 form is synthesized by intestinal bacteria, deficiency of the vitamin in adults is rare. However, long term antibiotic treatment can lead to deficiency in adults. The intestine of newborn infants is sterile, therefore, vitamin K deficiency in infants is possible if lacking from the early diet. The primary symptom of a deficiency in infants is a hemorrhagic syndrome.

7

Minerals

There are two kinds of minerals: **macrominerals** and **trace minerals.** Macro means "large" in Greek (and your body needs **larger** amounts of macrominerals than trace minerals). The macromineral group is made up of calcium, phosphorus, magnesium, sodium, potassium, chloride, and sulfur. A trace of something means that there is only a little of it. So even though your body needs trace minerals, it needs just a tiny bit of each one. Scientists aren't even sure how much of these minerals you need each day. Trace minerals includes iron, manganese, copper, iodine, zinc, cobalt, fluoride, and selenium.

Dietary minerals are the chemical elements required by living organisms, other than the four elements Carbon, Hydrogen, Nitrogen, and Oxygen which are ubiquitous in organic molecules.

These can be naturally occurring in food or added in elemental or mineral form, such as calcium carbonate or sodium chloride. Some of these additives come from natural sources such as ground oyster shells. Sometimes minerals are added to the diet separately from food, as vitamin and mineral supplements and in dirt eating, called pica or geophagy.

Appropriate intake levels of each dietary mineral must be sustained to maintain physical health. Excessive intake of a dietary mineral may either lead to illness directly or indirectly because of the competitive nature between mineral levels in the body. For example, large doses of zinc are not really harmful unto themselves, but will lead to a harmful copper deficiency

Soils in different geographic areas contain varying quantities of minerals.

Food sources

- Dairy products and green leafy vegetables for Calcium
- Nuts, soy beans, and cocoa for Magnesium
- Table salt (sodium chloride, the main source), milk and spinach for Sodium
- Legumes, whole grains, and bananas for Potassium
- Table salt is its main dietary source for Chlorine
- Meat, eggs, and legumes for Sulfur
- Red meat, leafy vegetables for iron

A large body of research suggests that humans often can benefit from mineral supplementation. Vitamins and minerals are interdependent, requiring the presence of one another for full benefit; taking a multivitamin without minerals is not nearly as effective as taking one with minerals. Extensive university research also demonstrates that the most bioavailable form of supplemental mineral is the chelated mineral (one that is bonded to a specific-size amino acid).

Iron

The body needs iron to transport oxygen from your lungs to the rest of your body. Your entire body needs oxygen to stay healthy and alive. Iron helps because it's important in the formation of hemoglobin (say: **hee**-muh-glo-bun), which is the part of your **red blood cells** that carries oxygen throughout the body.

Which foods are rich in iron?

- meat, especially red meat, such as beef
- tuna and salmon
- eggs
- beans
- baked potato with skins
- dried fruits, like raisins
- leafy green vegetables, such as broccoli
- whole and enriched grains, like wheat or oats

Iron has the longest and best described history among all the micronutrients. It is a key element in the metabolism of almost all living organisms. In humans, iron is an essential component of hundreds of proteins and enzymes.

Function

1. **Oxygen transport and storage**
   Hemoglobin is the primary protein found in red blood cells and represents about two thirds of the body's iron. The vital role of hemoglobin in transporting oxygen from the lungs to the rest of the body is derived from its unique ability to acquire oxygen rapidly during the short time it spends in contact with the lungs and to release oxygen as needed during its circulation through the tissues. Myoglobin functions in the transport and short-term storage of oxygen in muscle cells, helping to match the supply of oxygen to the demand of working muscles.

2. **Electron transport and energy metabolism**
   Cytochromes are heme-containing compounds that are critical to cellular energy production. They play important roles in mitochondrial electron transport.

3. **Antioxidant and beneficial pro-oxidant functions**
   Catalase and peroxidases are heme-containing enzymes that protect cells against the accumulation of hydrogen peroxide, a potentially damaging reactive oxygen species (ROS), by catalyzing a reaction that converts hydrogen peroxide to to water and oxygen. As part of the immune response, some white blood cells engulf bacteria and expose them to ROS in order to kill them. The synthesis of one such ROS, hypochlorous acid, by neutrophils is catalyzed by the heme-containing enzyme myeloperoxidase.

4. **Oxygen sensing**
   Inadequate oxygen (hypoxia), such as that experienced by those who live at high altitudes or those with chronic lung disease, induces compensatory physiologic responses, including increased red blood cell formation, increased blood vessel

growth (angiogenesis) and increased production of enzymes utilized in anaerobic metabolism.

5. **DNA synthesis**

   Ribonucleotide reductase is an iron-dependent enzyme that is required for DNA synthesis. Thus, iron is required for a number of vital functions, including growth, reproduction, healing, and immune function.

Regulation of intracellular iron

Iron response elements are short sequences of nucleotides found in the messenger RNA (mRNA) that codes for key proteins in the regulation of iron storage and metabolism. Iron regulatory proteins (IRP) can bind to iron response elements and affect mRNA translation, thereby regulating the synthesis of specific proteins.

It has been proposed that when the iron supply is high, more iron binds to IRPs and prevents them from binding to iron response elements on mRNA. When the iron supply is low, less iron binds to IRPs, allowing increased binding of iron response elements. Thus, when less iron is available, translation of mRNA that codes for the iron storage protein, ferritin, is reduced because iron is not available for storage. Translation of mRNA that codes for the key regulatory enzyme of heme synthesis in immature red blood cells is also reduced to conserve iron. In contrast, IRP binding to iron response elements in mRNA that codes for transferrin receptors inhibits mRNA degradation, resulting in increased synthesis of transferrin receptors and increased iron transport to cells (4).

Nutrient interactions

1. Vitamin A deficiency may exacerbate iron deficiency anaemia. Vitamin A supplementation has been shown to have beneficial effects on iron deficiency anemia and improve iron status among children and pregnant women. The combination of vitamin A and iron seems to ameliorate anaemia more effectively than either iron or vitamin A alone.
2. Copper is required for iron transport to the bone marrow for red blood cell formation. Adequate copper nutritional status appears to be necessary for normal iron metabolism and red blood cell formation.

3. High doses of iron supplements taken together with Zinc supplements on an empty stomach can inhibit the absorption of zinc.
4. When taken with food, supplemental iron does not appear to inhibit zinc absorption. Iron-fortified foods have no effect on zinc absorption.
5. When consumed together in a single meal, Calcium has been found to decrease the absorption of iron.

Deficiency

Iron deficiency is the most common nutrient deficiency in the world. Three levels of iron deficiency are generally identified.

Iron deficiency anaemia: There is inadequate iron to support normal red blood cell formation, resulting in anaemia. The anaemia of iron deficiency is characterized as microcytic and hypochromic, meaning red blood cells are measurably smaller than normal and their hemoglobin content is decreased. At this stage of iron deficiency, symptoms may be a result of inadequate oxygen delivery due to anemia and/or sub-optimal function of iron-dependent enzymes. It is important to remember that iron deficiency is not the only cause of anaemia, and that the diagnosis or treatment of iron deficiency solely on the basis of anaemia may lead to misdiagnosis or inappropriate treatment of the underlying cause.

Individuals at increased risk of iron deficiency

1. A full-term infant's iron stores are usually sufficient to last for 6 months. High iron requirements are due to the rapid growth rates sustained during this period.
2. Early adolescence is another period of rapid growth. In females, the blood loss that occurs with menstruation adds to the increased iron requirement of adolescence.
3. Increased iron utilization by the developing fetus and placenta, as well as blood volume expansion significantly, increase the iron requirement during pregnancy . Chronic bleeding or acute blood loss may result in iron deficiency.
4. One milliliter (ml) of blood with a hemoglobin concentration of 150 grams/liter contains 0.5 mg of iron. Thus, chronic loss

of very small amounts of blood may result in iron deficiency. A common cause of chronic blood loss and iron deficiency in developing countries is intestinal parasitic infection.

5. Individuals who donate blood frequently, especially menstruating women, may need to increase their iron intake to prevent deficiency because each 500 ml of blood donated contains between 200 and 250 mg of iron.
6. Celiac disease (celiac sprue) is an autoimmune disorder estimated to occur in 1% of the population. When people with celiac disease consume foods or products that contain gluten, the immune system response damages the intestinal villi, which may result in nutrient malabsorption and iron deficiency anemia.
7. Daily iron losses have been found to be greater in athletes involved in intense endurance training. This may be due to increased microscopic bleeding from the gastrointestinal tract or increased fragility and hemolysis of red blood cells.

The Recommended Dietary Allowance (RDA)

The U.S. Food and Nutrition Board (FNB) estimates that the average requirement for iron may be 30% higher for those who engage in regular intense exercise. The FNB has estimated that the bioavailability of iron from a vegetarian diet is only 10%, while it is 18% from a mixed diet. Therefore, the recommended dietary allowance (RDA) for iron from a completely vegetarian diet should be adjusted as follows: 14 mg/day for adult men and postmenopausal women, 33 mg/day for premenopausal women, and 26 mg/day for adolescent girls.

Recommended Dietary Allowance (RDA) for Iron

Life Stage	*Age*	*Males (mg / day)*	*Females (mg / day)*
Infants	0-6 months	0.27 (AI)	0.27 (AI)
Infants	7-12 months	11	11
Children	1-3 years	7	7
Children	4-8 years	10	10

(Contd.)

(Contd. Table)

Life Stage	*Age*	*Males (mg/day)*	*Females (mg/day)*
Children	9-13 years	8	8
Adolescents	14-18 years	11	15
Adults	19-50 years	8	18
Adults	51 years and older	8	8
Pregnancy	all ages	-	27
Breastfeeding	18 years and younger	-	10
Breastfeeding	19 years and older	-	9

Disease Prevention

The following health problems and diseases may be prevented through the treatment or prevention of iron deficiency- Impaired intellectual development in children, Lead toxicity, Pregnancy complications poor pregnancy outcomes. Impaired immune function.

Disease Treatment

Restless legs syndrome

Restless legs syndrome (RLS) is a neurologic movement disorder that is often associated with sleep problems. People with RLS experience unpleasant sensations resulting in an irresistible urge to move their legs. These sensations are more common at rest and often interfere with sleep. RLS occurs in some people with iron deficiency and some RLS patients benefit from iron supplementation.

Food Sources

The average dietary iron intake is 16-18 mg/day in men, 12 mg/day in pre- and postmenopausal women, and about 15 mg/day in pregnant women. The iron content of some relatively iron-rich foods is listed in milligrams (mg) in the table below:-

Food	*Serving*	*Iron content (mg)*
Beef	3 ounces*, cooked	2.31
Chicken, dark meat	3 ounces, cooked	1.13

(Contd.)

(Contd. Table)

Food	*Serving*	*Iron content (mg)*
Oysters	6 medium	5.04
Shrimp	8 large, cooked	1.36
Tuna, light	3 ounces, canned	1.30
Black-strap molasses	1 tablespoon	3.50
Raisin bran cereal	1 cup, dry	5.00
Raisins, seedless	1 small box (1.5 ounces)	0.89
Prune juice	6 fluid ounces	2.27
Prunes, dried	5 prunes (1.5 ounces)	1.06
Potato, with skin	1 medium potato, baked	2.75
Kidney beans	1/2 cup, cooked	2.60
Lentils	1/2 cup, cooked	3.30
Tofu, firm	1/4 block (~1/2 cup)	6.22
Cashew nuts	1 ounce	1.70

Supplements

Iron supplements are indicated for the prevention and treatment of iron deficiency. Individuals who are not at risk of iron deficiency (e.g., adult men and postmenopausal women) should not take iron supplements without an appropriate medical evaluation for iron deficiency. A number of iron supplements are available, and different forms provide different proportions of elemental iron.

Adverse effects

At therapeutic levels for iron deficiency, iron supplements may cause gastrointestinal irritation, nausea, vomiting, diarrhoea, or constipation. Stools will often appear darker in color. Iron-containing liquids can temporarily stain teeth, but diluting the liquid helps to prevent this effect. Taking iron supplements with food instead of on an empty stomach may relieve gastrointestinal effects

Drug Interactions

Medications that decrease stomach acidity, such as antacids, histamine (H_2) receptor antagonists (e.g., cimetidine, ranitidine), and proton pump inhibitors (e.g., omeprazole, lansoprazole), may impair iron absorption. Taking iron supplements at the same time as the following medications may result in decreased absorption and efficacy of the medication: levodopa, levothyroxine, methyldopa, penicillamine, quinolones, tetracyclines, and bisphosphonates. Therefore, it is best to take these medications two hours apart from iron supplements.

Natural Sources

Bananas, black molasses, prunes, raisins, whole rye, walnuts, kelp, lentils, liver, kidney, heart, red meat, oysters, and raw clams.

Calcium

Calcium is the most common mineral in the human body. About 99% of the calcium in the body is found in bones and teeth, while the other 1% is found in the blood and soft tissue. Calcium is the top macromineral when it comes to your bones. This mineral helps build strong bones, so you can do everything from standing up straight to scoring that winning goal. It also helps build strong, healthy teeth, for chomping on tasty food. Calcium levels in the blood and fluid surrounding the cells (extracellular fluid) must be maintained within a very narrow concentration range for normal physiological functioning. The physiological functions of calcium are so vital to survival that the body will demineralize bone to maintain normal blood calcium levels when calcium intake is inadequate. Thus, adequate dietary calcium is a critical factor in maintaining a healthy skeleton.

Calcium is a major structural element in bones and teeth. The mineral component of bone consists mainly of hydroxyapatite $[Ca_{10}(PO_4)_6(OH)_2]$ crystals, which contain large amounts of calcium and phosphate. Bone is a dynamic tissue that is remodeled throughout life. Bone cells called osteoclasts begin the process of remodeling by dissolving or resorbing bone. Bone-forming cells called osteoblasts then synthesize new bone to replace the bone that was resorbed. During normal growth, bone formation exceeds bone resorption. Osteoporosis may result when bone resorption exceeds formation.

Functions of Calcium

1. Most calcium in the body is contained in the bones, but about 1% is used for nerve impulses and muscle contractions

(including heart, kidney, and other organs) that sustain life and provide movement. Calcium participates in the protein structuring of RNA and DNA .

2. Calcium plays a role in mediating the constriction and relaxation of blood vessels (vasoconstriction and vasodilation), nerve impulse transmission, muscle contraction, and the secretion of hormones, such as insulin. Excitable cells, such as skeletal muscle and nerve cells, contain voltage-dependent calcium channels in their cell membranes that allow for rapid changes in calcium concentrations.

3. **Cofactor for enzymes and proteins**

   Calcium is necessary to stabilize or allow for optimal activity of a number of proteins and enzymes. The binding of calcium ions is required for the activation of the seven "vitamin K-dependent" clotting factors in the coagulation cascade. The term, "coagulation cascade," refers to a series of events, each dependent on the other that stops bleeding through clot formation.

4. **Regulation of calcium levels**

   Calcium concentrations in the blood and fluid that surrounds cells are tightly controlled in order to preserve normal physiological functioning. When blood calcium decreases (e.g. in the case of inadequate calcium intake), calcium-sensing proteins in the parathyroid glands send signals resulting in the secretion of parathyroid hormone (PTH). PTH stimulates the conversion of vitamin D to its active form, calcitriol, in the kidneys. Calcitriol increases the absorption of calcium from the small intestine. Together with PTH, calcitriol stimulates the release of calcium from bone by activating osteoclasts (bone resorbing cells), and decreases the urinary excretion of calcium by increasing its reabsorption in the kidneys. When blood calcium rises to normal levels, the parathyroid glands stop secreting PTH and the kidneys begin to excrete any excess calcium in the urine. Although this complex system allows for rapid and tight control of blood calcium levels, it does so at the expense of the skeleton.

Deficiency of Calcium :

The deficiency symptoms of Calcium include heart palpitations, insomnia,muscle cramps , nervousness, arm/leg numbness , tooth decay. A low blood calcium level usually implies abnormal parathyroid function, and is rarely due to low dietary calcium intake since the skeleton provides a large reserve of calcium for maintaining normal blood levels. Other causes of abnormally low blood calcium levels include chronic kidney failure, vitamin D deficiency, and low blood magnesium levels that occur mainly in cases of severe alcoholism. Magnesium deficiency results in a decrease in the responsiveness of osteoclasts to PTH. A chronically low calcium intake in growing individuals may prevent the attainment of optimal peak bone mass. Once peak bone mass is achieved, inadequate calcium intake may contribute to accelerated bone loss and ultimately the development of osteoporosis.

Nutrient interactions

Vitamin D

1. Vitamin D is required for optimal calcium absorption. Several other nutrients (and non-nutrients) influence the retention of calcium by the body and may affect calcium nutritional status.
2. Deficiencies of calcium and magnesium have been linked by researchers to high blood pressure. Calcium also helps in reducing the symptoms of premenstrual syndrome, and even in protection against colon cancer.
3. If daily calcium intake is inadequate the body steals bone calcium so that you won't die. In other words, your Blood Serum Calcium and Bone Calcium levels are constantly adjusting to maintain your most vital body functions.
4. A variety of calcium supplements exist, but absorption will vary greatly depending on the type of calcium, added cofactor nutrients that enhance calcium uptake, and individual bioabsorption (mainly adequate digestive acids to dissolve the calcium by the time it reaches the small intestines).
5. Chelated calcium forms like gluconate, citrate, fulvate, and amino acid chelates are metal-free. The citrate malate form is the most bioavailable form of calcium ever researched.

Therapeutic Uses

Calcium is used in the treatment of arthritis, osteoporosis, heart palpitations, aging symptoms, backache, bone pain, finger tremors, foot/leg cramps, insomnia, menstrual cramps, menopause problems, nervousness, overweight, premenstrual tension, rheumatism.

Cell signaling

Sodium

Increased sodium intake results in increased loss of calcium in the urine, possibly due to competition between sodium and calcium for reabsorption in the kidney or by an effect of sodium on parathyroid hormone (PTH) secretion. Each 2.3-gram increment of sodium (6 grams of salt; NaCl) excreted by the kidney has been found to draw about 24-40 milligrams (mg) of calcium into the urine. Because urinary losses account for about half of the difference in calcium retention among individuals, dietary sodium has a large potential to influence bone loss. In adult women, each extra gram of sodium consumed per day is projected to produce an additional rate of bone loss of 1% per year if all of the calcium loss comes from the skeleton.

Protein

As dietary protein intake increases, the urinary excretion of calcium also increases. Weaver and colleagues have calculated that each additional gram of protein results in an additional loss of 1.75 mg of calcium/day. Because only 30% of dietary calcium is generally absorbed, each one-gram increase in protein intake/day would require an additional 5.8 mg of calcium/day to offset the calcium loss.

Phosphorus

Phosphorus, which is typically found in protein-rich foods, tends to decrease the excretion of calcium in the urine. However, phosphorus-rich foods also tend to increase the calcium content of digestive secretions, resulting in increased calcium loss in the faeces. Thus, phosphorus does not offset the net loss of calcium associated with increased protein intake. Diets high in phosphorus and low in calcium have been found to increase parathyroid hormone (PTH) secretion, as have diets low in calcium.

Caffeine

Caffeine in large amounts increases urinary calcium content for a short time. However, caffeine intakes of 400 mg/day did not significantly change urinary calcium excretion over 24 hours in premenopausal women when compared to a placebo. On average, one 8-ounce cup of coffee decreases calcium retention by only 2-3 mg.

The Adequate Intake (AI)

Updated Adequate Intake level (AI) rather than a Recommended Dietary Allowance (RDA) recommendations for calcium intake based on the optimization of bone health were released by the Food and Nutrition Board (FNB) of the Institute of Medicine, USA in 1997 is as follows :-

Adequate Intake (AI) for Calcium

Life Stage	*Age*	*Males (mg/day)*	*Females (mg/day)*
Infants	0-6 months	210	210
Infants	7-12 months	270	270
Children	1-3 years	500	500
Children	4-8 years	800	800
Children	9-13 years	1,300	1,300
Adolescents	14-18 years	1,300	1,300
Adults	19-50 years	1,000	1,000
Adults	51 years and older	1,200	1,200
Pregnancy	18 years and younger	-	1,300
Pregnancy	19 years and older	-	1,000
Breastfeeding	18 years and younger	-	1,300
Breastfeeding	19 years and older	-	1,000

Disease Prevention

1. **Colorectal Cancer**

   Increased calcium intake is found to be only weakly associated with a decreased risk of colorectal cancer. Colorectal cancer is one of the most common gastrointestinal cancer. These weak associations might be explained by the presence of groups within the population that differ in their response to calcium.

2. **Osteoporosis**

Calcium is the nutrient consistently found to be most important for attaining peak bone mass and preventing osteoporosis, adequate vitamin D intake is also required for optimal calcium absorption.

Supplemental calcium alone cannot usually restore lost bone in individuals with osteoporosis. However, optimal treatment of osteoporosis with any drug therapy also requires adequate intake of calcium (1,200 mg/day) and vitamin D (600 IU/day).

3. **Kidney stones**

Most kidney stones are composed of calcium oxalate or calcium phosphate. Abnormaily elevated urinary calcium (hypercalciuria) increases the risk of developing calcium stones.

Pregnancy-induced hypertension (preeclampsia)

Pregnancy-induced hypertension (PIH) occurs in 10% of pregnancies, and is a major health risk for pregnant women and their unborn children. Calcium metabolism appears to play a role.

A systematic review of randomized placebo-controlled studies found that calcium supplementation reduced the incidence of high blood pressure in pregnant women at high risk of PIH, as well as in pregnant women with low dietary calcium intake.

Lead toxicity

Adequate calcium intake also prevents exposure to lead mobilized from the skeleton during bone demineralization. A recent study of blood lead levels during pregnancy found that women with inadequate calcium intake during the second half of pregnancy were more likely to have elevated blood lead levels, probably related to increased bone demineralization with the release of accumulated lead into the blood.

Which foods are rich in calcium?

- dairy products, such as milk, cheese, and yogurt
- canned salmon and sardines with bones

- leafy green vegetables, such as broccoli
- calcium-fortified foods - from orange juice to cereals and crackers
- Salmon, esame seeds

Dairy products represent rich and absorbable sources of calcium, but certain vegetables and grains also provide calcium. However, the bioavailability of that calcium must be taken into consideration. While the calcium rich plants in the kale family (broccoli, bok choy, cabbage, mustard, and turnip greens) contain calcium that is as bioavailable as that in milk, some food components have been found to inhibit the absorption of calcium. Oxalic acid, also known as oxalate, is the most potent inhibitor of calcium absorption, and is found in high concentrations in spinach and rhubarb and somewhat lower concentrations in sweet potato and dried beans. Phytic acid is a less potent inhibitor of calcium absorption than oxate. Yeast possess an enzyme (phytase) which breaks down phytic acid in grains during fermentation, lowering the phytic acid content of breads and other fermented foods. Only concentrated sources of phytate such as wheat bran or dried beans substantially reduce calcium absorption.

The table below lists a number of calcium rich foods, along with their calcium content, and the number of servings of that food required to equal the absorbable calcium from one glass of milk.

Food	*Serving*	*Calcium (mg)*	*Servings needed to equal the absorbable calcium in 8 oz of milk*
Milk	8 ounces	300	1.0
Yogurt	8 ounces	300	1.0
Cheddar cheese	1.5 ounces	303	1.0
Cheese food	1.5 ounces	241	1.2
Pinto beans	1/2 cup, cooked	45	8.1
Red beans	1/2 cup, cooked	41	9.7
White beans	1/2 cup, cooked	113	3.9

(Contd.)

(Contd. Table)

Food	*Serving*	*Calcium (mg)*	*Servings needed to equal the absorbable calcium in 8 oz of milk*
Tofu, calcium set	1/2 cup	258	1.2
Bok choy	1/2 cup, cooked	79	2.3
Kale	1/2 cup, cooked	61	3.2
Chinese cabbage	1/2 cup, cooked	239	1.0
Broccoli	1/2 cup, cooked	35	4.5
Spinach	1/2 cup, cooked	115	16.3
Rhubarb	1/2 cup, cooked	174	9.5
Fruit punch with calcium citrate malate	8 ounces	300	0.62

Supplements

Most experts recommend obtaining as much calcium as possible from foods because calcium in foods is accompanied by other important nutrients that assist the body in utilizing calcium.

Calcium preparations used as supplements include calcium carbonate, calcium lactate, calcium gluconate, calcium citrate, and calcium citrate malate. Calcium carbonate is generally the most economical calcium supplement. To maximize absorption, take not more than 500 mg of elemental calcium at one time. Most calcium supplements should be taken with meals, although calcium citrate and calcium citrate malate can be taken anytime.

Toxicity

Mild hypercalcemia may be without symptoms, or may result in loss of appetite, nausea, vomiting, constipation, abdominal pain, dry mouth, thirst, and frequent urination. More severe hypercalcemia may result in confusion, delirium, coma, and if not treated, death. Hypercalcemia has been reported only with the consumption of large quantities of calcium supplements usually in combination with antacids, particularly in the days when peptic ulcers were treated with large quantities of milk, calcium carbonate (antacid) and sodium bicarbonate (absorbable alkalai).

Although the risk of forming kidney stones is increased in individuals with abnormally elevated urinary calcium (hypercalciuria), this condition is not usually related to calcium intake, but rather to increased excretion of calcium by the kidneys. Overall, increased dietary calcium has been associated with a decreased risk of kidney stones.

The Food and Nutrition Board of the Institute of Medicine,USA set the tolerable upper level (UL) of intake for calcium in adults at 2,500 milligrams (mg) of calcium/day.

Tolerable Upper Intake Level (UL) for Calcium

Age Group	*UL (mg / day)*
Infants 0-12 months	Not possible to establish*
Children 1-13 years	2500
Adolescents 14-18 years	2500
Adults 19 years and older	2500

Do high calcium intakes increase the risk of prostate cancer?

Recent epidemiological studies have raised concern that high calcium intakes are associated with increased risk of prostate cancer.

Drug Interactions

Taking calcium supplements in combination with thiazide diuretics (e.g., hydrochlorthiazide) increases the risk of developing hypercalcemia due to increased reabsorption of calcium in the kidneys. High doses of supplemental calcium could increase the likelihood of abnormal heart rhythms in people taking digitalis (digoxin) for heart failure. Calcium supplements may also decrease the efficacy of calcium channel blockers. Calcium may decrease the absorption of tetracycline and quinolone class of antibiotics, bisphosphonates, and levothyroxine, so it is advisable to separate doses of these medications and calcium rich foods or supplements by two hours.

Nutrient Interactions

The presence of calcium decreases iron absorption from nonheme sources (i.e., most supplements and food sources other than meat). However, up to 12 weeks of calcium supplementation has not been found to change iron nutritional status, probably due to a compensatory increase in iron absorption. Individuals taking iron supplements should take them two hours apart from calcium rich foods or supplements to maximize iron absorption.

Sodium

Salt (sodium chloride) is essential for life. Sodium is one of the three main electrolytes in the body. Without electrolytes, the body would completely stop working.The tight regulation of the body's sodium and chloride concentrations is so important that multiple mechanisms work in concert to control them. Although scientists agree that a minimal amount of salt is required for survival, the health implications of excess salt intake represent an area of considerable controversy among scientists, clinicians, and public health experts.

Function of Sodium

Sodium (Na^+) and chloride (Cl^-) are the principal ions in the fluid outside of cells (extracellular fluid), which includes blood plasma. As such, they play critical roles in a number of life-sustaining processes.

1. **Maintenance of membrane potential**
   Sodium and chloride are electrolytes that contribute to the maintenance of concentration and charge differences across cell membranes. Potassium is the principal positively charged ion (cation) inside of cells, while sodium is the principal cation in extracellular fluid. Potassium concentrations are about 30 times higher inside than outside cells, while sodium concentrations are more than 10 times lower inside than outside cells. The concentration differences between potassium and sodium across cell membranes create an electrochemical gradient known as the membrane potential.

2. **Nutrient absorption and transport**
Absorption of sodium in the small intestine plays an important role in the absorption of chloride, amino acids, glucose, and water. Similar mechanisms are involved in the reabsorption of these nutrients after they have been filtered from the blood by the kidneys. Chloride, in the form of hydrochloric acid (HCl), is also an important component of gastric juice, which helps in the digestion and absorption of many nutrients.
3. **Maintenance of blood volume and blood pressure**
Because sodium is the primary determinant of extracellular fluid volume, including blood volume, a number of physiological mechanisms that regulate blood volume and blood pressure work by adjusting the body's sodium content. In the circulatory system, pressure receptors (baroreceptors) sense changes in blood pressure and send excitatory or inhibitory signals to the nervous system and/or endocrine glands to affect sodium regulation by the kidneys. In general, sodium retention results in water retention and sodium loss results in water loss.

Deficiency

Sodium (and chloride) deficiency does not generally result from inadequate dietary intake, even in those on very low-salt diets. **Deficiency symptoms include** excessive sweating, chronic diarrhoea, nausea, respiratory failure, heat exhaustion, impaired carbohydrate digestion.

Hyponatremia

Hyponatremia is defined as a serum sodium concentration of less than 136 mmol/liter, and may result from increased fluid retention (dilutional hyponatremia) or increased sodium loss. Dilutional hyponatremia may be due to inappropriate anti-diuretic hormone (ADH) secretion, which is associated with disorders affecting the central nervous system and a number of drugs and in some cases, excessive water intake may also lead to dilutional hyponatremia. Conditions that increase the loss of sodium and chloride include severe or prolonged vomiting or diarrhea, excessive and persistent sweating, the use of some diuretics, and some forms of kidney disease. Symptoms of hyponatremia include headache, nausea, vomiting, muscle cramps, fatigue, disorientation, and fainting. Complications of severe and rapidly developing hyponatremia may include cerebral oedema (swelling of the brain), seizures, coma, and brain damage. Acute or severe hyponatremia may be fatal without prompt and appropriate medical treatment.

Prolonged endurance exercise and hyponatremia

Hyponatremia has recently been recognized as a potential problem in individuals competing in very long endurance exercise events, such as marathons, ultramarathons.

Adequate intake (AI) for sodium and sodium chloride (salt)

In 2004, the Food and Nutrition Board of the Institute of Medicine, USA established an adequate intake level (AI) for sodium and sodium chloride (salt) based on the amount needed to replace losses through sweat in moderately active people.

Adequate Intake (AI) for Sodium and Sodium Chloride (Salt)

Life Stage	*Age*	*Males and Females Sodium (g/day)*	*Males and FemalesSalt (g/ day)*
Infants	0-6 months	0.12	0.30
Infants	7-12 months	0.37	0.93
Children	1-3 years	1.0	2.5
Children	4-8 years	1.2	3.0
Children	9-13 years	1.5	3.8
Adolescents	14-18 years	1.5	3.8
Adults	19-50 years	1.5	3.8
Adults	51-70 years	1.3	3.3
Adults	71 years and older	1.2	3.0
Pregnancy	14-50 years	1.5	3.8
Breastfeeding	14-50 years	1.5	3.8

Disease Prevention (Dietary Salt Reduction)

Gastric cancer

Epidemiological studies, conducted mainly in Asian countries, indicate that high intakes of salted, smoked, and pickled foods increase the risk of gastric cancer. Although these foods are high in salt, they may also contain carcinogens, such as nitrosamines. Additionally, populations with high intakes of salted foods tend to have low intakes of fruits and vegetables, which are also associated with increased risk of gastric cancer. The risk of developing stomach cancer is increased by chronic inflammation of the stomach and infection by the bacteria, *helicobacter pylori*. High concentrations of salt may damage the cells lining the stomach, potentially increasing the risk of *H. pylori* infection and cancer-promoting genetic damage to cells by carcinogens in the stomach.

Osteoporosis

Increased salt intake has been found to increase urinary excretion of calcium. Each 2.3 gram increment of sodium (5.8 grams of salt) excreted by the kidney has been found draws about 24-40 milligrams (mg) of calcium into the urine.

Kidney stones

A large prospective study that followed more than 90,000 women over a 12-year period found that women with a sodium intake averaging 4.9 grams/day (12.6 grams/day of salt) had a 30% higher risk of developing symptomatic kidney stones than women whose sodium intake averaged 1.5 grams/day (4.0 grams/day of salt).

Disease Treatment (Dietary Salt Reduction)

Therapeutic Uses in sun stroke , heat prostration, muscular weakness, mental apathy.

Hypertension (high blood pressure)

Many research studies have suggested that increased salt consumption is associated with increased blood pressure.

Salt and target organ damage

Salt intake has been significantly correlated with left ventricular hypertrophy, an abnormal thickening of the heart muscle, which is implicated in increased mortality from cardiovascular diseases. Recent research indicates that high salt intake may contribute to organ damage in ways that are independent of its effects on blood pressure.

The Food and Nutrition Board of the Institute of Medicine,USA recently recommended that adults consume not more than 5.8 grams/day of salt.

The tables below list the sodium content of some foods that are high in salt and some that are relatively low in salt in milligrams (mg).

High-Salt Foods

Food	*Serving*	*Sodium (g)*	*Salt (g)*
Hot dog (beef)	1	0.46	1.2
Dill pickle	1 medium	0.83	2.1
Tomato juice canned (salt added)	1 cup (8 fl. ounces)	0.88	2.2
Fish sandwich w/ tartar sauce & cheese	1 sandwich	0.94	2.4
Corn dog	1	0.97	2.4
Corned beef hash	1 cup	1.0	2.5
Ham	3 ounces	1.0	2.5
Pretzels, salted	2 ounces (10 pretzels)	1.0	2.5
Canned, chicken noodle soup	1 cup	1.1	2.8
Macaroni and cheese, canned	1 cup	1.3	3.3
Potato chips, salted	8 ounces (1 bag)	1.3	3.3

Low-Salt Foods

Food	*Serving*	*Sodium (g)*	*Salt (g)*
Olive oil	1 tablespoon	0.000	0.000
Pear, raw	1 medium	0.000	0.000

(Contd.)

(Contd. Table)

Low-Salt Foods *Food*	*Serving*	*Sodium (g)*	*Salt (g)*
Popcorn, air	1 cup	0.000	0.000
Almonds (unsalted)	1 cup	0.001	0.003
Brown rice -popped (unsalted)	1 cup, cooked	0.002	0.005
Orange juice (frozen)	1 cup (8 fl ounces)	0.003	0.008
Mango	1 fruit	0.004	0.010
Tomato	1 medium	0.011	0.028
Fruit cocktail, canned	1 cup	0.015	0.038
Potato chips, unsalted	8 ounces (1 bag)	0.018	0.045
Carrot	1 medium	0.021	0.053
Tomato juice, canned (no salt added)	1 cup (8 fl ounces)	0.024	0.060

Toxicity

Excessive intakes of sodium chloride lead to an increase in extracellular fluid volume as water is pulled from cells to maintain normal sodium concentrations. However, as long as water needs can be met, normally functioning kidneys can excrete the excess sodium and restore the system to normal. Ingestion of large amounts of salt may lead to nausea, vomiting, diarrhoea, and abdominal cramps. Abnormally high plasma sodium concentrations (hypernatremia) generally develop from excess water loss, frequently accompanied by an impaired thirst mechanism or lack of access to water. Symptoms of hypernatremia in the presence of excess fluid loss may include dizziness or fainting, low blood pressure, and diminished urine production. Severe hypernatremia may result in oedema (swelling), hypertension, rapid heart rate, difficulty breathing, convulsions, coma, and death. Hypernatremia is rarely caused by excessive sodium intake (e.g. the ingestion of large amounts of seawater or intravenous infusion of concentrated saline solution). In end-stage renal failure (kidney failure), impaired urinary sodium excretion may lead to fluid retention, resulting in oedema, high blood pressure, or congestive heart failure if salt and water intake are not restricted.

Adverse effects

In 2004, the Food and Nutriton Board of the Institute of Medicine established an upper level of sodium intake (UL).

Tolerable Upper Intake Level (UL) for Sodium and Sodium Chloride (Salt)

Age Group (g/day)	*UL for Sodium (g/day)*	*UL for Salt*
Infants 0-12 months	Not Determined*	Not Determined*
Children 1-3 years	1.5	3.8
Children 4-8 years	1.9	4.8
Children 9-13 years	2.2	5.5
Adolescents 14-18 years	2.3	5.8
Adults 19 years and older	2.3	5.8

Drug Interactions

The following drugs may increase the risk of hyponatremia (abnormally low blood sodium concentration):

Families of Medications Associated with Hyponatremia

Medication Family	*Examples*
Diuretics	Hydrochlorthiazide, Furosemide (Lasix)
Non-steroidal anti-inflammatory drugs (NSAIDs)	Ibuprofen (Advil, Motrin), Naproxen sodium (Alleve)
Opiate derivatives	Codeine, Morphine
Phenothiazines	Prochlorperazine (Compazine), Promethazine (Phenergan)

(Contd.)

(Contd. Table)

Medication Family	*Examples*
Serotonin-reuptake inhibitors (SSRIs)	Fluoxetine (Prozac), Paroxetine (Paxil)
Tricyclic antidepressants (Tofranil)	Amitriptyline (Elavil), Imipramine
Individual Medications Associated with Hyponatremia	
Carbamazepine (Tegretol)	
Chlorpropamide (Diabinese)	
Clofibrate (Atromid-S)	
Cyclophosphamide (Cytoxan)	
Desmopressin (DDAVP; nasal or oral)	
Oxytocin (Pitocin)	
Vincristine (Oncovin)	

Potassium

Potassium keeps your muscles and nervous system working properly. Did you know your blood and body tissues, such as muscles, contain water? They do, and potassium helps make sure the amount of water is just right. Potassium is an essential dietary mineral that is also known as an electrolyte. The term electrolyte refers to a substance that dissociates into ions (charged particles) in solution making it capable of conducting electricity. The normal functioning of our bodies depends on the tight regulation of potassium concentrations both inside and outside of cells.

Potassium is an electrolyte that interacts with sodium to conduct nerve impulses and many other functions in the cells. In the past, high potassium foods used to dominate, but unfortunately through evolution, our food has become saturated with sodium. The processing of food fills it with sodium and reverses the high potassium/low sodium ratio. This reversal in the potassium/sodium ratio has increased the incidence of high blood pressure; but studies show that increasing dietary potassium intake will lower blood pressure. Many research studies have shown that systolic blood pressure was lowered by a significant amount in the patients who received the potassium supplements.

A limited number of enzymes require the presence of potassium for their activity. The activation of sodium, potassium-ATPase requires the presence of sodium and potassium. The presence of potassium is also required for the activity of pyruvate kinase, an important enzyme in carbohydrate metabolism.

Deficiency

Deficiency Symptoms include acne, continuous thirst, dry skin, constipation, general weakness, insomnia , muscle damage, nervousness, slow irregular heartbeat, weak reflexes.

An abnormally low plasma potassium concentration is referred to as hypokalemia. Hypokalemia is most commonly a result of excessive loss of potassium, e.g., from prolonged vomiting, the use of some diuretics, some forms of kidney disease, or disturbances of metabolism. The symptoms of hypokalemia are related to alterations in membrane potential and cellular metabolism. They include fatigue, muscle weakness and cramps, and intestinal paralysis, which may lead to bloating, constipation, and abdominal pain. Severe hypokalemia may result in muscular paralysis or abnormal heart rhythms (cardiac arrhythmias) that can be fatal.

Conditions that increase the risk of hypokalemia.

- The use of potassium-wasting diuretics (e.g., thiazide diuretics or furosemide)
- Alcoholism
- Severe vomiting or diarrhoea
- Overuse or abuse of laxatives
- Anorexia nervosa or bulimia
- Magnesium depletion
- Congestive heart failure (CHF)

Adequate Intake (AI)

In 2004, the Food and Nutrition Board of the Institute of Medicine established an adequate intake level (AI) for potassium based on intake levels that have been found to lower blood pressure, reduce salt sensitivity, and minimize the risk of kidney stones.

Adequate Intake (AI) for Potassium

Life Stage	*Age*	*Males (mg / day)*	*Females (mg / day)*
Infants	0-6 months	400	400
Infants	7-12 months	700	700
Children	1-3 years	3000	3000
Children	4-8 years	3800	3800
Children	9-13 years	4500	4500
Adolescents	14-18 years	4700	4700
Adults	19 years and older	4700	4700
Pregnancy	14-50 years	-	4700
Breastfeeding	14-50 years	-	5100

Disease Prevention

The relative deficiency of dietary potassium in the modern diet may play a role in the pathology of some chronic diseases.

Stroke

Several large epidemiological studies have suggested that increased potassium intake is associated with decreased risk of stroke.

Osteoporosis

Four cross-sectional studies have reported significant positive associations between dietary potassium intake and bone mineral density (BMD) in populations of premenopausal, perimenopausal, and postmenopausal women and elderly men. Increased consumption of fruits and vegetables reduces the net acid content of the diet and may preserve calcium in bones, which might otherwise be mobilized to maintain normal pH.

Kidney stones

Increasing dietary potassium (and alkalai) intake by increasing fruit and vegetable intake or by taking potassium bicarbonate supplements has been found to decrease urinary calcium excretion. Additionally, potassium deprivation has been found to increase urinary calcium excretion (17, 18).

Disease Treatment

Therapeutic Uses of potassium include acne, alcoholism, allergies, burns, colic in infants, diabetes, high blood pressure, heart disease, angina, heart attack, high blood pressure (hypertension).

Food sources of Potassium

The richest sources of potassium are fruits and vegetables. People who eat large amounts of fruits and vegetables have a high potassium intake (8-11 grams/day). A recent dietary survey in the U.S. indicated that the average dietary potassium intake is about 2,300 mg/day for adult women and 3,100 mg/day for adult men. The potassium content of some relatively potassium-rich foods is listed in milligrams (mg) in the table below.

Food	*Serving*	*Potassium (mg)*
Banana	1 medium	467
Potato, baked with skin	1 medium	721
Prune juice	6 fluid ounces	530
Prunes, dried	1/2 cup	633
Orange juice	6 fluid ounces	354
Orange	1 medium	237
Tomato juice	6 fluid ounces	400
Tomato	1 medium	273
Raisins	1/2 cup	598
Raisin bran cereal	1 ounce	437
Artichoke, cooked	1 medium	425
Lima beans, cooked	1/2 cup	478
Acorn squash, cooked	1/2 cup (cubes)	448
Spinach, cooked	1/2 cup	419
Sunflower seeds	1 ounce	241
Almonds	1 ounce	211
Molasses	1 tablespoon	293

Supplements

Potassium supplements are available as a number of different salts, including potassium chloride, citrate, gluconate, bicarbonate, aspartate and orotate (26). Because of the potential for serious side effects the decision to use a potent potassium supplement should be made in consultation with one's health care provider. Individuals with kidney diseases or complications should not take supplemental potassium. Also, potassium taken on an empty stomach can cause nausea.

Toxicity

Abnormally elevated serum potassium concentrations are referred to as hyperkalemia. Hyperkalemia occurrs when potassium intake exceeds the capacity of the kidneys to eliminate it. Acute or chronic renal (kidney) failure, the use of potassium-sparing diuretics, and insufficient aldosterone secretion (hypoaldosteronism) may result in the accumulation of excess potassium due to decreased urinary potassium excretion. Oral doses greater than 18 grams taken at one time may lead to severe hyperkalemia, even in those with normal kidney function. The most serious complication of hyperkalemia is the development of an abnormal heart rhythm (cardiac arrhythmia), which can lead to cardiac arrest.

Adverse reactions to potassium supplements

Gastrointestinal symptoms are the most common side effects of potassium supplements, including nausea, vomiting, abdominal discomfort, and diarrhoea. Intestinal ulceration has been reported after the use of enteric-coated potassium chloride tablets. Taking potassium with meals or taking a microencapsulated form of potassium may reduce gastrointestinal side effects. The most serious adverse reaction to potassium supplementation is hyperkalemia.

Drug interactions

The following classes of medication are known to increase the risk of hyperkalemia:-

Medications Associated with Hyperkalemia

Medication Family	*Specific medications*
Potassium-sparing agents	Spironolactone, triamterene, amiloride

(Contd.)

(Contd. Table)

Medication Family	*Specific medications*
Angiotensin converting enzyme (ACE) inhibitors	Captopril, enalapril, fosinopril
Nonsteroidal anti-inflammatory agents (NSAID)	Indomethacin, ibuprofen, ketorolac
Anti-infective agents	Trimethoprim-sulfamethoxazole, pentamidine
Anticoagulant	Heparin
Cardiac glycoside	Digitalis
Anti-hypertensive agents	Beta-blockers, alpha- and beta-blockers
Angiotensin receptor blockers	Losartan, valsartan, irbesartan, candesartan

The following medications are known to increase the risk of hypokalemia (low serum potassium).

Medications Associated with Hypokalemia

Medication family	*Specific medications*
Beta-adrenergic agonists	Epinephrine
Decongestants	Psuedoephedrine, phyenylpro panolamine
Bronchodilators	Albuterol, terbutaline, pirbuterol, isoetharine, fenoterol, ephedrine, isoporterenol, metaproternenol, theophylline
Tocolytic (labor suppressing) agents	Ritodrine, nylidrin
Diuretics	Acetazolamide, thiazides, chlorthalidone, indapamide, metolazone, quinethazone, bumetanide, ethycrinic acid, furosemide, torsemide
Mineralocorticoids	Fludrocortisone

(Contd.)

(Contd. Table)

Medication family	*Specific medications*
Substances with mineralocorticoid effects	Licorice, carbenoxolone, gossypol
High-dose glucocorticoids	
High-dose antibiotics	Penicillin, nafcillin, carbenicillin
Other	Caffeine, phenopthalein, sodium polystyrene sulfonate

Which foods are rich in potassium?

- bananas
- broccoli
- tomatoes
- potatoes with skins
- leafy green vegetables, such as broccoli
- citrus fruits, like oranges
- dried fruits
- legumes, such as beans, peas, lentils, and peanuts

Natural Sources of potassium

Green leafy vegetables, bananas, tomatoes, water cress, and whole grains.

Iodine

Iodine required by humans for the synthesis of thyroid hormones. You need dietary iodine to make your thyroid hormones. Because they control all energy in the body, you better get it right. Inadequate iodine causes the thyroid in the neck to grow massive (goiter). Goiters affect over 200 million people throughout the world, and 96% of it is caused by iodine deficiency.

Iodine deficiency is an important health problem throughout the world. Most of the Earth's iodine is found in its oceans. Mountainous regions, such as the Himalayas, the Andes, and the Alps, and flooded river valleys, such as the Ganges, are among the most severely iodine deficient areas in the world.

Function

Iodine is an essential component of the thyroid hormones, triiodothyronine (T_3) and thyroxine (T_4) and is therefore, essential for normal thyroid function. To meet the body's demand for thyroid hormones, the thyroid gland traps iodine from the blood and converts it into thyroid hormones that are stored and released into the circulation when needed. In target tissues, such as the liver and the brain, T_3, the physiologically active thyroid hormone, can bind to thyroid receptors in the nuclei of cells and regulate gene expression. T_4, the most abundant circulating thyroid hormone, can be converted to T_3 by enzymes known as deiodinases in target tissues. In this manner, thyroid hormones regulate a number of physiologic processes, including growth, development, metabolism, and reproductive function .

The regulation of thyroid function is a complex process that involves the brain (hypothalamus) and pituitary gland. In response to thyrotropin-releasing hormone (TRH) secretion by the hypothalamus, the pituitary gland secretes thyroid-stimulating hormone (TSH), which stimulates iodine trapping, thyroid hormone synthesis, and release of T_3 and T_4 by the thyroid gland. The presence of adequate circulating T_4 decreases the sensitivity of the pituitary gland to TRH, limiting its secretion of TSH. When circulating T_4 levels decrease, the pituitary increases its secretion of TSH, resulting in increased iodine trapping, as well as increased production and release of T_3 and T_4. Iodine deficiency results in inadequate production of T_4. In response to decreased blood levels of T_4, the pituitary gland increases its output of TSH. Persistently elevated TSH levels may lead to hypertrophy (enlargement) of the thyroid gland, also known as goiter.

Iodine has also its role in energy production, metabolism (excess fat), physical and mental development.

Deficiency

Iodine deficiency is now accepted as the most common cause of preventable brain damage in the world. According to the World Health Organization (WHO), iodine deficiency disorders (IDD) affect 740 million people throughout the world, and nearly 50 million people suffer from some degree of IDD-related brain damage. The spectrum of IDD includes mental retardation, hypothyroidism, goiter, and varying degrees of other growth and developmental abnormalities. Nearly 2.2 million people throughout the world live in areas of iodine deficiency and risk its consequences. Major international efforts have produced dramatic improvements in the correction of iodine deficiency in the 1990's mainly through the use of iodized salt and iodized vegetable oil in iodine deficient countries.

Thyroid enlargement, or goiter, is one of the earliest and most visible signs of iodine deficiency. The thyroid enlarges in response to persistent stimulation by TSH. In mild iodine deficiency, this adaptation response may be enough to provide the body with sufficient thyroid hormone. However, more severe cases of iodine deficiency result in hypothyroidism. Adequate iodine intake will generally reduce the size of goiters, but the reversibility of the effects of hypothyroidism depends on an individual's stage of development. Iodine deficiency has adverse effects in all stages of development, but is most damaging to the developing brain. In addition to regulating many aspects of growth and development, thyroid hormone is important for the myelination of the central nervous system, which is most active before and shortly after birth.

Nutrient Interactions

Selenium deficiency can exacerbate the effects of iodine deficiency. Iodine is essential for the synthesis of thyroid hormone, but selenium-dependent enzymes (iodothyronine deiodinases) are also required for the conversion of thyroxine (T_4) to the biologically active thyroid hormone, triiodothyronine (T_3). Deficiencies of vitamin A or iron may also exacerbate the effects of iodine deficiency.

Goitrogens

Some foods contain substances that interfere with iodine utilization or thyroid hormone production, known as goitrogens. The occurrence of goiter in the Democratic Republic of Congo has been related to the consumption of casava, which contains a compound that is metabolized to thiocyanate and blocks thyroidal uptake of iodine. Some species of millet and cruciferous vegetables (for example, cabbage, broccoli, cauliflower, and Brussel sprouts) also contain goitrogens. The soybean isoflavones, genistein and daidzein, have also been found to inhibit thyroid hormone synthesis. Most of these goitrogens are not of clinical importance unless they are consumed in large amounts or there is coexisting iodine deficiency. Recent findings also indicate that tobacco smoking may be associated with an increased risk of goiter in iodine deficient areas.

Iodine deficiency symptoms include dry hair, goiter, intellectual disability, growth retardation, irritability, nervousness, obesity.

The Recommended Dietary Allowance (RDA)

The RDA for iodine was reevaluated by the Food and Nutrition Board (FNB) of the Institute of Medicine,USA in 2001.

Recommended Dietary Allowance (RDA) for Iodine

Life Stage	*Age*	*Males (mcg / day)*	*Females (mcg / day)*
Infants	0-6 months	110 (AI)	110 (AI)
Infants	7-12 months	130 (AI)	130 (AI)
Children	1-3 years	90	90
Children	4-8 years	90	90
Children	9-13 years	120	120
Adolescents	14-18 years	150	150
Adults	19 years and older	150	150
Pregnancy	all ages	-	220
Breastfeeding	all ages	-	290

Disease Prevention

Radiation-induced thyroid cancer

Radioactive iodine, especially I^{131} may be released into the environment as a result of nuclear reactor accidents. Thyroid accumulation of radioactive iodine increases the risk of developing thyroid cancer, especially in children. The increased iodine trapping activity of the thyroid gland in iodine deficiency results in increased thyroid accumulation of radioactive iodine. Thus, iodine deficient individuals are at increased risk of developing radiation-induced thyroid cancer because they will accumulate greater amounts of radioactive iodine. Potassium iodide administered in pharmacologic doses (50-100 mg for adults) within 48 hours before or 8 hours after radiation exposure from a nuclear reactor accident can significantly reduce thyroid uptake of I^{131} and decrease the risk of radiation-induced thyroid cancer. The prompt and widespread use of potassium iodide prophylaxis in Poland after the 1986 Chernobyl nuclear reactor accident may explain the lack of a significant increase in childhood thyroid cancer in Poland compared to fallout areas where potassium iodide prophylaxis was not widely used.

Disease Treatment

Therapeutic Uses of iodine include arteriosclerosis , hair problems, goiter, hypothyroidism, Fibrocystic breast condition.

Fibrocystic breast condition is a benign (non-cancerous) condition of the breasts, characterized by lumpiness and discomfort in one or both breasts.

Food sources

The food source of iodine include Kelp, seafood, fish liver oils, egg yolks, citrus fruits, and garlic.

The iodine content of most foods depends on the iodine content of the soil in which it was raised. Seafood is rich in iodine because marine animals can concentrate the iodine from seawater.

The table below lists the iodine content of some iodine-rich foods in micrograms (mcg).

Food	*Serving*	*Iodine (mcg)*
Salt (iodized)	1 gram	77
Cod	3 ounces*	99
Shrimp	3 ounces	35
Fish sticks	2 fish sticks	35
Tuna, canned in oil	3 ounces (1/2 can)	17
Milk (cow's)	1 cup (8 fluid ounces)	56
Egg, boiled	1 large	29

(Contd.)

(Contd. Table)

Food	*Serving*	*Iodine (mcg)*
Navy beans, cooked	1/2 cup	35
Potato with peel, baked	1 medium	63
Turkey breast, baked	3 ounces	34
Seaweed	1 ounce, dried	Variable; may be greater than 18,000 mcg (18 mg)

Supplements

Potassium iodide is available as a nutritional supplement, typically in combination products, such as multivitamin/ multimineral supplements. Iodine makes up approximately 77% of the total weight of potassium iodide. A multivitamin/multimineral supplement that contains 100% of the daily value (DV) for iodine provides 150 mcg of iodine.

Acute toxicity with Iodine :

Acute iodine poisoning is rare and usually occurs only with doses of many grams. Symptoms of acute iodine poisoning include burning of the mouth, throat, and stomach, fever, nausea, vomiting, diarrhoea, a weak pulse, and coma.

In iodine deficiency: Iodine supplementation programmes in iodine-deficient populations have been associated with an increased incidence of iodine-induced hyperthyroidism (IHH), mainly in older people and those with multinodular goiter. Iodine intakes of 150-200 mcg/day have been found to increase the incidence of IHH in iodine-deficient populations. Iodine deficiency increases the risk of developing autonomous thyroid nodules that are unresponsive to the normal thyroid regulation system, resulting in hyperthyroidism after iodine supplementation. IHH is considered by some experts to be an iodine deficiency disorder. In general, the large benefit of iodization programes outweighs the small risk of IHH in iodine-deficient populations.

The Food and Nutrition Board (FNB) of the Institute of Medicine,USA set a tolerable upper level of intake (UL) for iodine at 1,100 mcg/day for adults.

Tolerable Upper Intake Level (UL) for Iodine

Age Group	*UL (mg / day)*
Infants 0-12 months	Not possible to establish*
Children 1-3 years	200 mcg/day
Children 4-8 years	300 mcg/day
Children 9-13 years	600 mcg/day
Adolescents 14-18 years	900 mcg/day
Adults 19 years and older	1,100 mcg/day (1.1 mg/day)

Drug interactions

Amiodarone, a medication used to prevent abnormal heart rhythms, contains high levels of iodine and may affect thyroid function. Medications used to treat hyperthyroidism, such as propylthiuracil (PTU) and methimazole may increase the risk of hypothyroidism. The use of lithium in combination with pharmacologic doses of potassium iodide may result in hypothyroidism. The use of pharmacologic doses of potassium iodide may decrease the anticoagulant effect of warfarin (coumarin).

Zinc

Zinc is an essential trace element for all forms of life. The significance of zinc in human nutrition and public health was recognized relatively recently. Clinical zinc deficiency in humans was first described in 1961, when the consumption of diets with low zinc bioavailability due to high phytic acid content was associated with "adolescent nutritional dwarfism" in the Middle East. Since then, zinc deficiency has been described by a number of experts as an important public health issue, especially in developing countries.

Zinc is a part of every cell in the body and forms part of over 200 enzymes that have functions ranging from proper action of body hormones to cell growth. Because the body readily uses zinc for many different functions, it constantly needs to be replaced. Sufficient levels of zinc are very important for the body's immunity and strength. Zinc helps your immune system, which is your body's system for fighting off illnesses and infections. It also helps with cell growth and helps heal wounds, such as cuts.

Zinc plays a vital role during pregnancy, and because of that, the dosage taken during pregnancy should be increased. It has been proven that low zinc levels are associated with premature births, low birth weight, growth retardation, and preeclampsia—a serious condition of pregnancy associated with elevations in blood pressure, fluid retention, and loss of protein in the urine. Zinc also works wonders on the immune system, especially for fighting the common cold. Zinc works like vitamin C and uses its antiviral activity against several viruses that cause the common cold. A double-blind clinical trial demonstrated zinc-containing lozenges significantly reduced the average duration of common colds by 7 days.

Male sexual function can also be linked back to zinc. Male hormone metabolism, sperm formation, and sperm motility are all associated with levels of zinc. Several studies have proven the success of zinc supplementation in cases of infertility and sterility.

Zinc can also help fight every teenagers worst nightmare—acne. In several studies, zinc has demonstrated similar results to tetracycline in superficial acne and superior results in deeper acne. For those who want blemish-free skin, try taking extra zinc.

Zinc is needed for blood, brain, heart, prostrate gland.,burn and wound healing, carbohydrate digestion, prostrate gland function, reproductive organ growth and maturity, vitamin B1, and phosphorus and protein metabolism. Zinc is also needed for bone growth. Zinc is often found deficient in those with arthritis.

In HIV disease, the most poignant observation may be that zinc supplementation has been observed to improve "accretion of lean tissue rather than fat after dietary zinc supplementation in children recovering from malnutrition" (Cavan *et al*, 1993).

Function

Numerous aspects of cellular metabolism are zinc-dependent. Zinc plays important roles in growth and development, the immune response, neurological function, and reproduction. On the cellular level, the function of zinc can be divided into three categories: 1. catalytic, 2. structural, and 3. regulatory.

1. **Catalytic role**

   From 70 to over 100 enzymes in the human body are reported to require zinc; "zinc is a part of more enzyme systems than the rest of the trace elements combined". These enzymes/ proteins include many from both the immune and digestive systems. Thus low levels of zinc interfere with digestion of our food, as well as our immune function. Immune dysfunction from zinc deficiency has been called "profound", and "severe deficiency is produced easily and rapidly" (Beisel, 1982).

   Nearly 100 different enzymes depend on zinc for their ability to catalyze vital chemical reactions. Zinc-dependent enzymes can be found in all known classes of enzymes.

2. **Structural role**

   Zinc plays an important role in the structure of proteins and cell membranes. A finger-like structure, known as a zinc finger motif, stabilizes the structure of a number of proteins. For example, copper provides the catalytic activity for the antioxidant enzyme copper-zinc superoxide dismutase (CuZnSOD), while zinc plays a critical structural role. The structure and function of cell membranes are also affected by zinc. Loss of zinc from biological membranes increases their susceptibility to oxidative damage and impairs their function.

3. **Regulatory role**

   Zinc finger proteins have been found to regulate gene expression by acting as transcription factors (binding to DNA and influencing the transcription of specific genes). Zinc also plays a role in cell signaling and has been found to influence hormone release and nerve impulse transmission. Recently zinc has been found to play a role in apoptosis (gene-directed cell death), a critical cellular regulatory process with implications for growth and development, as well as a number of chronic diseases.

Nutrient Interactions

Copper

Taking large quantities of zinc (50 mg/day or more) over a period of weeks can interfere with copper bioavailability. High intake of zinc induces the intestinal synthesis of a copper-binding protein called metallothionein. Metallothionein traps copper within intestinal cells and prevents its systemic absorption. More typical intakes of zinc do not affect copper absorption and high copper intakes do not affect zinc absorption.

Iron

Supplemental (38-65 mg/day of elemental iron) but not dietary levels of iron may decrease zinc absorption. This interaction is of concern in the management of iron supplementation during pregnancy and lactation and has led some experts to recommend zinc supplementation for pregnant and lactating women taking more than 60 mg/day of elemental iron.

Calcium

Increasing the calcium intake of postmenopausal women by 890 mg/day in the form of milk or calcium phosphate (total calcium intake 1,360 mg/day) reduced zinc absorption and zinc balance in postmenopausal women, but increasing the calcium intake of adolescent girls by 1,000 mg/day in the form of calcium citrate malate (total calcium intake 1,667 mg/day) did not affect zinc absorption or balance. Calcium in combination with phytic acid reduces zinc absorption. This effect is particularly relevant to individuals consuming a diet that is highly dependent on tortillas made with lime (calcium oxide).

Folic acid

The bioavailability of dietary folate is increased by the action of a zinc-dependent enzyme, suggesting a possible interaction between zinc and folic acid.

Deficiency

Zinc deficiency symptoms include delayed sexual maturity, fatigue, loss of taste, poor appetite, prolonged wound healing, retarded growth, sterility.

Severe zinc deficiency

The symptoms of severe zinc deficiency include the slowing or cessation of growth and development, delayed sexual maturation, characteristic skin rashes, chronic and severe diarrhea, immune system deficiencies, impaired wound healing, diminished appetite, impaired taste sensation, night blindness, swelling and clouding of the corneas, and behavioral disturbances.

Mild zinc deficiency

More recently, it has become apparent that milder zinc deficiency contributes to a number of health problems, especially common in children who live in developing countries. Mild zinc deficiency contributes to impaired physical and neuropsychological development, and increased susceptibility to life-threatening infections in young children

Individuals at risk of zinc deficiency:

- Infants and children
- Pregnant and lactating (breastfeeding) women, especially teenagers
- Patients receiving total parenteral nutrition (intravenous feedings)
- Malnourished individuals, including those with protein-energy
- malnutrition and anorexia nervosa
- Individuals with severe or persistent diarrhea
- Individuals with malabsorption syndromes, including celiac disease and short bowel syndrome
- Individuals with inflammatory bowel disease, including Crohn's disease and ulcerative colitis
- Individuals with alcoholic liver disease have increased urinary zinc excretion and low liver zinc levels
- Individuals with sickle cell anemia
- Older adults (65 years and older)
- Strict vegetarians: The requirement for dietary zinc may be as much as fifty percent greater for strict vegetarians whose major food staples are grains and legumes because high levels of phytic acid in these foods reduce the absorption of zinc.

The Recommended Dietary Allowance (RDA)

The U.S. recommended dietary allowances (RDA) for zinc are listed for all age groups because infants, children, and pregnant and lactating women are at increased risk of zinc deficiency.

The Recommended Dietary Allowance (RDA) for Zinc

Life Stage	*Age*	*Males (mg/day)*	*Females (mg/day)*
Infants	0-6 months	2 (AI)	2 (AI)
Infants	7-12 months	3	3
Children	1-3 years	3	3
Children	4-8 years	5	5
Children	9-13 years	8	8
Adolescents	14-18 years	11	9
Adults	19 years and older	11	8
Pregnancy	18 years and younger	-	12
Pregnancy	19 years and older	-	11
Breastfeeding	18 years and younger	-	13
Breastfeeding	19 years and older	-	12

Prevention of diseases related to zinc deficiency

Growth retardation

Significant delays in linear growth and weight gain, known as growth retardation or failure to thrive, are common features of mild zinc deficiency in children.

Delayed neurological and behavioral development in young children

Low maternal zinc nutritional status has been associated with diminished attention in the newborn infant and poorer motor function at 6 months of age. Zinc supplementation has been associated with improved motor development in very low-birth-weight infants, more vigorous activity in Indian infants and toddlers. Additionally, zinc supplementation was associated with better neuropsychologic functioning (e.g., attention).

Impaired immune system function

Adequate zinc intake is essential in maintaining the integrity of the immune system and zinc deficient individuals are known to experience increased susceptibility to a variety of infectious agents.

Increased susceptibility to infectious disease in children

The adverse effects of zinc deficiency on immune system function are likely to increase the susceptibility of children to infectious diseases like diarrhoea, pneumonia, malaria.

Immune response in the elderly

Age-related declines in immune function are similar to those associated with zinc deficiency, and the elderly represent a group that is vulnerable to mild zinc deficiency.

Pregnancy complications

It has been estimated that 82% of pregnant women worldwide are likely to have inadequate zinc intakes. Poor maternal zinc nutritional status has been associated with a number of adverse outcomes of pregnancy, including low birth weight, premature delivery, and labour and delivery complications.

Disease Treatment

Therapeutic Uses of Zinc include alcoholism, alzheimers, arteriosclerosis, baldness, cirrhosis, arthritis, osteoporosis, diabetes mellitus, internal/external wound/injury healing, high cholesterol, infertility, fatigue, common cold.

HIV/AIDS

Sufficient zinc is essential in maintaining immune system function and HIV infected individuals are particularly susceptible to zinc deficiency. Decreased serum zinc levels have been associated with more advanced disease and increased mortality in HIV patients. In one of the few zinc supplementation studies conducted in AIDS patients, 45 mg/day of zinc for one month resulted in a decreased incidence in opportunistic infections compared to placebo. However, the HIV virus also requires zinc, and excessive zinc intake may stimulate the progression of HIV infection. In an observational study of HIV-infected men, increased zinc intake was associated with more rapid disease progression and any intake of zinc supplements was associated with poorer survival. These results indicate that further research is necessary to determine optimal zinc intakes for HIV-infected individuals.

Food sources

The following foods are rich in zinc?

- beef
- pork
- lamb
- legumes, such as beans, peas, lentils, and peanuts

Shellfish, beef, and other red meats are rich sources of zinc. Nuts and legumes are relatively good plant sources. Zinc bioavailability (the fraction of zinc retained and used by the body) is relatively high in meat, eggs, and seafood because of the relative absence of compounds that inhibit zinc absorption and the presence of certain amino acids (cysteine and methionine) that improve zinc absorption. The zinc in whole grain products and plant proteins is less bioavailable due to their relatively high content of phytic acid, a compound that inhibits zinc absorption. The enzymatic action of yeast reduces the level of phytic acid in foods. Therefore, leavened whole grain breads have more bioavailable zinc than unleavened whole grain breads.

Recently, national dietary surveys in the U.S. estimated that the average dietary zinc intake was 9 mg/day for adult women and 13 mg/day for adult men. The zinc content of some relatively zinc-rich foods is listed in milligrams (mg) in the table below.

Food	*Serving*	*Zinc (mg)*
Oysters	6 medium (cooked)	43.4
Crab, Dungeness	3 ounces (cooked)	4.6
Beef	3 ounces* (cooked)	5.8
Pork	3 ounces (cooked)	2.2
Chicken (dark meat)	3 ounces (cooked)	2.4
Turkey (dark meat)	3 ounces (cooked)	3.5

(Contd.)

(Contd. Table)

Food	*Serving*	*Zinc (mg)*
Yogurt, fruit	1 cup (8 ounces)	1.8
Cheese, cheddar	1 ounce	0.9
Milk	1 cup (8 ounces)	1.0
Cashews	1 ounce	1.6
Almonds	1 ounce	1.0
Peanuts	1 ounce	0.9
Beans, baked	1/2 cup	1.8
Chickpeas (garbanzo beans)	1/2 cup	1.3

Supplements

A number of zinc supplements are available, including zinc acetate, zinc gluconate, zinc picolinate, and zinc sulfate. Zinc picolinate has been promoted as a more absorbable form of zinc, but there is little data to support this idea in humans

Acute toxicity

Isolated outbreaks of acute zinc toxicity have occurred as a result of the consumption of food or beverages contaminated with zinc released from galvanized containers. Signs of acute zinc toxicity are abdominal pain, diarrhoea, nausea, and vomiting. Single doses of 225 to 450 mg of zinc usually induce vomiting. Milder gastrointestinal distress has been reported at doses of 50 to 150 mg/day of supplemental zinc

Adverse effects

The major consequence of long-term consumption of excessive zinc is copper deficiency. Total zinc intakes of 60 mg/day (50 mg supplemental and 10 mg dietary zinc) have been found to result in signs of copper deficiency. In order to prevent copper deficiency, the U.S. Food and Nutrition Board set the tolerable upper level of intake (UL) for adults at 40 mg/day, including dietary and supplemental zinc.

Drug Interactions

Concomitant administration of zinc supplements and certain antibiotics, specifically tetracyclines and quinolones, may decrease absorption of the antibiotic with potential reduction of its efficacy. Taking zinc supplements and these antibiotics at least two hours apart should prevent this interaction. The therapeutic use of metal chelating (binding) agents like penicillamine (used to treat copper overload in Wilson's disease) and diethylenetriamine pentaacetate or DTPA (used to treat iron overload) has resulted in severe zinc deficiency. Anticonvulsant drugs, especially sodium valproate, may also precipitate zinc deficiency. Prolonged use of diuretics may increase urinary zinc excretion, resulting in increased loss of zinc. The tuberculosis medication, ethambutol, has metal chelating properties and has been shown to increase zinc loss in rats.

Tolerable Upper Intake Level (UL) for Zinc

Age Group	*UL (mg / day)*
Infants 0-6 months	4
Infants 7-12 months	5
Children 1-3 years	7
Children 4-8 years	12
Children 9-13 years	23
Adolescents 14-18 years	34
Adults 19 years and older	40

Copper

Copper is an essential trace mineral involved in many functions in the human body. It helps build bones and make blood. It is also important in forming elastin and collagen, which are the connective tissues of skin, muscles, heart, blood vessels, and lungs. Copper is involved in the healing process, energy production, hair and skin coloring, and taste sensitivity. It is also needed for healthy nerves and joints. Interestingly the highest tissue concentrations of copper are found in the brain.

Copper (Cu) is an essential trace element for humans and animals. In the body, copper shifts between the cuprous (Cu^{1+}) and the cupric (Cu^{2+}) forms, though the majority of the body's copper is in the Cu^{2+} form. The ability of copper to easily accept and donate electrons explains its important role in oxidation-reduction (redox) reactions and the scavenging of free radicals. Although Hippocrates is said to have prescribed copper compounds to treat diseases as early as 400 B C.

Function

Copper has got important roles in blood, bones, brain, connective tissues, skin, and nerves, development of hair and skin color, healing processes of body, haemoglobin and red blood cell formation. Copper is a critical functional component of a number of essential enzymes, known as cuproenzymes.

Energy production

The copper-dependent enzyme, cytochrome *c* oxidase, plays a critical role in cellular energy production. By catalyzing the reduction of molecular oxygen (O_2) to water (H_2O), cytochrome *c* oxidase generates an electrical gradient used by the mitochondria to create the vital energy-storing molecule, ATP.

Connective tissue formation

Another cuproenzyme, lysyl oxidase, is required for the cross-linking of collagen and elastin, which are essential for the formation of strong and flexible connective tissue. The action of lysyl oxidase helps maintain the integrity of connective tissue in the heart and blood vessels and plays a role in bone formation.

Iron metabolism

Two copper-containing enzymes, ceruloplasmin (ferroxidase I) and ferroxidase II have the capacity to oxidize ferrous iron (Fe2+) to ferric iron (Fe3+), the form of iron that can be loaded onto the protein transferrin for transport to the site of red blood cell formation. Although the ferroxidase activity of these two cuproenzymes has not yet been proven to be physiologically significant, the fact that iron mobilization from storage sites is impaired in copper deficiency supports their role in iron metabolism.

Central nervous system

A number of reactions essential to normal function of the brain and nervous system are catalyzed by cuproenzymes.

Neurotransmitter synthesis

Dopamine-b-monooxygenase catalyzes the conversion of dopamine to the neurotransmitter norepinephrine.

Metabolism of neurotransmitters

Monoamine oxidase (MAO) plays a role in the metabolism of the neurotransmitters norepinephrine, epinephrine, and dopamine. MAO also functions in the degradation of the neurotransmitter serotonin, which is the basis for the use of MAO inhibitors as antidepressants.

Formation and maintenance of myelin

The myelin sheath is made of phospholipids whose synthesis depends on cytochrome *c* oxidase activity.

Melanin formation

The cuproenzyme, tyrosinase, is required for the formation of the pigment melanin. Melanin is formed in cells called melanocytes and plays a role in the pigmentation of the hair, skin, and eyes.

Antioxidant functions

Superoxide dismutase

Superoxide dismutase (SOD) functions as an antioxidant by catalyzing the conversion of superoxide radicals (free radicals or ROS) to hydrogen peroxide, which can subsequently be reduced to water by other antioxidant enzymes. Two forms of SOD contain copper:

1. copper/zinc SOD is found within most cells of the body, including red blood cells,
2. extracellular SOD is a copper containing enzyme found in high levels in the lungs and low levels in blood plasma.

Ceruloplasmin

Ceruloplasmin may function as an antioxidant in two different ways. Free copper and iron ions are powerful catalysts of free radical damage. By binding copper, ceruloplasmin prevents free copper ions from catalyzing oxidative damage. The ferroxidase activity of ceruloplasmin (oxidation of ferrous iron) facilitates iron loading onto its transport protein, transferrin, and may prevent free ferrous ions (Fe^{2+}) from participating in harmful free radical generating reactions.

Regulation of gene expression

Copper-dependent transcription factors regulate transcription of specific genes. Thus, cellular copper levels may affect the synthesis of proteins by enhancing or inhibiting the transcription of specific genes. Genes regulated by copper-dependent transcription factors include genes for copper/zinc superoxide dismutase (Cu/Zn SOD), catalase (another antioxidant enzyme), and proteins related to the cellular storage of copper.

Nutrient interactions

Iron

Adequate copper nutritional status appears to be necessary for normal iron metabolism and red blood cell formation. Anaemia is a clinical sign of copper deficiency, and iron has been found to accumulate in the livers of copper deficient animals, indicating that copper (probably in the form of ceruloplasmin) is required for iron transport to the bone marrow for red blood cell formation. Infants fed a high iron formula absorbed less copper than infants fed a low iron formula, suggesting that high iron intakes may interfere with copper absorption in infants.

Zinc

High supplemental zinc intakes of 50 mg/day or more for extended periods of time may result in copper deficiency. High dietary zinc increases the synthesis of an intestinal cell protein called metallothionein, which binds certain metals and prevents their absorption by trapping them in intestinal cells. Metallothionein has a stronger affinity for copper than zinc, so high levels of metallothionein induced by excess zinc cause a decrease in intestinal copper absorption. High copper intakes have not been found to affect zinc nutritional status.

Deficiency

Copper deficiency symptoms include Cardiovascular Disease, High LDL Cholesterol, aneurysms ruptures, artery wall damage, general weakness, low energy,brain disturbances, early aging signs, impaired immune function, anemia, baldness, slow healing sores, joint dysfunction and pain. Clinically evident or frank copper deficiency is relatively uncommon. Serum copper levels and ceruloplasmin levels may fall to 30% of normal in cases of severe copper deficiency. One of the most common clinical signs of copper deficiency is an anaemia that is unresponsive to iron therapy but corrected by copper supplementation. Less common features of copper deficiency may include loss of pigmentation, neurological symptoms, and impaired growth.

Individuals at risk of deficiency

High-risk individuals include: premature infants, especially those with low-birth weight, infants with prolonged diarrhoea, infants and children recovering from malnutrition, individuals with malabsorption syndromes, including celiac disease, sprue, and short bowel syndrome due to surgical removal of a large portion of the intestine. Individuals receiving intravenous total parenteral nutrition or other restricted diets may also require supplementation with copper and other trace elements. Recent research indicates that cystic fibrosis patients may also be at increased risk of copper insufficiency.

Therapeutic uses of Copper

Therapeutic Uses of Copper include heart disease, high cholesterol, artery wall damage, chronic fatigue, arthritis, osteoporosis, skin dryness/unelasticity, Alzheimer's disease, immune dysfunctionality, anemia, baldness.

The Recommended Dietary Allowance (RDA)

The recommended dietary allowance (RDA) for copper is as follows:-.

Recommended Dietary Allowance (RDA) for Copper

Life Stage	*Age*	*Males (mcg/day)*	*Females (mcg/day)*
Infants	0-6 months	200 (AI)	200 (AI)

(Contd.)

(Contd. Table)

Life Stage	*Age*	*Males (mcg/day)*	*Females (mcg/day)*
Infants	7-12 months	220 (AI)	220 (AI)
Children	1-3 years	340	340
Children	4-8 years	440	440
Children	9-13 years	700	700
Adolescents	14-18 years	890	890
Adults	19 years and older	900	900
Pregnancy	all ages	-	1,000
Breastfeeding	all ages	-	1,300

Disease Prevention

Cardiovascular disease

Research studies have suggested that copper deficiency rather than excess copper increases the risk of cardiovascular diseases.

Epidemiological studies

Several epidemiological studies have found increased serum copper levels to be associated with increased risk of cardiovascular disease.

Immune system function

Copper is known to play an important role in the development and maintenance of immune system function.

Osteoporosis

The copper-dependent enzyme, lysyl oxidase, is required for the maturation (cross-linking) of collagen, a key element in the organic matrix of bone. Osteoporosis has been observed in infants and adults with severe copper deficiency.

Food sources

Copper is found in a wide variety of foods and is most plentiful in organ meats, shellfish, nuts, and seeds. Wheat bran cereals and whole grain products are also good sources of copper. The copper content of some foods that are relatively rich in copper is listed in micrograms (mcg) in the table below.

Food	*Serving*	*Copper (mcg)*
Liver (beef), cooked	1 ounce	1,265
Oysters, cooked	1 medium oyster	670
Clams, cooked	3 ounces	585
Crab meat, cooked	3 ounces	624
Cashews	1 ounce	629
Sunflower seeds	1 ounce	519
Hazelnuts	1 ounce	496
Almonds	1 ounce	332
Peanut butter (chunky)	2 tablespoons	165
Lentils, cooked	1 cup	497
Mushrooms, raw	1 cup (sliced)	344
Shredded wheat cereal	2 biscuits	143
Chocolate (semisweet)	1 ounce	198
Hot cocoa mix	1 ounce (1 packet)	169

Supplements

Copper supplements are available as cupric oxide, copper gluconate, copper sulfate, and copper amino acid chelates.

Toxicity

Copper toxicity is rare in the general population. The U.S. Food and Nutrition Board (FNB) recently set the tolerable upper level of intake (UL) for copper at 10 mg/day from food and supplements.

Tolerable Upper Intake Level (UL) for Copper

Age Group	*UL (mcg / day)*
Infants 0-12 months	Not possible to establish*
Children 1-3 years	1,000
Children 4-8 years	3,000
Children 9-13 years	5,000
Adolescents 14-18 years	8,000
Adults 19 years and older	10,000

Drug Interactions

Relatively little is known about the interaction of copper with drugs.

Natural Sources

Beef liver, organ meats, oysters and other shellfish, almonds, beans and legumes, prunes, and green leafy vegetables.

Phosphorus

Phosphorus is an essential mineral that is required by every cell in the body for normal function. The majority of the phosphorus in the body is found as phosphate (PO_4). Approximately 85% of the body's phosphorus is found in bone.Out of the 800 grams of phosphorous in your body, about 88% is in your bones. The other 12% is used for many other important processes in the body including the metabolism of red blood cells, and the production of adenosine triphosphate (ATP) in the energy cycle. Phosphorus is found in many foods, so most people have a sufficient intake of this mineral.

Function

Phosphorus is a major structural component of bone in the form of a calcium phosphate salt called hydroxyapatite. Phospholipids (e.g., phosphatidylcholine) are major structural components of cell membranes. All energy production and storage are dependent on phosphorylated compounds, such as adenosine triphosphate (ATP) and creatine phosphate. Nucleic acids (DNA and RNA), responsible for the storage and transmission of genetic information, are long chains of phosphate-containing molecules. A number of enzymes, hormones, and cell signaling molecules depend on phosphorylation for their activation. Phosphorus also helps to maintain normal acid-base balance (pH) in its role as one of the body's most important buffers. The phosphorus-containing molecule 2,3-diphosphoglycerate (2,3-DPG) binds to hemoglobin in red blood cells and affects oxygen delivery to the tissues of the body.

Nutrient interactions:

Fructose

A recent study of 11 adult men found that a diet high in fructose (20% of total calories) resulted in increased urinary loss of phosphorus and a negative phosphorus balance (i.e., daily loss of phosphorus was higher than daily intake

Calcium and vitamin D

Dietary phosphorus is readily absorbed in the small intestine, and any excess phosphorus absorbed is excreted by the kidneys. The regulation of blood calcium and phosphorus levels is interrelated through the actions of parathyroid hormone (PTH) and vitamin D. A slight drop in blood calcium levels (e.g., in the case of inadequate calcium intake) is sensed by the parathyroid glands resulting in their increased secretion of PTH. PTH stimulates increased conversion of vitamin D to its active form (calcitriol) in the kidneys. Increased calcitriol levels result in increased intestinal absorption of both calcium and phosphorus. The increased urinary excretion of phosphorus is advantageous in bringing blood calcium levels up to normal because high blood levels of phosphate suppress the conversion of vitamin D to its active form in the kidneys.

Is high phosphorus intake detrimental to bone health?

Nowadays, there is increasing amounts of phosphates in the diet which can be attributed to phosphoric acid in soft drinks and phosphate additives in a number of commercially prepared foods. Phosphorus is not as tightly regulated by the body as calcium. Serum phosphate levels can rise slightly with a high phosphorous diet, especially after meals. High blood phosphate levels reduce the formation of the active form of vitamin D (calcitriol) in the kidneys, reduce blood calcium, and lead to increased PTH release by the parathyroid glands. However, high serum phosphorus levels also lead to decreased urinary calcium excretion. If sustained, elevated PTH levels could have an adverse effect on bone mineral content, but this effect has only been observed in humans on diets that were high in phosphorus and low in calcium.

Deficiency

Inadequate phosphorus intake results in abnormally low serum phosphate levels (hypophosphatemia). The effects of hypophosphatemia may include loss of appetite, anaemia, muscle weakness, bone pain, rickets (in children), osteomalacia (in adults), increased susceptibility to infection, numbness and tingling of the extremities, and difficulty in walking. Severe hypophosphatemia may result in death. Because phosphorus is so widespread in food, dietary phosphorus deficiency is usually seen only in cases of near total starvation

The Recommended Dietary Allowance (RDA)

The recommended dietary allowance (RDA) for phosphorus was based on the maintenance of normal serum phosphate levels in adults, which was felt to represent adequate phosphorus intake to meet cellular and bone formation needs.

Recommended Dietary Allowance (RDA) for Phosphorus

Life Stage	*Age*	*Males (mg/day)*	*Females (mg/day)*
Infants	0-6 months	100 (AI)	100 (AI)
Infants	7-12 months	275 (AI)	275 (AI)
Children	1-3 years	460	460
Children	4-8 years	500	500
Children	9-13 years	1,250	1,250
Adolescents	14-18 years	1,250	1,250
Adults	19 years and older	700	700
Pregnancy	18 years and younger	-	1,250
Pregnancy	19 years and older	-	700
Breastfeeding	18 years and younger	-	1,250
Breastfeeding	19 years and older	-	700

Food sources

Phosphorus is found in most foods because it is a critical component of all living organisms. Dairy products, meat, and fish are particularly rich sources of phosphorus. Phosphorus is also a component of many polyphosphate food additives, and is present in most soft drinks as phosphoric acid. The table below lists a number of phosphorus rich foods along with their phosphorus content in milligrams (mg).

Food	*Serving*	*Phosphorus (mg)*
Milk, skim	8 ounces	247
Yogurt, plain nonfat	8 ounces	383
Cheese, mozarella; part skim	1 ounce	131
Egg	1 large, cooked	104
Beef	3 ounces, cooked*	173
Chicken	3 ounces, cooked*	155
Turkey	3 ounces, cooked*	173
Fish, halibut	3 ounces, cooked*	242
Fish, salmon	3 ounces, cooked*	252
Bread, whole wheat	1 slice	64
Bread, enriched white	1 slice	24
Carbonated cola drink	12 ounces	44
Almonds#	1 ounce	139
Peanuts#	1 ounce	101
Lentils#	1/2 cup, cooked	356

*Phosphorus from nuts, seeds, and grains is about 50% less bioavailable than phosphorus from other sources.

Supplements

Sodium phosphate and potassium phosphate salts are used for the treatment of hypophosphatemia, and their use requires medical supervision. Calcium phosphate salts are sometimes used as calcium supplements.

Toxicity

The most serious adverse effect of abnormally elevated blood levels of phosphate (hyperphosphatemia) is the calcification of non-skeletal tissues, most commonly the kidneys. Such calcium phosphate deposition can lead to organ damage, especially kidney damage. Because the kidneys are very efficient at eliminating excess phosphate from the circulation, hyperphosphatemia from dietary causes is a problem mainly in people with kidney failure (end-stage renal disease) or hypoparathyroidism. When kidney function is only 20% of normal, even typical levels of dietary phosphorus may lead to hyperphosphatemia. Pronounced hyperphosphatemia has also occurred due to increased intestinal absorption of phosphate salts taken by mouth, as well as due to colonic absorption of the phosphate salts in enemas. The Food and Nutrition Board ,USA set a tolerable upper intake level (UL) for oral phosphorus intake in generally healthy individuals.

Tolerable Upper Intake Level (UL) for Phosphorus

Age Group	*UL (mg/day)*
Infants 0-12 months	Not possible to establish*
Children 1-3 years	3,000 (3.0 g)
Children 4-8 years	3,000 (3.0 g)
Children 9-13 years	4,000 (4.0 g)
Adolescents 14-18 years	4,000 (4.0 g)
Adults 19-70 years	4,000 (4.0 g)
Adults 70 years and older	3,000 (3.0 g)
Pregnancy	3,500 (3.5 g)
Breastfeeding	4,000 (4.0 g)

*Source of intake should be from food and formula only.

Drug Interactions

Aluminum-containing antacids reduce the absorption of dietary phosphorus by forming aluminum phosphate, which is unabsorbable. When consumed in high doses, aluminum containing antacids can produce abnormally low blood phosphate levels (hypophosphatemia), as well as aggravate phosphate deficiency due to other causes. As little as one ounce of aluminum hydroxide gel three times a day for several weeks can diminish serum phosphate levels and lead to increased urinary calcium loss. Excessively high doses of calcitriol, the active form of vitamin D, or its analogs may result in hyperphosphatemia.

Potassium supplements or potassium-sparing diuretics taken together with a phosphate may result in high blood levels of potassium (hyperkalemia). Hyperkalemia can be a serious problem, resulting in life threatening heart rhythm abnormalities (arrythmias).

Magnesium

Magnesium plays important roles in the structure and the function of the human body. The adult human body contains about

25 grams of magnesium. Over 60% of all the magnesium in the body is found in the skeleton, about 27% is found in muscle, while 6 to 7% is found in other cells, and less than 1% is found outside of cells.

Magnesium functions in more than 300 enzymatic reactions. Magnesium is essential for the conversion of vitamin D to its biologically active form that then helps the body absorb and utilize of calcium. The highest magnesium concentration is found in the tissues that are most metabolically active including the brain, heart, liver, and kidney.

Every 30 seconds someone will die from cardiovascular disease. Magnesium supplements can improve energy production within the heart, improve delivery of oxygen to the heart, reduce demand on the heart, inhibit the formation of blood clots, and improve heart rate. Magnesium supplementation has been used in many of these applications for over 50 years.

Magnesium is also effective with Chronic Fatigue Syndrome. People with CFS have low red blood cell magnesium levels.

Body Components and Functions — Arteries, bones, heart, muscles, nerves, and teeth. An important nutrient—out of the known 11 nutrients—for building bone. Acid/alkaline balance, blood sugar, metabolism (energy), and metabolism (calcium and vitamin C). Needed to balance with calcium.

Function

Magnesium is involved in more than 300 essential metabolic reactions, some of which are discussed below.

Energy production

Magnesium is required by the adenosine triphosphate (ATP) synthesizing protein in mitochondria. ATP, the molecule that provides energy for almost all metabolic processes, exists primarily as a complex with magnesium (MgATP).

Synthesis of essential molecules

Magnesium is required at a number of steps during the synthesis of nucleic acids (DNA and RNA) and proteins. A number of enzymes participating in the synthesis of carbohydrates and lipids require magnesium for their activity. Glutathione, an important antioxidant, requires magnesium for its synthesis.

Structural roles

Magnesium plays a structural role in bone, cell membranes, and chromosomes.

Ion transport across cell membranes

Magnesium is required for the active transport of ions like potassium and calcium across cell membranes. Through its role in ion transport systems, magnesium affects the conduction of nerve impulses, muscle contraction and the normal rhythm of the heart.

Cell signaling

Cell signaling requires MgATP for the phosphorylation of proteins and the formation of the cell signaling molecule, cyclic adenosine monophosphate (cAMP). cAMP is involved in many processes, including the secretion of parathyroid hormone (PTH) from the parathyroid glands.

Cell migration

Calcium and magnesium levels in the fluid surrounding cells affect the migration of a number of different cell types. Such affects on cell migration may be important in wound healing.

Nutrient Interactions

Zinc

High doses of zinc in supplement form appear to interfere with the absorption of magnesium.

Fibre

Large increases in the intake of dietary fibre have been found to decrease magnesium utilization in experimental studies.

Protein

Dietary protein may affect magnesium absorption.

Vitamin D and Calcium

The active form of vitamin D (calcitriol) may increase the intestinal absorption of magnesium to a small extent.

Deficiency

Magnesium deficiency symptoms include confusion, disorientation,easily aroused anger, nervousness, rapid pulse, tremors, tiredness/fatigue,

Magnesium deficiency in healthy individuals who are consuming a balanced diet is quite rare.

- Gastrointestinal disorders: Prolonged diarrhoea, Crohn's disease, malabsorption syndromes, celiac disease, surgical removal of a portion of the intestine, and intestinal inflammation due to radiation may all lead to magnesium depletion.
- Renal disorders (magnesium wasting): Diabetes mellitus and long-term use of certain diuretics may result in increased urinary loss of magnesium.
- Chronic alcoholism: Poor dietary intake, gastrointestinal problems, and increased urinary loss of magnesium may all contribute to magnesium depletion, which is frequently encountered in alcoholics.
- Age: Suboptimal dietary magnesium intake may increase the risk of magnesium depletion in the elderly.

The RDA

In 1997, the Food and Nutrition Board of the Institute of Medicine, USA increased the recommended dietary allowance (RDA) for magnesium, based on the results of recent, tightly controlled balance studies that utilized more accurate methods of measuring magnesium.

Recommended Dietary Allowance (RDA) for Magnesium

Life Stage	*Age*	*Males (mg/day)*	*Females (mg/day)*
Infants	0-6 months	30 (AI)	30 (AI)

(Contd.)

(Contd. Table)

Life Stage	*Age*	*Males (mg/day)*	*Females (mg/day)*
Infants	7-12 months	75 (AI)	75 (AI)
Children	1-3 years	80	80
Children	4-8 years	130	130
Children	9-13 years	240	240
Adolescents	14-18 years	410	360
Adults	19-30 years	400	310
Adults	31 years and older	420	320
Pregnancy	18 years and younger	-	400
Pregnancy	19-30 years	-	350
Pregnancy	31 years and older	-	360
Breastfeeding	18 years and younger	-	360
Breastfeeding	19-30 years	-	310
Breastfeeding	31 years and older	-	320

Disease Prevention

Hypertension (high blood pressure)

Many studies have suggested that low serum magnesium levels may play a modest role in the development of hypertension.

Cardiovascular disease

A number of studies have found decreased mortality from cardiovascular diseases in populations who routinely consume "hard" water.

Disease Treatment

Therapeutic Uses of magnesium include alcoholism, heart attack, erratic heart beat, high cholesterol, heart conditions, depression, kidney stones, nervousness, prostrate troubles, sensitivity to noise, chronic fatigue, stomach acidity, tooth decay, overweight, Magnesium.

Preeclampsia-eclampsia (toxaemia of pregnancy)

For many years, high dose intravenous magnesium sulfate has been the treatment of choice for preventing eclamptic seizures that may occur in association with preeclampsia-eclampsia late in pregnancy or during labour. Magnesium is believed to relieve cerebral blood vessel spasm, increasing blood flow to the brain.

Cardiovascular Disease

Myocardial infarction (heart attack)

Results of a meta-analysis of randomized placebo-controlled trials indicated that an intravenous (IV) magnesium infusion given early after suspected myocardial infarction (MI) could decrease the risk of death.

Endothelial dysfunction

Recent research indicates that pharmacologic doses of oral magnesium may improve endothelial function in individuals with cardiovascular disease.

Diabetes mellitus

Magnesium depletion is commonly associated with both insulin dependent (IDDM) and non-insulin dependent (NIDDM) diabetes mellitus. Between 25% and 38% of diabetics have been found to have decreased serum levels of magnesium (hypomagnesemia). Dietary magnesium supplements (400 mg/day) were found to improve glucose tolerance in elderly individuals. A few studies suggest that correcting magnesium depletion in elderly and diabetic individuals may improve glucose tolerance.

Osteoporosis

Magnesium comprises about 1% of bone mineral and is known to influence both bone matrix and bone mineral metabolism. As the magnesium content of bone mineral decreases, bone crystals become larger and more brittle.

Migraine headaches

Individuals who suffer from recurrent migraine headaches have been found to have lower intracellular magnesium levels than individuals who do not experience migraines.

Food sources

Green leafy vegetables are rich in magnesium because magnesium is part of chlorophyll, the green pigment in plants.

Unrefined grains and nuts also have high magnesium content. Meats and milk have an intermediate magnesium content, while refined foods generally have the lowest magnesium content.

Food	***Serving***	***Magnesium (mg)***
100% Bran Cereal (e.g., All Bran)	½ cup	128.7
Oat bran	½ cup dry	96.4
Shredded wheat	2 biscuits	54.3
Brown rice	1 cup cooked	83.8
Almonds	1 ounce (22 almonds)	81.1
Hazelnuts	1 ounce	49.0
Peanuts	1 ounce	49.8
Lima beans	½ cup cooked	62.9
Black-eyed peas	½ cooked	42.8
Spinach, chopped	½ cup cooked	78.3
Swiss chard, chopped	½ cup cooked	75.2
Okra, sliced	½ cup cooked	45.6
Molasses, blackstrap	1 tablespoon	43.0
Banana	1 medium	34.2
Milk 1% fat	8 fluid ounces	33.7

Supplements

Magnesium supplements are available as magnesium oxide, magnesium gluconate, magnesium chloride, and magnesium citrate salts, as well as a number of amino acid chelates, including magnesium aspartate. Magnesium hydroxide is used as an ingredient in a number of antacids.

Toxicity

The initial symptom of excess magnesium supplementation is diarrhoea, a well-known side effect of magnesium that is used therapeutically as a laxative. Individuals with impaired kidney function are at higher risk for adverse effects from magnesium supplementation, and symptoms of magnesium toxicity have occurred in people with impaired kidney function taking moderate doses of magnesium-containing laxatives or antacids. Elevated serum levels of magnesium (hypermagnesemia) may result in a fall in blood pressure (hypotension). Some of the later effects of magnesium toxicity, such as lethargy, confusion, disturbances in normal cardiac rhythm, and deterioration of kidney function, are related to severe hypotension. As hypermagnesemia progresses, muscle weakness and difficulty breathing may occur. Severe hypermagnesemia may result in cardiac arrest.

The Food and Nutrition Board (FNB) of the Institute of Medicine,USA set the tolerable upper level (UL) for supplemental magnesium intake in generally healthy adolescents and adults at 350 mg/day.

Tolerable Upper Intake Level (UL) for Supplemental Magnesium

Age Group	*UL (mg / day)*
Infants 0-12 months	Not possible to establish*
Children 1-3 years	65
Children 4-8 years	110
Children 9-13 years	350
Adolescents 14-18 years	350
Adults 19 years and older	350

*Source of intake should be from food and formula only.

Drug Interactions

Magnesium interferes with the absorption of digoxin (a heart medication), nitrofurantoin (an antibiotic), and certain anti-malarial drugs, potentially reducing their efficacy. Bisphosphonates (e.g., alendronate and etidronate), drugs used to treat osteoporosis, and magnesium should be taken two hours apart so the absorption of the bisphosphonate is not inhibited. Magnesium has also been found to reduce the efficacy of chlorpromazine (a tranquilizer), penicillamine, oral anticoagulants, and the quinolone and tetracycline classes of antibiotics. Because intravenous magnesium has increased the effects of certain muscle relaxing medications used during anesthesia for surgery.

Manganese

Manganese plays an essential part of proper bone and cartilage formation, and glucose metabolism. Manganese helps build and support strong bones in your body, but many people are deficient in this mineral because as much as 75 percent of all manganese is lost in the refining of wheat to white flour. Manganese is a mineral element that is both nutritionally essential and potentially toxic. The derivation of its name from the Greek word for magic remains appropriate because scientists are still working to understand the diverse effects of manganese deficiency and manganese toxicity in living organisms.

Manganese forms bone and fragile ear and joint cartilage, brain, thyroid and mammary glands, muscles, and nerves. Manganese plays a role in enzyme activation, reproduction and growth, sex hormone production, and tissue respiration. Manganese is needed for normal bone growth.

Function

Manganese (Mn) plays an important role in a number of physiologic processes as a constituent of some enzymes and an activator of other enzymes.

Antioxidant function

Manganese superoxide dismutase (MnSOD) is the principal antioxidant enzyme of mitochondria. Because mitochondria consume over 90% of the oxygen used by cells, they are especially vulnerable to oxidative stress.

Metabolism

A number of manganese-activated enzymes play important roles in the metabolism of carbohydrates, amino acids, and cholesterol. Pyruvate carboxylase, a manganese-containing enzyme, and phosphoenolpyruvate carboxykinase (PEPCK), a manganese-activated enzyme, play critical roles in gluconeogenesis— the production of glucose from non-carbohydrate precursors. Arginase, another manganese-containing enzyme, is required by the liver for the urea cycle, a process that detoxifies ammonia generated during amino acid metabolism.

Bone development

Manganese is the preferred cofactor of enzymes called glycosyltransferases, which are required for the synthesis of proteoglycans that are needed for the formation of healthy cartilage and bone.

Wound healing

Manganese is required for the activation of prolidase, an enzyme that functions to provide the amino acid, proline, for collagen formation in human skin cells. A genetic disorder known as prolidase deficiency results in abnormal wound healing among other problems, and is characterized by abnormal manganese metabolism Glycosaminoglycan synthesis, which requires manganese-activated glycosyltranserases, may also play an important role in wound healing.

Nutrient interactions

Iron

There are some research findings to suggest that iron and manganese can share common absorption and transport pathways. Absorption of manganese from a meal is reduced as the meal's iron content is increased. Iron supplementation (60 mg/day for 4 months) was associated with decreased blood manganese levels. Intestinal absorption of manganese is increased during iron deficiency, and increased iron stores (ferritin levels) are associated with decreased manganese absorption.

Magnesium

Supplemental magnesium (200 mg/day) decreased manganese bioavailability slightly, either by decreasing manganese absorption or by increasing its loss in healthy adults.

Calcium

In one set of studies, supplemental calcium (500 mg/day) resulted in slightly lower manganese bioavailability in healthy adults.

Deficiency

Manganese deficiency symptoms include ataxia(muscle coordination failure), dizziness, ear noises, hearing loss.

The Adequate Intake (AI)

Because there was not enough information on manganese requirements to set a Recommended Dietary Allowance (RDA), the

Food and Nutrition Board (FNB) of the Institute of Medicine set an adequate intake level (AI).

Adequate Intake (AI) for Manganese

Life Stage	*Age*	*Males (mg / day)*	*Females (mg / day)*
Infants	0-6 months	0.003	0.003
Infants	7-12 months	0.6	0.6
Children	1-3 years	1.2	1.2
Children	4-8 years	1.5	1.5
Children	9-13 years	1.9	1.6
Adolescents	14-18 years	2.2	1.6
Adults	19 years and older	2.3	1.8
Pregnancy	all ages	-	2.0
Breastfeeding	all ages	-	2.6

Disease Prevention

Low dietary manganese or low levels of manganese in blood or tissue have been associated with several chronic diseases such as osteoporosis, diabetes mellitus, epilepsy seizures .

Therapeutic Uses of Manganese include allergies, asthma, diabetes, fatigue, osteoporosis.

Food sources

Rich sources of manganese include whole grains, nuts, leafy vegetables, and teas. Foods high in phytic acid, such as beans, seeds, nuts, whole grains, and soy products, or foods high in oxalic acid, such as cabbage, spinach, and sweet potatoes, may slightly inhibit manganese absorption.

Food	*Serving*	*Manganese (mg)*
Pineapple, raw	1/2 cup, diced	1.28
Pineapple juice	1/2 cup (4 ounces)	1.24
Almonds	1 ounce	0.74

(Contd.)

(Contd. Table)

Food	Serving	Manganese (mg)
Peanuts	1 ounce	0.59
Instant oatmeal (prepared with water)	1 packet	1.20
Raisin bran cereal	1 cup	1.88
Brown rice, cooked	1/2 cup	0.88
Whole wheat bread	1 slice	0.65
Spinach, cooked	1/2 cup	0.84
Sweet potato, cooked	1/2 cup, mashed	0.55
Tea (green)	1 cup (8 ounces)	0.41-1.58
Tea (black)	1 cup (8 ounces)	0.18-0.77

Supplements

Several forms of manganese are found in supplements, including manganese gluconate, manganese sulfate, manganese ascorbate, and amino acid chelates of manganese.

Safety Toxicity

Inhaled manganese

The symptoms of manganese toxicity generally appear slowly over a period of months to years. In its worst form, manganese toxicity can result in a permanent neurological disorder with symptoms similar to those of Parkinson's disease, including tremors, difficulty in walking, and facial muscle spasms. This syndrome is sometimes preceded by psychiatric symptoms, such as irritability, aggressiveness, and even hallucinations.

Methylcyclopentadienyl manganese tricarbonyl (MMT)

MMT is a manganese-containing compound used in gasoline as an anti-knock additive. The impact of long-term exposure to low levels of MMT combustion products has not been thoroughly evaluated and will require additional study.

Individuals with increased susceptibility to manganese toxicity

- Chronic liver disease: Manganese is eliminated from the body mainly in bile. Thus, impaired liver function may lead to decreased manganese excretion. Manganese accumulation in individuals with cirrhosis or liver failure may contribute to neurological problems and Parkinson's disease-like symptoms.

- Newborns: The newborn brain may be more susceptible to manganese toxicity due to a greater expression of receptors for the manganese transport protein (transferrin) in developing nerve cells and the immaturity of the liver's bile elimination system.

Due to the severe implications of manganese neurotoxicity the Food and Nutrition Board (FNB) of the Institute of Medicine,USA set very conservative upper levels of intake (UL) for manganese, which are listed in the table below.

Tolerable Upper Intake Level (UL) for Manganese

Age Group	*UL (mg/day)*
Infants 0-12 months	Not possible to establish*
Children 1-3 years	2
Children 4-8 years	3
Children 9-13 years	6
Adolescents 14-18 years	9
Adults 19 years and older	11

*Source of intake should be from food and formula only.

Drug interactions

Magnesium-containing antacids and laxatives and the antibiotic medication, tetracycline, may decrease the absorption of manganese if taken together with manganese-containing foods or supplements.

Flouride

Fluoride is considered a trace element because only small amounts are present in the body (about 2.6 grams in adults), and because the daily requirement for maintaining dental health is only a few milligrams a day. About 95% of the total body fluoride is found in bones and teeth. Although its role in the prevention of dental caries (tooth decay) is well established, fluoride is not generally considered an essential mineral element because humans do not require it for growth or to sustain life . However, if one considers the prevention of chronic disease (dental caries), an important criterion in determining essentiality, then fluoride might well be considered an essential trace element .

Fluoride is essential for both teeth and bones. Calcium by itself won't build a molecule of bone. To use the calcium, your body has to have adequate supplies of at least 9 other minerals; and flouride is one of those minerals.

Function

Fluoride is absorbed in the stomach and small intestine. Once in the blood stream it rapidly enters mineralized tissue (bones and developing teeth). At usual intake levels, fluoride does not accumulate in soft tissue. The predominant mineral elements in bone are crystals of calcium and phosphate, known as hydroxyapatite crystals. Fluoride's high chemical reactivity and small radius allow it to either displace the larger hydroxyl (-OH) ion in the hydroxyapatite crystal, forming fluoroapatite, or to increase crystal density by entering spaces within the hydroxyapatite crystal. Fluoroapatite hardens tooth enamel and stabilizes bone mineral.

Nutrient interactions

Both calcium and magnesium form insoluble complexes with fluoride and are capable of significantly decreasing fluoride absorption when present in the same meal. However, the absorption of fluoride in the form of monofluorophosphate (unlike sodium fluoride) is unaffected by calcium. A diet low in chloride (salt) has been found to increase fluoride retention by reducing urinary excretion of fluoride.

Deficiency symtpoms of flouride include appetite loss , fatigue, irregular breathing, nervous disorders, overweight, weight loss.

In humans, the only clear effect of inadequate fluoride intake is an increased risk of dental caries (tooth decay) for individuals of all ages.

The Adequate Intake (AI)

The Food and Nutrition Board (FNB) of the Institute of Medicine, USA recommended the Adequate Intake of Flouriode as follows :-

Adequate Intake (AI) for Fluoride

Life Stage	*Age*	*Males (mg/day)*	*Females (mg/day)*
Infants	0-6 months	0.01	0.01
Infants	7-12 months	0.5	0.5
Children	1-3 years	0.7	0.7
Children	4-8 years	1.0	1.0
Children	9-13 years	2.0	2.0
Adolescents	14-18 years	3.0	3.0
Adults	19 years and older	4.0	3.0
Pregnancy	all ages	-	3.0
Breastfeeding	all ages	-	3.0

Disease Prevention

Dental caries (cavities and tooth decay)

Increased fluoride intake, most commonly through water fluoridation, has been found to decrease dental caries in children and adults. The role of fluoride in preventing dental caries is well established. When enamel is partially demineralized by organic acids, fluoride in the saliva can enhance the remineralization of enamel through its interactions with calcium and phosphate. In the presence of fluoride, remineralized enamel contains more fluoride and is more resistant to demineralization. In salivary concentrations associated with optimum fluoride intake, fluoride has been found to inhibit bacterial enzymes, resulting in reduced acid production by cariogenic bacteria.

Disease Treatment

Therapeutic Uses of Flouride include tooth decay, bone growth, arthritis, stunting growth in children, tooth/gum disorders, fatigue.

Osteoporosis

Pharmacologic doses of fluoride are capable of producing large increases in the BMD of the lumbar spine.

Sources

Water fluoridation

When water is fluoridated, it is adjusted to between 0.7 and 1.2 milligrams (mg) of fluoride per liter or 0.7-1.2 ppm. This concentration has been found to decrease the incidence of dental caries while minimizing the risk of dental fluorosis and other adverse effects.

Food sources

The natural sources of flouride include dairy products, whole grains, seeds and nuts, egg, fish, and poultry.

The table below provides a range of fluoride contents for a few fluoride-rich foods.

Food	*Serving*	*Fluoride (mg)*
Tea	100 ml (3.5 fluid ounces)	0.1-0.6
Canned sardines (with bones)	100 g (3.5 ounces)	0.2-0.4
Fish (without bones)	100 g (3.5 ounces)	0.01-0.17
Chicken	100g (3.5 ounces)	0.06-0.10

Toothpaste

Fluoridated toothpastes add considerably to fluoride intake of children, especially young children who are more likely to swallow them.

Acute toxicity

Fluoride is toxic when consumed in excessive amounts, so concentrated fluoride products should be used and stored with caution to prevent the possibility of acute fluoride poisoning, especially in children and other vulnerable individuals.

Dental fluorosis

The mildest form of dental fluorosis is detectable only to the trained observer, and is characterized by small opaque white flecks or spots on the enamel of the teeth. Moderate dental fluorosis is characterized by mottling and mild staining of the teeth, and severe dental fluorosis results in marked staining and pitting of the teeth. In its moderate to severe forms, dental fluorosis becomes a cosmetic concern when it affects the incisors and canines (front teeth). Dental fluorosis is a result of excess fluoride intake prior to the eruption of the first permanent teeth (generally before 8 years of age).

Tolerable Upper Intake Level (UL) for Fluoride

Age Group	*UL (mg / day)*
Infants 0-6 months	0.7
Infants 7-12 months	0.9
Children 1-3 years	1.3
Children 4-8 years	2.2
Children 9-13 years	10.0
Adolescents 14-18 years	10.0
Adults 19 years and older	10.0

Skeletal fluorosis

Intake of fluoride at excessive levels for long periods of time may lead to changes in bone structure known as skeletal fluorosis. The early stages of skeletal fluorosis are characterized by increased bone mass, detectable by x-ray. If very high fluoride intake persists over many years, joint pain and stiffness may result from the skeletal changes. The most severe form of skeletal fluorosis is known as "crippling skeletal fluorosis," which may result in calcification of ligaments, immobility, muscle wasting, and neurological problems related to spinal cord compression.

Drug Interactions

Calcium supplements, as well as calcium and aluminum containing antacids, can decrease the absorption of fluoride. It is best to take these products two hours before or after fluoride supplements.

Selenium

Selenium is a trace element that is essential in small amounts, but can be toxic in larger amounts. Humans and animals require selenium for the function of a number of selenium-dependent enzymes, also known as *selenoproteins*. During selenoprotein synthesis, selenocysteine is incorporated into a very specific location in the amino acid sequence in order to form a functional protein. Selenium works as an antioxidant with vitaman E to destroy hydroperoxides, free radicals that damage cell membranes. Selenium is a antioxidant weapon that must be in any health arsenal for battling cancer, cardiovascular disease, diabetes, and arthritis. In fact several of these major diseases have been proven to be associated with selenium deficiency.

Low selenium intakes or decreased selenium concentrations in the blood stream are associated with increased risk of cancer in humans. Although low levels of selenium are linked with many forms of cancer, respiratory and gastrointestinal tract cancers are affected the most by selenium.

Selenium levels are correlated with heart disease and strokes. Researchers have found that rates for heart disease are highest where selenium intakes are lowest. The eye lens depends on adequate levels and activity of superoxide dismutase, catalase, and glutathione peroxidase; and adequate levels of the accessory antioxidants vitamins E and C and selenium. The human lens glutathione peroxidase is selenium-dependent.

Body Components and Functions — Blood, membranes, cells, organs, prostrate gland, liver, and testicles. Powerful antioxidant that protects cellular and organelle membranes from free radical damage, helps the body handle hydrogenated and polyunsaturated (trans) fats, slows the aging process of skin and organs.

Function

Selenoproteins

At least 11 selenoproteins have been characterized, and there is evidence that additional selenoproteins exist.

Glutathione peroxidases

Four selenium-containing glutathione peroxidases (GPx) have been identified: **cellular or classical GPx, plasma or extracellular GPx, phospholipid hydroperoxide GPx,** and **gastrointestinal GPx**. Although each GPx is a distinct selenoprotein, they are all antioxidant enzymes that reduce potentially damaging reactive oxygen species (ROS), such as hydrogen peroxide and lipid hydroperoxides, to harmless products like water and alcohols by coupling their reduction with the oxidation of glutathione.

Thioredoxin reductase

In conjunction with the compound thioredoxin, thioredoxin reductase participates in the regeneration of several antioxidant systems, possibly including vitamin C. Maintenance of thioredoxin in a reduced form by thioredoxin reductase is important for regulating cell growth and viability.

Iodothyronine deiodinases (thyroid hormone deiodinases)

The thyroid gland releases very small amounts of biologically active thyroid hormone (triiodothyronine or T_3) and larger amounts of an inactive form of thyroid hormone (thyroxine or T_4) into the circulation. Most of the biologically active T_3 in the circulation and inside cells is created by the removal of one iodine atom from T_4 in a reaction catalyzed by selenium-dependent iodothyronine deiodinase enzymes. Through their actions on T_3, T_4, and other thyroid hormone metabolites, three different selenium-dependent iodothyronine deiodinases (types I, II, and III) can both activate and inactivate thyroid hormone, making selenium an essential element for normal development, growth, and metabolism through the regulation of thyroid hormones.

Selenoprotein P

Selenoprotein P is found in plasma and also associated with vascular endothelial cells (cells that line the inner walls of blood vessels).

Selenoprotein W

Selenoprotein W is found in muscle. Although its function is presently unknown, it is thought to play a role in muscle metabolism.

Selenophosphate synthetase

Incorporation of selenocysteine into selenoproteins is directed by the genetic code and requires the enzyme selenophosphate synthetase. A selenoprotein itself, selenophosphate synthetase catalyzes the synthesis of monoselenium phosphate, a precursor of selenocysteine which is required for the synthesis of selenoproteins.

Nutrient interactions

Antioxidant nutrients

As an integral part of the glutathione peroxidases and thioredoxin reductase, selenium probably interacts with every nutrient that affects the pro-oxidant/antioxidant balance of the cell. Selenium as gluthathione peroxidase also appears to support the activity of vitamin E (a-tocopherol) in limiting the oxidation of lipids. Thioredoxin reductase also maintains the antioxidant function of vitamin C by catalyzing its regeneration.

Iodine

Selenium deficiency may exacerbate the effects of iodine deficiency. Iodine is essential for the synthesis of thyroid hormone. Selenium supplementation in a small group of elderly individuals decreased plasma T_4, indicating increased deiodinase activity with increased conversion to T_3.

Deficiency Symptoms of Selenium include heart disease, heart attack, stroke, early aging signs, age spots, muscular dysfunction, myalgia, organ failures, immune system problems. Insufficient selenium intake results in decreased activity of the glutathione peroxidases. Even when severe, isolated selenium deficiency does not usually result in obvious clinical illness. However, selenium deficient individuals appear to be more susceptible to additional physiological stresses.

Individuals at increased risk of selenium deficiency

Clinical selenium deficiency has been observed in chronically ill patients who were receiving total parenteral nutrition (TPN) without added selenium for prolonged periods of time. Muscular weakness, muscle wasting, and cardiomyopathy (inflammation and damage to the heart muscle) have been observed in these patients.

TPN solutions are now supplemented with selenium to prevent such problems. People who have had a large portion of the small intestine surgically removed or those with severe gastrointestinal problems, such as Crohn's disease, are also at risk for selenium deficiency due to impaired absorption.

Keshan disease

Keshan disease is a cardiomyopathy that affects young women and children in a selenium deficient region of China. The acute form of the disease is characterized by the sudden onset of cardiac insufficiency, while the chronic form results in moderate to severe heart enlargement with varying degrees of cardiac insufficiency.

Kashin-Beck Disease

Kashin-Beck disease is characterized by the degeneration of the articular cartilage between joints (osteoarthritis) and is associated with poor selenium status in areas of northern China, North Korea, and eastern Siberia. The disease affects children between the ages 5 and 13 years. Severe forms of the disease may result in joint deformities and dwarfism, due to degeneration of cartilage forming cells

The Recommended Dietary Allowance (RDA)

The most recent RDA is based on the amount of dietary selenium required to maximize the activity of the antioxidant enzyme glutathione peroxidase in blood plasma. The RDA revised in 2000 by the Food and Nutrition Board (FNB) of the Institute of Medicine was as follows:-

Recommended Dietary Allowance (RDA) for Selenium

Life Stage	*Age*	*Males (mcg/day)*	*Females (mcg/day)*
Infants	0-6 months	15 (AI)	15 (AI)
Infants	7-12 months	20 (AI)	20 (AI)
Children	1-3 years	20	20

(Contd)

(Contd. Table)

Life Stage	*Age*	*Males (mcg/day)*	*Females (mcg/day)*
Children	4-8 years	30	30
Children	9-13 years	40	40
Adolescents	14-18 years	55	55
Adults	19 years and older	55	55
Pregnancy	all ages	-	60
Breastfeeding	all ages	-	70

Disease Prevention

Immune function

Selenium deficiency has been associated with impaired function of the immune system. Moreover, selenium supplementation in individuals who are not overtly selenium deficient appears to stimulate the immune response.

Viral infection

Selenium deficiency appears to enhance the virulence or progression of some viral infections. The increased oxidative stress resulting from selenium deficiency may induce mutations or changes in the expression of some viral genes.

Cancer

Epidemiological studies

Geographic studies have consistently shown that a relatively low selenium intakes to have higher cancer mortality rates. Chronic infection with viral hepatitis B or C significantly increases the risk of liver cancer.

Therapeutic Uses of selenium include slow the aging process , cardiovascular disease, heart attack, stroke, myalgia, muscular dystrophy, organ dsyfunction, cancer, Alzheimer's disease, immune system.

HIV/AIDS

There appears to be a unique interaction between selenium and the human immunodeficiency viruses (HIV) that cause acquired immunodeficiency syndrome (AIDS). Declining selenium levels in HIV-infected individuals are sensitive markers of disease progression and severity, even before malnutrition becomes a factor. Low levels of plasma selenium have also been associated with a significantly increased risk of death from HIV. Adequate selenium nutritional status may increase resistance to HIV infection by enhancing the function of important immune system cells known as T cells and modifying their production of intracellular messengers known as cytokines. In HIV infection, increased oxidative stress appears to favour viral replication, possibly by activating specific transcription pathways. As an integral component of glutathione peroxidase and thioredoxin reductase, selenium plays an important role in decreasing oxidative stress in HIV-infected cells and possibly suppressing the rate of HIV replication. Recent research indicates that HIV may be capable of incorporating host selenium into viral selenoproteins that have glutathione-peroxidase activity. Though the significance of these findings requires further clarification, they suggest that both the human immune system and the activity of the virus are affected by selenium nutritional status.

Only a few trials of selenium supplementation in HIV-infected individuals have been published. Two uncontrolled trials of selenium supplementation (one using 400 mcg/day of selenium-enriched yeast and the other 80 mcg/day of sodium selenite plus 25 mg/day of vitamin C) reported subjective improvement, but did not demonstrate any improvement in biological parameters related to AIDS progression. Another trial followed 15 HIV-infected patients supplemented with 100 mcg/day of sodium selenite and 22 unsupplemented patients for 1 year and found evidence of decreased oxidative stress and a significant decrease in a biological marker of immunologic activation and HIV progression in the selenium supplemented patients. However, there were no differences in CD4 T cell count (an important biological marker of the progress of HIV infection) or mortality between the supplemented and unsupplemented patients . At least two double-blind placebo-controlled trials of selenium supplementation in HIV-positive individuals are presently under way.

Sources

Food sources

The richest food sources of selenium are organ meats and seafood, followed by muscle meats. In general, there is wide variation in the selenium content of plants and grains because plants do not appear to require selenium. Thus, the incorporation of selenium into plant proteins is dependent only on soil selenium content. The table below lists some good food sources of selenium and their selenium content in micrograms (mcg).

Food	*Serving*	*Selenium (mcg)*
Brazil nuts (from selenium-rich soil)	1 ounce (6-8 kernels)	839*
Shrimp	3 ounces (10-12)	34
Crab meat	3 ounces	40
Salmon	3 ounces	40
Halibut	3 ounces	40
Noodles, enriched	1 cup, cooked	35
Rice, brown	1 cup, cooked	19
Chicken (light meat)	3 ounces	20
Pork	3 ounces	33
Beef	3 ounces	17
Whole wheat bread	2 slices	15
Milk	8 ounces (1 cup)	5
Walnuts, black	1 ounce, shelled	5

*Above the tolerable upper intake level (UL) of 400 mcg/day.

Supplements

Selenium supplements are available in several forms. Sodium selenite and sodium selenate are inorganic forms of selenium.

Toxicity

Although selenium is required for health, high doses can be toxic. Acute and fatal toxicities have occurred with accidental or suicidal ingestion of gram quantities of selenium.

The Food and Nutrition Board (FNB),USA recently set the tolerable upper level (UL) for selenium at 400 mcg/day in adults.

Tolerable Upper Intake Level (UL) for Selenium

Age Group	*UL (mcg / day)*
Infants 0-6 months	45
Infants 6-12 months	60
Children 1-3 years	90
Children 4-8 years	150
Children 9-13 years	280
Adolescents 14-18 years	400
Adults 19 years and older	400

Chromium

Chromium is an extremely important nutrient- it is essential for normal glucose metabolism, insulin metabolism, fatty acid metabolism, and muscle growth.

The two most common forms of chromium are trivalent chromium (III) and hexavalent chromium (VI). Chromium (III) is the principal form in foods, as well as the form utilized by the body. Chromium (VI) is derived from chromium (III) by heating at alkaline pH and is used as a source of chromium for industrial purposes. It is a strong irritant and is recognized as a carcinogen when inhaled. At low levels, chromium (VI) is readily reduced to chromium (III) by reducing substances in foods and the acidic environment of the stomach, which serve to prevent the ingestion of chromium (VI).

Chromium was identified in 1957 by researchers Walter Mertz and Kenneth Swartz as the active component of the "glucose tolerance factor (GTF)."

Deficiency Symptoms include arteriosclerosis, glucose intolerance in diabetics, diabetic symptoms. Signs of chromium deficiency mirror the symptoms of Type II Adult Onset Diabetes. Recent studies found that chromium helps raise HDL cholesterol, the "good" kind that escorts bad cholesterol out of your body.

Many studies have been done on the muscle-enhancing and fat-reducing effects of chromium picolinate. In one study, patients were given chromium picolinate in one of the following three doses daily for 2 1/2 months: 0 microgram (placebo), 200 micrograms, or 400 micrograms. The fifteen patients taking the 200 mcg and 400 mcg dose lost an average of 4.2 pounds of fat. The group taking the placebo lost only 0.4 pounds. Even more impressive was the chromium group's muscle gain (1.4 versus 0.2 pounds) versus that of the placebo group. The results were most striking in elderly subjects and men. The men taking chromium picolinate lost more than 7 times the body fat as those taking the placebo (7.7 versus 1 pound).

Body Components and Functions — Arteries, and blood. Part of glucose and insulin metabolism (energy). Weight-loss aid while increasing lean body mass.

Therapeutic Uses include diabetes, hypoglycemia, elevated blood cholesterol, triglyceride levels, weight loss, acne,

Natural Sources

Brewers yeast, whole grains, raw cane sugar, meat, shell fish, chicken, clams, and corn oil.

Function

A biologically active form of chromium participates in glucose metabolism by enhancing the effects of insulin. Insulin is secreted by specialized cells in the pancreas in response to increased blood glucose levels, for example, after a meal. Insulin binds to insulin receptors on the surface of cells, activating those receptors and stimulating glucose uptake by cells. Through its interaction with insulin receptors, insulin provides cells with glucose for energy and prevents blood glucose levels from becoming elevated. In addition to its effects on carbohydrate (glucose) metabolism, insulin also influences the metabolism of fat and protein. A decreased response to insulin or decreased insulin sensitivity may result in impaired glucose tolerance or type 2 diabetes, also known as non-insulin dependent diabetes mellitus (NIDDM). Type 2 diabetes is characterized by elevated blood glucose levels and insulin resistance.

Recent research suggests that a low-molecular-weight chromium-binding substance (LMWCr) may enhance the response of the insulin receptor to insulin. First, the inactive form of the insulin receptor is converted to the active form by binding insulin. The binding of insulin by the insulin receptor stimulates the movement of chromium into the cell and results in binding of chromium to apoLMWCr, a form of the LMWCr that lacks chromium. Once it binds chromium the LMWCr binds to the insulin receptor and enhances its activity. The ability of the LMWCr to activate the insulin receptor is dependent on its chromium content. When insulin levels drop due to normalization of blood glucose levels, the LMWCr may be released from the cell in order to terminate its effects.

Nutrient interactions

Iron

Chromium competes for one of the binding sites on the iron transport protein, transferrin.

Vitamin C

Chromium uptake is enhanced in animals when given at the same time as vitamin C

Carbohydrates

Diets high in simple sugars (e.g., sucrose), compared to diets high in complex carbohydrates (e.g., whole grains), increase urinary chromium excretion in adults. This effect may be related to increased insulin secretion in response to the consumption of simple sugars compared to complex carbohydrates.

Deficiency

Patients with chromium deficiency developed evidence of abnormal glucose utilization and increased insulin requirements that responded to chromium supplementation.

The Adequate Intake (AI)

The Food and Nutrition Board, USA has set an adequate intake level (AI) based on the chromium content in normal diets.

Adequate Intake (AI) for Chromium

Life Stage	*Age*	*Males (mcg/day)*	*Females (mcg/day)*
Infants	0-6 months	0.2	0.2

(Contd.)

(Contd. Table)

Life Stage	*Age*	*Males (mcg/day)*	*Females (mcg/day)*
Infants	7-12 months	5.5	5.5
Children	1-3 years	11	11
Children	4-8 years	15	15
Children	9-13 years	25	21
Adolescents	14-18 years	35	24
Adults	19-50 years	35	25
Adults	51 years and older	30	20
Pregnancy	18 years and younger	-	29
Pregnancy	19 years and older	-	30
Breastfeeding	18 years and younger	-	44
Breastfeeding	19 years and older	-	45

Disease Prevention

Disease Treatment

Type 2 diabetes mellitus

Individuals with type 2 diabetes have been found to have higher rates of urinary chromium loss than healthy individuals, especially those with diabetes of more than 2 years duration.

Gestational diabetes

Few studies have examined the effects of chromium supplementation on gestational diabetes. Women with gestational diabetes whose diets were supplemented with 4 mcg of chromium per kilogram of body weight daily as chromium picolinate for 8 weeks had decreased fasting blood glucose and insulin levels compared with those who took a placebo. However, insulin therapy rather than chromium picolinate was required to normalize severely elevated blood glucose levels.

Food sources

Processed meats, whole grain products, ready-to-eat bran cereals, green beans, broccoli, and spices are relatively rich in chromium. The chromium content of some foods is listed below in micrograms (mcg).

Food	*Serving*	*Chromium (mcg)*
Broccoli	1/2 cup	11.0
Green beans	1/2 cup	1.1
Potatoes	1 cup, mashed	2.7
Grape juice	8 fl. ounces	7.5
Orange juice	8 fl. ounces	2.2
Beef	3 ounces	2.0
Turkey breast	3 ounces	1.7
Turkey ham (processed)	3 ounces	10.4
Waffle	1 (~2.5 ounces)	6.7
Bagel	1	2.5
English muffin	1	3.6
Apple w/ peel	1 medium	1.4
Banana	1 medium	1.0

Supplements

Chromium (III) is available as a supplement in several forms: chromium chloride, chromium nicotinate, chromium picolinate, and high-chromium yeast. They are available as stand-alone supplements or in combination products. Doses typically range from 50 to 200 mcg of elemental chromium. Chromium nicotinate and chromium picolinate may be more bioavailable than chromium chloride.

Toxicity

Hexavalent chromium or chromium (VI) is a recognized carcinogen. Exposure to chromium (VI) in dust is associated with increased incidence of lung cancer and is known to cause inflammation of the skin (dermatitis).

Molybdenum

Molybdenum is an essential trace element for virtually all life forms. It functions as a cofactor for a number of enzymes that catalyze important chemical transformations in the global carbon, nitrogen, and sulfur cycles. Thus, molybdenum-dependent enzymes are not only required for the health of the human beings but for the health of its ecosystems as well.

Molybdenum functions as a component in several enzymes that are involved in alcohol detoxification, uric acid formation, and sulfur metabolism. Researchers have also found a that low molybdenum levels is an associated condition accompanying cancer. Studies in China concluded that where soil molybdenum levels are low, the rate of esophageal cancer is higher. Presumably the anticancer effects of molybdenum stem from its role in the detoxification of cancer-causing chemicals. Molybdenum is also correlated with cavity prevention and tooth decay. It is possible that molybdenum enhances flouride, causing less tooth decay.

Function

The biological form of molybdenum present in almost all molybdenum-containing enzymes (molybdoenzymes) is an organic molecule known as the molybdenum cofactor. In humans, molybdenum is known to function as a cofactor for three enzymes.

- **Sulfite oxidase** catalyzes the transformation of sulfite to sulfate, a reaction that is necessary for the metabolism of sulfur-containing amino acids, such as cysteine.
- **Xanthine oxidase** catalyzes the breakdown of nucleotides (precursors to DNA and RNA) to form uric acid, which contributes to the antioxidant capacity of the blood.
- **Aldehyde oxidase** and xanthine oxidase catalyze hydroxylation reactions involving a number of different molecules with similar structures. Xanthine oxidase and aldehyde oxidase also play a role in the metabolism of drugs and toxins.

Of these three enzymes, only sulfite oxidase is known to be crucial for human health.

Nutrient Interactions

Copper

Excess dietary molybdenum has been found to result in copper deficiency in grazing animals (ruminants). In ruminants, the formation of compounds containing sulfur and molybdenum, known as thiomolybdates, appears to prevent the absorption of copper. This interaction between thiomolybdates and copper does not occur to a significant degree in humans. Dietary molybdenum deficiency has never been observed in healthy people.

The Recommended Dietary Allowance (RDA)

The recommended dietary allowance (RDA) for molybdenum was revised in January 2001. The RDA values for molybdenum are listed in the table below in micrograms (mcg)/day by age and gender.

Recommended Dietary Allowance (RDA) for Molybdenum

Life Stage	*Age*	*Males (mcg / day)*	*Females (mcg / day)*
Infants	0-6 months	2 (AI)	2 (AI)
Infants	7-12 months	3 (AI)	3 (AI)
Children	1-3 years	17	17
Children	4-8 years	22	22
Children	9-13 years	34	34
Adolescents	14-18 years	43	43
Adults	19 years and older	45	45
Pregnancy	all ages	-	50
Breastfeeding	all ages	-	50

Disease Prevention

Gastroesophageal cancer

Linxian is a small region in northern China where the incidence of cancer of the esophagus and stomach is very high (10 times higher than the average in China and 100 times higher than the average in the U.S.). The soil in this region is low in molybdenum and other mineral elements, so dietary molybdenum is also low.

Food sources

Legumes, such as beans, lentils, and peas, are the richest sources of molybdenum. Grain products and nuts are considered good sources, while animal products, fruits, and many vegetables are generally low in molybdenum.

Supplements

Molybdenum in nutritional supplements is generally in the form of sodium molybdate or ammonium molybdate.

Toxicity

The toxicity of molybdenum compounds appears to be relatively low in humans.

Tolerable Upper Intake Level (UL) for Molybdenum

Age Group	*UL (mcg / day)*
Infants 0-12 months	Not possible to establish*
Children 1-3 years	300
Children 4-8 years	600
Children 9-13 years	1,100 (1.1 mg/day)
Adolescents 14-18 years	1,700 (1.7 mg/day)
Adults 19 years and older	2,000 (2.0 mg/day)

*Source of intake should be from food and formula only.

Body Components and Functions — Blood. Integral part of enzymes involved in oxidation processes.

Therapeutic Uses include copper poisoning, improper carbohydrate metabolism.

Natural Sources

Brown rice, millet, buck wheat, legumes, leafy vegetables, and whole cereals.

Boron

Prior to 1981 boron was thought to be unimportant in human nutrition. Since then numerous animal and human studies have established it as essential for normal growth and for hormones involved in bone metabolism, and for normal balanced levels of estrogen and testosterone.

A 1988 study by Neilsen and Prasad "Essential and Toxic Trace Elements in Human Health and Disease," found that boron is essential for the manufacture of several hormones. Boron helps the body to maintain normal levels. Of course without those normal levels many facets of enjoyable living will suffer.

Body Components and Functions - Bones — cofactor for mineral uptake into bone matrix structure, Hormones — including estrogen and testosterone, insomnia, muscle cramps.

Deficiency Symptoms- bone pain, backache, PMS and menstrual cramps, menopause problems.

Therapeutic Uses- arthritis, fatigue, migraine headaches, nervousness, fluid retention, depression, hot flashes, backache.

Natural Sources-Cheese, sardines, salmon, dark leafy vegetables, and sesame seeds.

RDA: Not yet established. Researched Supplement Range: 1.5 mg to 6.0 mg, Average Daily Intake: 0.35 to 0.42 mg, Notes: never above 45 mg per day, interferes with riboflavin and phosphorus uptake.

Cobalt

Cobalt is one of the essential trace minerals that has been taken out of our soils by replacement of only NPK. Until the 1940's, most farmers returned essential minerals to the soil by mulching, manuring, and crop rotation. At the end of the Second World War, drug conglomerates making nitrates and phosphates for explosives, were frantic for new markets, and began selling NPK fertilizers at incredibly low prices that made traditional farming methods uneconomic. So therefore, the American soils have been reduced to only Nitrogen, Potassium, and Phosphorus, leaving out all the other essential trace minerals.

Human bodies need essential minerals to grow, cobalt is one that forms an essential part of vitamin B^{12}. It is also a necessary cofactor for making the thyroid hormone.

Body Components and Functions — Blood. Aids in hemoglobin formation.

Deficiency Symptoms include slow growth and development,

Therapeutic Uses include anemia, retardation.

Natural Sources

All green leafy vegetables, clams, liver, oysters, milk, and red meat.

RDA: 3 mcg to 4 mcg

Sulfur

Sulfur is a structural part of most proteins and thereby participates in many life-sustaining enzymatic, antibody, and tissue activities. It also is found in the anticoagulant heparin and in chondroitin sulfate and glucosamine sulfate. Deficiency of sulfur results in degeneration of collagen, cartilage, ligaments, and tendons.

Body Components and Functions — Hair, skin, nails, and nerves. Collagen synthesis and body tissue formation.

Therapeutic Uses include arthritis, eczema, dermatitis, psoriasis

Natural Sources

Radish, onions, kale, and water cress

RDA: Not established

Researched Supplement Range: Not set to date

Average Daily Intake: Unavailable

Germanium

Germanium carries oxygen to the cells. This helps to fight pain, keep the immune system functioning properly, and rid the body of toxins and poisons. A Japanese scientist, Kazuhiko Asai, found that individuals taking 100-300 mg of germanium improved many illnesses including rheumatoid arthritis, food allergies, elevated cholesterol, chronic viral infections, cancer and AIDS.

Body Components and Functions — All cells. A relatively new mineral. Builds immune cells, gives energy, and has rejuvenate properties. A powerful antioxidant that also relieves pain.

Therapeutic Uses include anaemia , arthritis,

Natural Sources

Garlic, aloe, comfrey, chorella, ginseng, and water cress

RDA: Not established

Researched Supplement Range: Not set to date

Average Daily Intake: Unavailable

Lithium

Body Components and Functions — Nerves, muscles, and brain. Helps transport sodium metabolism to brain nerves and muscles.

Deficiency Symptoms include nerves , mental disorders

Therapeutic Uses include paranoid schizophrenic

Natural Sources

Kelp, dulse, and seafood

RDA: Not established

Researched Supplement Range: Not set to date

Average Daily Intake: Unavailable

Silicon

Second to oxygen, silicon is the most abundant element on earth, but it wasn't regarded as an essential nutrient for health until 1972. All the publicity about the toxicity of silicon breast implants should not be confused with silicon as a nutrient. Silicon (the nutrient) is important for normal bone growth, and for proper integrity of the skin.

One study of 50 women with signs of aging skin, hair and nails produced very significant results. After 90 days of taking daily oral doses of 10 milliliters of colloidal silicic acid and applying colloidal silicic acid twice daily to the face, improvements were made in the thickness of skin, strength of skin, wrinkles, and health of the hair and nails.

Body Components and Functions — Bones, hair, nails, and teeth. Helps healing process and builds immune system.

Deficiency Symptoms include aging symptoms of skin (wrinkles), thinning/loss of hair, poor bone development, soft or brittle nails

Therapeutic Uses include hair loss, irritations in mucous membranes, skin disorders, insomnia.

Natural Sources

Flaxseed, oats, nuts, seeds, apples, and beets.

RDA: Not established

Researched Supplement Range: 5 mg to 20 mg

Average Daily Intake: 329 mg

Notes: generally regarded as being nontoxic, but increased levels of silicon have been detected in Alzheimer's disease patients

Vanadium

According to an article in the Journal of the American Dietetic Association, vanadium has an essential role in human nutrition. Vanadium research has shown that this nutrient improves insulin action and even mimicks the functionality of insulin.Most research on vanadium has been done on animals, but most researchers would agree that vanadium would produce similar effect on humans. In one study on goats, researchers discovered that after a 3-year vanadium restricted diet, female goats gave birth to kids with serious birth defects. Some of the kids were born with a reversible bone deformity, some died within 3 days, some could not stand after birth, and the mothers produced significantly less milk.

Body Components and Functions — Heart and blood vessels. Inhibits formation of cholesterol in blood vessels.

Deficiency Symptoms include high blood pressure, hardening of arteries.

Therapeutic Uses include heart attack prevention, high blood pressure, arteriosclerosis, diabetes.

Natural Sources :-Fish : Recommended Daily Allowance - 10 mcg to 60 mcg. Researched Supplement Range: 10 mcg to 100 mcg, Excessive amounts lead to cramping and diarrhoea.

8

Viral Hepatitis and HIV

Taking Care of Your Liver

Whether you have liver damage because of a viral hepatitis infection or for any other reason, talk with your healthcare provider about liver health and consider the following:

- Get vaccinated against hepatitis A and hepatitis B if you don't already have the antibodies.
- Don't share: drug paraphernalia (needles, syringes, cookers, cotton, water, snorting straws); toothbrushes, razors, manicure implements, and other items that can retain blood.
- Consider reducing or stopping your alcohol intake. Alcohol significantly increases the risk of developing cirrhosis and liver cancer.
- If you have chronic HBV or HCV, find a doctor who understands viral hepatitis — a gastroenterologist (digestive system specialist) and some infectious disease and primary care physicians. If you're considering treatment, a team approach, including access to a psychiatrist, is best.
- Get regular health check-ups, including liver enzyme tests. Keep track of all appropriate test results — liver enzyme levels, viral load, and genotype.
- Eat a balanced diet of fresh vegetables, fruits, beans, whole grains, and lean meats.
- Cut down on foods with high salt, sugar or fat content: cheese, fast food, fried food, and processed foods (cookies, cakes, frozen dinners, packaged foods with long shelf lives, "instant" foods).

- Get a healthy balance of protein in your diet — too much protein can stress your liver.
- Drink lots of fluids — especially water — to flush toxins from your body.
- Get regular exercise and develop a stress reduction plan.
- Acetaminophen (Tylenol and other non-aspirin pain relievers), particularly in large amounts (2,000/mg day), are toxic to the liver. Acetaminophen is in many medications, so read the labels carefully. Acetaminophen and alcohol together can cause severe liver damage.
- Avoid high doses of vitamins A, D, E, and K.
- Herbs and herbal products that are sometimes used to promote liver health include: milk thistle (silymarin), astragalus, dandelion, bupleurum, garlic, licorice root, artichoke, thioctic (alpha-lipoic) acid, and ginkgo biloba. All substances, including herbs, can have side effects and may interact with other drugs you are taking, including anti-HIV medications. Talk with your healthcare provider or pharmacist before using and complementary or alternative therapies — including over-the-counter ones.
- Avoid herbs that are known to be toxic to the liver: peppermint, mistletoe, yerba tea, sassafras, germander, chaparral, skull cap, nutmeg, valerian, Jin Bu Juan, comfrey (bush tea), pennyroyal, and tansy ragwortsenna.
- Don't take iron supplements unless advised to by your healthcare provider — too much iron can be hard on the liver.

What is Hepatitis-B ?

Hepatitis B is a serious disease caused by a virus that attacks the liver. The virus, which is called hepatitis B virus (HBV), can cause lifelong infection, cirrhosis (scarring) of the liver, liver cancer, liver failure, and death.

Hepatitis B vaccine is available for all age groups to prevent hepatitis B virus infection.

How do you know if you have hepatitis B?

Only a blood test can tell for sure.

How is HBV spread?

HBV is spread when blood from an infected person enters the body of a person who is not infected. For example, HBV is spread through having sex with an infected person without using a condom (the efficacy of latex condoms in preventing infection with HBV is unknown, but their proper use might reduce transmission), by sharing drugs, needles, or "works" when "shooting" drugs, through needlesticks or sharps exposures on the job, or from an infected mother to her baby during birth.

Hepatitis B is not spread through food or water, sharing eating utensils, breastfeeding, hugging, kissing, coughing, sneezing or by casual contact.

How long does it take for a blood test, such as HBsAg, to be positive after exposure to hepatitis B virus?

HBsAg will be detected in an infected person's blood on the average of 4 weeks (range 1-9 weeks) after exposure to the virus. About 1 out of 2 patients will no longer be infectious by 7 weeks after onset of symptoms and all patients, who do not remain chronically infected, will be HBsAg-negative by 15 weeks after onset of symptoms.

If a person has symptoms, how long does it take for symptoms to occur after exposure to hepatitis B virus?

If symptoms occur, they occur on the average of 12 weeks (range 9-21 weeks) after exposure to hepatitis B virus. Symptoms occur in about 70% of patients. Symptoms are more likely to occur in adults than in children.

What are the symptoms of hepatitis B?

Sometimes a person with HBV infection has no symptoms at all. The older you are, the more apt you are to have symptoms. You might be infected with HBV (and be spreading the virus) and not know it.

If you have symptoms, they might include:

- yellow skin or yellowing of the whites of your eyes (jaundice)
- tiredness
- loss of appetite

- nausea
- abdominal discomfort
- dark urine
- clay-colored bowel movements joint pain

What are the risk factors for hepatitis B?

You are at increased risk of HBV infection if you:

- have sex with someone infected with HBV
- have sex with more than one partner
- shoot drugs
- are a man and have sex with a man
- live in the same house with someone who has chronic (long-term) HBV infection
- have a job that involves contact with human blood
- are a client in a home for the developmentally disabled
- have hemophilia
- travel to areas where hepatitis B is common.

Is there a cure for hepatitis B?

There are no medications available for recently acquired (acute) HBV infection. Hepatitis B vaccine is available for the prevention of HBV infection. There are antiviral drugs available for the treatment of chronic HBV infection.

Can I donate blood if I have had any type of viral hepatitis?

If you had any type of viral hepatitis since aged 11 years, you are not eligible to donate blood. In addition, if you ever tested positive for hepatitis B or hepatitis C, at any age, you are not eligible to donate, even if you were never sick or jaundiced from the infection.

How long can HBV survive outside the body?

HBV can survive outside the body at least 7 days and still be capable of causing infection.

What do you use to remove HBV from environmental surfaces?

You should clean up any blood spills - including dried blood, which can still be infectious - using 1:10 dilution of one part household bleach to 10 parts of water for disinfecting the area.

Who should get vaccinated for Hepatitis-B ?

- All babies, at birth
- All children 0-18 years of age who have not been vaccinated
- People of any age whose behaviour or job puts them at high risk for HBV infection

What are the dosages and schedules for hepatitis B vaccines?

The vaccination schedule most often used for adults and children has been three intramuscular injections, the second and third administered on the 7th and 28th day after the first.

What should be done if there is an interruption between doses of hepatitis B vaccine?

If the vaccination series is interrupted after the first dose, the second dose should be administered as soon as possible. The second and third doses should be separated by an interval of at least 2 months. If only the third dose is delayed, it should be administered when convenient.

Can other vaccines be given at the same time that hepatitis B vaccine is given?

Yes. When hepatitis B vaccine has been administered at the same time as other vaccines, no interference with the antibody response of the other vaccines has been demonstrated.

Are hepatitis B vaccines safe?

Yes. Hepatitis B vaccines have been shown to be safe when administered to both adults and children. Is it harmful to have an extra dose(s) of hepatitis A or hepatitis B vaccine or to repeat the entire hepatitis A or hepatitis B vaccine series if you have forgotten whether or not you had the vaccine or do not have written documentation that was requested?

No. If necessary, getting extra doses of hepatitis A or hepatitis B vaccine is not harmful.

How long does hepatitis B vaccine protect you?

Recent studies indicate that immunologic memory remains intact for at least 23 years and confers protection against clinical illness and chronic HBV infection, even though anti-HBs levels might become low or decline below detectable levels.

Can hepatitis B vaccine be given after exposure to HBV?

Yes. After a person has been exposed to HBV, appropriate treatment, given in an appropriate time frame, can effectively prevent infection. The mainstay of post exposure immunoprophylaxis is hepatitis B vaccine, but in some settings the addition of HBIG will provide some increase in protection.

Should pre-vaccination testing be done?

Pre-vaccination testing is not routinely recommended. Pre-vaccination testing is not indicated for immunization programmes for children or adolescents because of the low rate of HBV infection and the relatively low cost of vaccine.

Who should get post-vaccination testing?

Testing for immunity is advised only for persons whose subsequent clinical management depends on knowledge of their immune status.

When should post-vaccination testing be done?

When necessary, post-vaccination testing, using the anti-HBs test, should be performed 1 to 2 months after completion of the vaccine series – EXCEPT for post-vaccination testing of infants born to HBsAg-positive mothers. Testing of these infants should be performed 3 to 9 months after the completion of the vaccination series

Are booster doses of hepatitis B vaccine needed routinely?

No, booster doses of hepatitis B vaccine are not recommended routinely for persons who are not immune compromised.

Can hepatitis B vaccine be given during pregnancy or when breastfeeding?

Yes, neither pregnancy nor breastfeeding should be considered a contraindication to vaccination of women.

Can hepatitis B vaccine be given to immune compromised people?

Yes, however larger vaccine doses or an increased number of doses are required to induce protective antibody in a high proportion of hemodialysis patients and might also be necessary for other immune compromised people.

Who should not receive the vaccine?

A serious allergic reaction to a prior dose of hepatitis B vaccine or a vaccine component is a contraindication to further doses of hepatitis b vaccine.

What does the term "chronic hepatitis B" mean?

Chronic infection with HBV means that you have a long-term HBV infection; your body did not get rid of the virus when you were first infected with HBV. The risk of progressing to chronic infection is age dependent (i.e., 2% to 6% of people over aged 5 years; 30% of children aged 1-5 years; and up to 90% of infants). People with chronic infection can infect others and are at increased risk of serious liver disease including cirrhosis and liver cancer.

What drugs are used to treat chronic hepatitis B?

There are at least six drugs used for the treatment of people with chronic hepatitis B: Adefovir dipivoxil, interferon alfa-2b, pegylated interferon alfa-2a, lamivudine, entecavir, and telbivudine.

What is the risk of getting HBV infection while traveling in other countries?

The risk of HBV infection for international travelers is generally low, except for certain travelers in countries where the prevalence of chronic HBV infection is high or intermediate (country listing).

Factors to consider in assessing risk include 1) the prevalence of chronic HBV infection in the local population, 2) the extent of direct contact with blood or other body fluids or of sex contact with potentially infected people, and 3) the duration of travel.

Hepatitis-C

What is hepatitis-C ?

Hepatitis C is a blood-borne, infectious, viral disease that is caused by a hepatotropic virus called *Hepatitis C virus* (**HCV**). The infection can cause liver inflammation that is often asymptomatic, but ensuing chronic hepatitis can result later in cirrhosis and liver cancer.

When it was discovered ?

In the mid 1970s, Harvey J. Alter, Chief of the Infectious Disease Section in the Department of Transfusion Medicine at the National Institutes of Health (NIH), USA and his research team demonstrated that most post-transfusion hepatitis cases were not due to hepatitis A and B viruses. In 1987, Michael Houghton, Qui-Lim Choo, and George Kuo at Chiron Corporation utilized molecular cloning to identify the unknown organism. In 1988, the virus was confirmed by Alter by verifying it. In April of 1989, the discovery of the virus, re-named hepatitis C virus, was published in two articles in the journal *Science.*

How is Hepatitis-C transmitted from one person to another

Several activities and practices have been identified as potential sources of exposure to the hepatitis C virus. Anyone who may have been exposed to HCV through one or more of these routes should be screened for hepatitis C.

Sharing of needles and syringes among Injection drug uses

Those who currently or have previously injected drugs are at increased risk for getting hepatitis C because they may be sharing needles or other drug paraphernalia (includes cookers, cotton, spoons, water, etc.), which may be contaminated with HCV-infected blood. An estimated 60% to 80% of all IV drug users in the Manipur have been infected with HCV.

Insuffulated drug use (Drugs which are "snorted")

Researchers have suggested that the transimssion of HCV may be possible through the insuffulation of illegal drugs such as cocaine and crank when straws are shared among users.

Blood products

Blood transfusion, blood products, or organ transplantation prior to implementation of HCV screening in India.

The virus was first isolated in 1989 and reliable tests to screen for the virus were not available until 1992. Therefore, those who received blood or blood products prior to the implementation of screening the blood supply for HCV may have been exposed to the virus. Blood products include clotting factors (taken by hemophiliacs), immuneglobulin, Rhogam, platelets, and plasma.

Iatrogenic medical or dental exposure

People can be exposed to HCV via inadequately or improperly sterilized medical or dental equipment.

Occupational exposure to blood

Medical and dental personnel, first responders (e.g., firefighters, paramedics, emergency medical technicians, law enforcement officers), and military combat personnel can be exposed to HCV through accidental exposure to blood through accidental needlesticks or blood spatter to the eyes. Universal precautions to protect against such accidental exposures significantly reduce the risk of exposure to HCV.

Recreational exposure to blood

Contact sports and other activities that may result in accidental blood-to-blood exposure are potential sources of exposure to HCV.

Sexual exposure to blood

Although HCV is not a sexually transmitted disease (STD), transmission can occur during unprotected sexual contact if the sexual activity involves blood-to-blood contact. It is important to note that the sexual spread of HCV is due to blood-blood contact rather than the presence of the virus in vaginal fluid or semen.

Body piercings and tattoos

Tattooing dyes, ink pots, stylets and piercing implements can transmit HCV-infected blood from one person to another if proper sterilization techniques are not followed. Tattoos or piercings done non-professionally are particularly concerning as sterile techniques in such settings may be lacking.

Shared personal care items

Personal care items such as razors, toothbrushes, cuticle scissors, and other manicuring or pedicuring equipment can easily be contaminated with blood. Sharing such items can potentially lead to exposure to HCV.

HCV is not spread through casual contact such as hugging, kissing, or sharing eating or cooking utensils.

Vertical transmission

Mother-to-child transmission of hepatitis C has been well described, but occurs relatively infrequently. Transmission occurs only among women who are HCV RNA positive at the time of delivery; the risk of transmission in this setting is approximately 6 out of 100. Among women who are both HCV and HIV positive at the time of delivery, the risk of HCV is increased to approximately 25 out of 100.

The risk of vertical transmission of HCV does not appear to be associated with method of delivery or breast feeding.

Epidemiology

Hepatitis C infects an estimated 170 million people worldwide.

Co-infection with HIV

Approximately 350,000, or 35% of patients in the USA infected with HIV are also infected with the hepatitis C virus, mainly because both viruses are blood-borne and present in similar populations. In other countries, co-infection is less common, this is possibly related to differing drug policies. HCV is the leading cause of chronic liver disease in the USA. It has been demonstrated in clinical studies that HIV infection causes a more rapid progression of chronic hepatitis C to cirrhosis and liver failure. This is not to say treatment is not an option for those living with co-infection.

What are the signs and symptoms of Acute Hepatitis C

Acute hepatitis C refers to the first 6 months after infection with HCV. Remarkably, 60% to 70% of people infected develop no symptoms during the acute phase. In the minority of patients who experience acute phase symptoms, they are generally mild and nonspecific, and rarely lead to a specific diagnosis of hepatitis C. Symptoms of acute hepatitis C infection include decreased appetite, fatigue, abdominal pain, jaundice, itching, and flu-like symptoms.

The hepatitis C virus is usually detectable in the blood within one to three weeks after infection, and antibodies to the virus are generally detectable within 3 to 12 weeks. Approximately 20-30% of persons infected with HCV clear the virus from their bodies during the acute phase as shown by normalization in liver function tests (LFTs) such as alanine transaminase (ALT) & aspartate transaminase (AST) normalization, as well as plasma HCV-RNA clearance (this is known as spontaneous viral clearance). The remaining 70-80% of patients infected with HCV develop chronic hepatitis C, i.e., infection lasting more than 6 months.

Previous practice was to not treat acute infections to see if the person would spontaneously clear; recent studies have shown that treatment during the acute phase of genotype 1 infections has a greater than 90% success rate with half the treatment time required for chronic infections, but that the majority of acute hepatitis C is cleared. [5]

What are the signs and symptoms of *Chronic* Hepatitis C

Chronic hepatitis C is defined as infection with the hepatitis C virus persisting for more than six months. Clinically, it is often asymptomatic (without jaundice) and it is mostly discovered accidentally.

The natural course of chronic hepatitis C varies considerably from one person to another. Virtually all people infected with HCV have evidence of inflammation on liver biopsy, however, the rate of progression of liver scarring (fibrosis) shows significant variability among individuals. Recent data suggests that among untreated patients, roughly one-third progress to liver cirrhosis in less than 20 years. Another third progress to cirrhosis within 30 years. The remainder of patients appear to progress so slowly that they are unlikely to develop cirrhosis within their lifetimes. Factors that have been reported to influence the rate of HCV disease progression include age (increasing age associated with more rapid progression), gender (males have more rapid disease progression than females), alcohol consumption (associated with an increased rate of disease progression), HIV coinfection (associated with a markedly increased rate of disease progression), and fatty liver (the presence of fat in liver cells has been associated with an increased rate of disease progression).

Generalized signs and symptoms associated with chronic hepatitis C include fatigue, flu-like symptoms, muscle pain, joint pain, intermittent low-grade fevers, itching, sleep disturbances, abdominal pain (especially in the right upper quadrant), appetite changes, nausea, dyspepsia, cognitive changes, depression, headaches, and mood swings.

Once chronic hepatitis C has progressed to cirrhosis, signs and symptoms may appear that are generally caused by either decreased liver function or increased pressure in the liver circulation, a condition known as portal hypertension. Possible signs and symptoms of liver cirrhosis include ascites (accumulation of fluid in the abdomen), bruising and bleeding tendency, bone pain, varices (enlarged veins, especially in the stomach and esophagus), fatty stools (steatorrhea), jaundice, and a syndrome of cognitive impairment known as hepatic encephalopathy.

Liver function tests show variable elevation of ALAT, AST and GGTP and periodically they might show normal results. Usually prothrombin and albumin results are normal.

Chronic hepatitis C more than other forms of hepatitis is diagnosed because of extrahepatic manifestations associated with the presence of HCV such as thyroiditis (inflammation of the thyroid) with hyperthyreosis or hypothyreosis, porphyria cutanea tarda, cryoglobulinemia (a form of vasculitis)[6] and glomerulonephritis (inflammation of the kidney), specifically membranoproliferative glomerulonephritis (MPGN). Hepatitis C is also associated with sicca syndrome, thrombocytopenia, lichen planus, diabetes mellitus and with B-cell lymphoproliferative disorders.

What is the diagnosis of hepatitis-C

The diagnosis of hepatitis C is rarely made during the acute phase of the disease because the majority of people infected experience no symptoms during this phase of the disease. Chronic hepatitis C may be suspected on the basis of the medical history, a history of tattoos, unexplained symptoms, or abnormal liver enzymes or liver function tests found during routine blood testing. Occasionally, hepatitis C is diagnosed as a result of targeted screening such as blood donation (blood donors are screened for numerous blood-borne diseases including hepatitis C) or contact tracing.

Hepatitis C testing begins with serological blood tests used to detect antibodies to HCV. Anti-HCV antibodies can be detected in 80% of patients within 15 weeks after exposure, in >90% within 5 months after exposure, and in >97% by 6 months after exposure. Overall, HCV antibody tests have a strong positive predictive value for exposure to the hepatitis C virus, but may miss patients who have not yet developed antibodies (seroconversion), or have an insufficient level of antibodies to detect .A small minority of people infected with HCV never develop antibodies to the virus and therefore, never test positive using HCV antibody screening.

Anti-HCV antibodies indicate exposure to the virus, but cannot determine if ongoing infection is present. All persons with positive anti-HCV antibody tests must undergo additional testing for the presence of the hepatitis C virus itself to determine whether current infection is present. The presence of the virus is tested for using molecular nucleic acid testing methods such as polymerase chain reaction (PCR), transcription mediated amplification (TMA), or branched DNA (b-DNA). All HCV nucleic acid molecular tests have the capacity to detect not only whether the virus is present, but also to measure the amount of virus present in the blood (the HCV viral load).

In people with confirmed HCV infection, genotype testing is generally recommended. There are six major genotypes of the hepatitis C virus, which are indicated numerically (e.g., genotype 1, genotype 2, etc.). HCV genotype testing is used to determine the required length and potential response to interferon-based therapy.

Prevention

The following guidelines may be most, but not least, effective way of preventing the disease

- Avoid unprotected sex
- Avoid sharing drug needles

- Avoid unsanitary tattoo methods
- Avoid unsanitary body piercing methods and acupuncture.
- Avoid needlestick injury
- Avoid sharing grooming utensils
- Avoid sharing personal items such as toothbrushes, razors, and nail clippers with an infected person

Treatment and prognosis

There is a very small chance of clearing the virus spontaneously (0.5 to 0.74% per year), and the majority of patients with chronic hepatitis C will not clear it without treatment.

Current treatment is a combination of (pegylated) interferon alpha (brand names Pegasys and PEG-Intron) and the antiviral drug ribavirin for a period of 24 or 48 weeks, depending on genotype. Indications for treatment include patients with proven hepatitis C virus infection and persistent abnormal liver function tests. Sustained cure rates (sustained viral response) of 75% or better occur in people with genotypes HCV 2 and 3 in 24 weeks of treatment, about 50% in those with genotype 1 with 48 weeks of treatment and 65% for those with genotype 4 in 48 weeks of treatment.

Treatment during the acute infection phase has much higher success rates (greater than 90%) with a shorter duration of treatment (but balance this against the 80% chance of spontaneous clearance without treatment).

Current combination therapy should be usually supervised by physicians in the fields of gastroenterology, hepatology or infectious disease.

In addition to the standard treatment with interferon and ribavirin, several studies have shown higher success rates when the antiviral drug amantadine (Symmetrel) is added to the regimen. Sometimes called "triple therapy", it involves the addition of 100mg of amantadine twice a day. Current guidelines strongly recommend that hepatitis C patients be vaccinated for hepatitis A and B if they have not yet been exposed to these viruses, as this would radically worsen their liver disease.

Alcoholic beverage consumption accelerates HCV associated fibrosis and cirrhosis, and makes liver cancer more likely; insulin resistance and metabolic syndrome may similarly worsen the hepatic prognosis.

During pregnancy and breastfeeding

If a pregnant woman has risk factors for hepatitis C, she should be tested for antibodies against HCV. About four out of every hundred infants born to HCV infected women become infected. The virus is spread to the baby at the time of birth. There is no treatment that can prevent this from happening.

In a mother that also has HIV, the rate of transmission can be as high as 19%. There is currently no data to determine whether antiviral therapy reduces perinatal transmission. Ribavirin and interferons are contraindicated during pregnancy. However, avoiding fetal scalp monitoring and prolonged labor after rupture of membranes may reduce the risk of transmission to the infant.

HCV antibodies from the mother may persist in infants until 15 months of age. If an early diagnosis is desired, testing for HCV RNA can be performed between the ages of 2 and 6 months, with a repeat test done independent of the first test result. If a later diagnosis is preferred, an anti-HCV test can performed after 15 months of age. Most infants infected with HCV at the time of birth have no symptoms and do well during childhood. There is no evidence that breast-feeding spreads HCV. To be cautious, an infected mother could avoid breastfeeding if her nipples are cracked and bleeding.

Alternative therapies

Several "alternative therapies" purport to reduce the liver's duties, rather than treat the virus itself, thereby slowing the course of the disease or keeping the quality of life of the person. As an example, extract of Silybum marianum and licorice are sold for their HCV related effects; the first is said to provide some generic help to hepatic functions, and the second to have a mild antiviral effect and to raise blood pressure. It is important to note that the current standard of treatment with pegylated-interferon and ribavirin is unsurpassed in its ability to control HCV replication.

9

Nutrition and ART

The introduction of highly active antiretroviral therapy (HAART) with the use of protease inhibitors (PIs) has resulted in significant reductions in morbidity and mortality from HIV infection in recent years. Although initial strong enthusiasm for HAART led to its widespread use early in HIV infection, practitioners have now become more cautious in early initiation of HAART in light of reports concerning serious and potentially irreversible toxicities associated with numerous antiretroviral drugs These toxicities include the development of diabetes mellitus, insulin resistance (IR) , hyperlipidemia, lipodystrophy, and lactic acidosis

Although Anti-retroviral drugs (ARVs) do not completely destroy HIV, they significantly reduce the replication of the virus in the blood, which slows down progression of the disease to AIDS.

ARVs and Breastfeeding

Breastfeeding is strongly encouraged and commonly practiced in resource limited settings, including by HIV positive women. WHO recommends that: "When replacement feeding is acceptable, feasible, affordable, sustainable, and safe, avoidance of all breastfeeding by HIV-infected mothers is recommended. Otherwise, exclusive breastfeeding is recommended during the first months of life. To minimize HIV transmission risk, breastfeeding should be discontinuedas soon as feasible, taking into account local circumstances, the individual woman's situation, and the risks of replacement feeding including infections other than HIV and malnutrition." Since some ARVs can affect fat metabolism, the effects of ARVs on breastmilk composition are not known. These effects may have implications for the health of infants as well as the health of HIV-positive mothers taking ARVs.

Modern medications can interact with food in four major ways . Proper dietary management interventions can help manage some of these negative effects and can help PLWHAs maintain adequate food intake and compensate for affected nutrients.

Types of Food-Medication Interactions Nutritional Issues Associated with ARVs and Other Modern Medications

1. Food (affects) medication efficacy absorption, metabolism efficiency distribution, excretion.
2. Medication (affects) nutrient absorption, metabolism, distribution, excretion.
3. Medication side effects (affects) food consumption, nutrient absorption.
4. Medication + certain foods (creates) unhealthy side effects.

Food Affects Medication Efficacy

Food can enhance or inhibit the absorption, metabolism, distribution, and excretion of medication and, therefore, affect the medication's efficacy. This type of interaction varies from drug to drug and requires tailored dietary responses, which can improve the efficacy of the drug as well as encourage clients to adhere to the prescribed drug regimen. For example:

- Food reduces the absorption of Isoniazid, which is used to treat TB, a common opportunistic infection. Therefore, Isoniazid should be taken at least one hour before or two hours after a meal.
- Rifampin is also used to treat TB and, like Isoniazid, its absorption is reduced by food. Rifampin should be taken one or two hours after a meal to increase the drug's absorption.

Food enhances absorption or metabolism of some ARVs and inhibits absorption or metabolism of others. For example, a high calorie, high fat, high protein meal decreases absorption of the protease inhibitor Indinavir. A high fat meal increases the bioavailability of Tenofovir and reduces the absorption of Zidovidune. Zidovidune should not be taken with high fat meals (i.e., more than 40 g of fat or three tablespoons of margarine or oil).

Medication Effects on Nutrient Absorption, Metabolism, Distribution, and Excretion

Certain modern medications can affect health and nutritional outcome by inhibiting or enhancing nutrient absorption, metabolism, and excretion. Dietary management may require nutrient supplements or increased food intake, if there is a need to compensate for a depleted nutrient.

Rifampin may increase vitamin D metabolism, resulting in weakened bones. Therefore, vitamin D supplementation may be required. Treatment of TB should be accompanied by a vitamin B6 or vitamin D supplement, depending on the type of antibiotic used. Some ARVs can lead to lipodystrophy syndrome or fat maldistribution, which is characterized by either fat accumulation (e.g.,breasts, upper back, visceral fat) or fat loss (e.g., face, extremities). Depending on the ARV drug, patients may experience changes in fat distribution in the body and levels of triglicerides and cholesterol in the blood. It is important to maintain a healthy weight, eat a variety of foods, reduce intake of refined sugar and excessive carbohydrates, increase intake of fibre, avoid alcoholic beverages and smoking, exercise regularly, and take medications to lower harmful fats in the blood. The effective management of lipodystrophy syndrome has not yet been established. Potential approaches include diet and exercise, use of medications, and change in the ARV regimen. Some protease inhibitors, such as Indinavir, may affect glucose or sugar metabolism and cause insulin resistance. Insulin resistance is associated with increased risk of diabetes. In case of diabetes, a specific carbohydrate controlled diet, reduced intake of refined sugar and saturated fat, exercise, and anti-diabetic medications are recommended.

The Side Effects of Modern Medications

Modern medications may have side effects that affect food intake and nutrient absorption. Many of these side effects may be managed by dietary responses. Proper nutritional management of these side effects will contribute to improved adherence to the regimen. When not properly managed, side effects of medications often lead to the interruption of treatment and contribute to poor adherence. Health workers and counsellors should provide clients with dietary guidance that is specific to local situations. Side effects of medication, such as taste changes, loss of appetite (i.e., anorexia), nausea, bloating, heartburn, constipation, vomiting, and diarrhoea, indirectly affect nutritional status by causing a reduction in food intake or nutrient absorption. Reduced food intake and poor nutrient absorption can lead to weight loss and continuing impairment of the immune system, which, in turn, allows HIV to more quickly progress to AIDS. Dietary management of these side effects can help maintain food intake, compensate for nutrient losses, and prevent weight loss. Some side effects of medications can be similar to certain AIDS-related symptoms and call for similar dietary management. (See Chapter 11 Nutrition Side effects and coping with complications of HIV/AIDS)

Multiple Medications

Treatment of AIDS may require taking many pills on a daily basis, which can make it difficult to maintain food intake. If medications make it difficult to eat, a person is less likely to strictly adhere to the drug regimen, which can create drug resistance, especially in the case of ARVs. It is vital that health workers explain the necessity of healthy eating to the furthest extent possible, while also adhering to the drug regimen. Multiple medications have multiple food-drug interactions and side effects that require setting specific timing, identifying recommended foods, and avoided foods for each drug. Health workers should spend enough time with the PLWHAs, to list all the drugs taken and counsel on the dietary management of the side effects and the interactions with food.

Drug-Drug Interactions

Drug interactions need to be managed adequately in order to ensure that the prescribed drug combination does not diminish drug efficacy, increase side effects, and affect nutritional status. For example, the ARV Didanosine reacts with antacid medications containing magnesium and aluminium, leading to increased side effects of Didanosine. Therefore, Didanosine should not be taken at the same time with the antacid medications containing magnesium and aluminium.

Medication and Food Can Cause Unhealthy Side Effects

The combination of some medications and food can create unhealthy side effects or reduce the positive impacts of the drugs.

Rifampin : Treatment of TB-Should be taken on an empty stomach one hour before or two hours after meals. May cause Nausea, vomiting, diarrhoea, loss of appetite

Isoniazid TB treatment- Food reduces absorption of Isoniazid. Do not take Isoniazid during meals. Take one hour before or two hours after meals. May affect vitamin B6 metabolism Daily consumption of food sources of vitamin B6 such as white beans, maize avocado, meat, and fish, or vitamin B6 (25 to 50 mg daily) supplementation is recommended .Increased risk of hepatitis when combined with alcohol Avoid alcohol. For anorexia (i.e., loss of appetite) eat small and frequent meals. Eat favourite foods. For diarrhoea -drink plenty of fluids and eat energy- and nutrient -rich food. Avoid fried foods.

Quinine Treatment of malaria-to be taken with food. May cause abdominal or stomach pain, diarrhoea, nausea, vomiting; lower blood sugar

Sulfadoxine and Pyrimethamine (Fansidar ®) Treatment of malaria Pyrimethamine is also used to treat toxoplasmosis. To be taken with food and consume large quantities of water. Supplement daily with folinic acid (leucovorin), the active form of folate (5-10 mg/ day) May cause diarrhoea , vomiting , taste loss and not recommended if folate deficient; not recommended for breastfeeding women.

Chloroquine Treatment of malaria –to be taken with food. May cause stomach pain, loss of appetite, nausea, vomiting; not recommended for breastfeeding women

Fluconazole : Treatment of thrush –to be taken with food Nausea, vomiting, diarrhoea; can be used during breastfeeding

Nystatin ® Treatment ofthrush : to be taken with food Infrequent occurrence of diarrhoea, vomiting, nausea

Antiretroviral drugs

Abacavir (ABC)

NNRTI

Antiretroviral Can be taken without regard to food. May cause nausea, vomiting, fever, allergic reaction, anorexia, abdominal pain, diarrhoea, anaemia, rash, hypotension, pancreatitis, dyspnoea, weakness and insomnia, cough, headache

Didanosine (ddl)

NNRTI

Antiretroviral- Take one hour before or two hours after eating with water only May cause anorexia, diarrhoea, nausea, vomiting, pain, headache, weakness, insomnia, rash, dry mouth, lost of taste, constipation, stomatitis, anaemia, fever, dizziness, pancreatitis; do not take with antacid containing aluminium or magnesium

Lamivudine (3TC)

NNRTI

Antiretroviral . Can be taken without regard to food. May cause nausea, vomiting, headache, dizziness, diarrhoea, abdominal pain, nasal symptoms, cough, fatigue, pancreatitis, anaemia, insomnia, muscle pain, and rash

Stavudine (d4T)

NNRTI

Antiretroviral- Can be taken without regard to food Limit alcohol . May cause nausea, vomiting, diarrhoea, peripheral neuropathy, chills and fever, anorexia, stomatitis, diarrhoea, anaemia, headaches, rash, bone marrow, and Pancreatitis

Tenefovir (TDF)

NNRTI

Antiretroviral-to be taken with food. Limit Alcohol. May cause abdominal pain, headache, fatigue, and dizziness.

Zidovudine (AZT)
NNRTI
Antiretroviral -Can may cause be taken with food, but do not take with a high fat meal Alcohol Anorexia, anaemia, nausea, vomiting, bone marrow suppression, headache, fatigue, constipation, fever dizziness, dyspnoea, insomnia, muscle pain, rash

Efavirenz
NRTI
Antiretroviral- Can be taken with food, but do not take with a high fat meal Limit Alcohol. May cause elevated blood cholesterol, levels, elevated triglycerides levels, rash, dizziness, anorexia, nausea, vomiting, diarrhoea, dyspepsia, abdominal pain, flatulence

Nevirapine (NVP)
NRTI
Antiretroviral-Can be taken without regard to food. May cause nausea, vomiting rash, fever, headache, skin reactions, fatigue, stomatitis, abdominal pain, drowsiness, paraesthesia; high hepatoxicity

Medication Purpose Nutrition
Indinavir (IDV)
PI
Antiretroviral -Take the drug one hour before or two hours after meal; drink at least 1,500 mL of water. May cause nausea, abdominal pain, headache, kidney stones, taste changes, vomiting, vomiting, diarrhoea, insomnia, ascites, weakness, dizziness; may increase the risk of lipodystrophy; do not consume grape fruit as it may lower the level of medicine in the blood

Lopinavir
PI
Antiretroviral- Can be taken without regard to ,food . May cause abdominal pain, diarrhoea, headaches, , weakness, nausea; may increase the risk of lipodystrophy and or diabetes

Nelfinavir
PI
Antiretroviral -Take with meal or light snack . May cause diarrhoea, flatulence, nausea, abdominal pain, rash; may increase the risk of lipodystrophy

Ritonavir

PI

Antiretroviral -Take with meal. May cause nausea, vomiting, diarrhoea, hepatitis, jaundice, weakness, anorexia, abdominal pain, fever, diabetes, headache, dizziness; may increase the risk of Lipodystrophy

Saquinavir

PI

Antiretroviral -Take with meal or light snack; take within two hours of a high fat meal and high calcium Meal Garlic supplements. May cause mouth ulceration, taste changes, nausea, vomiting, abdominal pain, diarrhoea, constipation, flatulence, weakness rash, headache; may increase the risk of lipodystrophy

What should a person taking ARV treatment do about food?

As for any person with HIV, someone taking ARV treatment should, as far as possible, eat a balanced diet. That means food that includes plenty of green vegetables, proteins, starches and fruit. Some fat is also necessary in the diet to help maintain health and to assist in absorbing some ARVs into the body . A person taking ARVs should seek advice from a support group, health worker or nutritionist to work out the best diet possible within their resources.

How does ARV treatment affect a person's eating?

- If a person is tired and lacks the energy to prepare meals, they might not eat enough of the right foods. If this happens, they should try to get support, from their family, friends or home based care worker.
- Several ARV drugs cause side effects that affect a person's ability to eat. Some of these effects might disappear quickly, but others might last a long time.
- If any side effects continue for a long time, a person should see their doctor or health worker. This is because the effects might be due to another health problem or require a change in the ARV treatment.
- Often, a person can take simple actions to combat the side effects of ARVs. For example:

How do ARV treatment and food interact?

- Different ARVs interact with food in different ways.
- Some ARVs must be taken with meals which contain some fat, because this makes them more effective. Some others must be taken before meals so that they are absorbed quickly before food gets in the way. Others have to be taken after meals because they can irritate the stomach. For some drugs, it does not matter.

Gas and Bloating and stomach pains
What is it?

Due to difficulties in digestion, gas (wind) develops in the gut. This causes:

- bloating, which is swelling of the abdomen and/or stomach;
- sharp 'griping' pains in the abdomen

Which ARVs can cause it?

Bloating and wind: protease inhibitors, especially Indinavir or Nelfinavir.

Stomach pains: Zidovudine, protease inhibitors at the start of treatment.

What should a person do?

For bloating and wind:

- Ask their doctor for advice.
- Drugs which alleviate bloating and gas can reduce absorption of other drugs in the intestine and reduce their effectiveness. So, they are not always recommended.

For stomach pains:

- Take antispasmodic drugs in early stages of ARV treatment, especially if using protease inhibitors.
- If strong pains suddenly occur during a treatment that is well tolerated, inform their doctor immediately.

How can a person prevent or reduce these effects?

For bloating and wind:

- Identify and avoid foods and drinks that make bloating worse (e.g. cabbage, onions, peppers, chillies, carbonated drinks, coffee, alcohol, very spicy food and, sometimes, milk).

- Eat while sitting down.
- Chew food well.
- If possible, take physical exercise, especially walking.

Diarrhoea - What is it? Some ARVs can stimulate the gut to move too quickly, resulting in diarrhoea

Which ARVs can cause it? Didanosine (tablets in particular), Nelfinavir, Indinavir. Diarrhoea is common at the start of ARV treatment, but it disappears after some weeks. It might continue when taking a drug such as Nelfinavir. Some opportunistic infections or HIV itself can also cause diarrhoea. If diarrhoes persists, consult a doctor.

What should a person do?

- Treat diarrhoea quickly, because it can cause dehydration. It can also cause loss of weight and loss of important nutrients from the body.
- If the diarrhoea happens when starting ARV treatment, use anti-diarrhoea medicine to stop it, such as loperamide. Such medicines should not be used for more than 3 days without consulting a doctor.
- If the diarrhoea continues even when taking anti-diarrhoea medicine, it might be caused by an infection, so a doctor might prescribe antibiotics.
- If an ARV causes persistent diarrhoea which cannot be controlled, a doctor might decide to change the ARV treatment.

How can a person prevent or reduce these effects?

- Drink 2-3 litres of liquids during the day. Have soups, and unchilled sugared carbonated drinks (sodas), because these will help to replace the minerals lost through diarrhoea. (Open soda some minutes before drinking to allow gas to escape,).· Avoid large amounts of tea, coffee, alcohol and milk, which make food pass more quickly through the gut.· Avoid fats and sugary foods.· Eat helpful foods such as oats, yoghurt, bananas, rice, rice water, cooked carrots.

Dry Mouth or Change in taste -What is it? Producing saliva is important for making it easier to chew food and to protect teeth from decay. A bad taste in the mouth can discourage eating.

Which ARVs can cause it? Dry mouth: Several drugs, including ARVs, can cause a decrease in the production of saliva. This increases the risk of tooth decay

Change in taste: ARVS, especially protease inhibitors, can sometimes change a person's ability to taste and give the impression of having a bad taste in the mouth.

What should a person do?

- For a dry mouth, consult the doctor – who might be able to prescribe a drug to increase secretion of saliva.

How can a person prevent or reduce these effects? For a dry mouth:

- Chew chewing gum to stimulate the production of saliva.
- Drink water frequently.

For change in taste:

- Eat menthol sweets or chew gum to change the taste in the mouth.

Loss of Appetite - What is it? A person on ARVs should eat properly, to recover quickly and make treatment work well.

Which ARVs can cause it? Loss of appetite can be caused by several ARVs, especially when starting or changing treatment.It can also happen if a person is depressed or has pains in the mouth which make it hard to eat.

What should a person do?

- Check with the doctor to find out if the loss of appetite might be due to the drugs that the person is taking
- Talk to a counsellor if depressed
- Do not stop taking ARVs

How can a person prevent or reduce these effects?

- Chose tasty food for a balanced diet.
- Avoid sweets and coffee.
- Eat smaller, more frequent, meals.

Nausea or Vomiting - What is it? Nausea and vomiting are common signs of illness or disturbance in the body. They can be caused by food, anxiety, or some medicines.

Which ARVs can cause it? Zidovudine, Combivir, Didanosine (caplets in particular), Indinavir, Nelfinavir.

What should a person do?

- Ask the doctor for advice.
- The doctor might prescribe anti-nausea medication such as metoclopramide. It is important not to take such drugs without advice and not to take more than prescribed.
- Do not take Prepulsid (an anti-nauseant) with protease inhibitors (Indinavir, Nelfinavir).

How can a person prevent or reduce these effects?

- Drink several mouthfuls of cold carbonated drink or lemon water in the morning when waking and before meals.
- Drink mint tea, or boiling water containing a small piece of peeled ginger.
- Eat small but more frequent meals.
- Eat more cold than hot meals.
- Avoid spicy or fatty foods.

- Limit consumption of coffee, cigarettes and alcohol.
- Do not go to bed immediately after eating.
- Keep a few dry biscuits next to the bed and eat one or two before getting up in the morning.

NB. If vomiting occurs some hours after taking a dose, do not repeat that that dose again - just take the next dose at the correct time.

Hepatic Problems - What is it? Inflammation and other disorders in the liver. Symptoms can include:

- Increase in transaminase enzymes in the blood.
- In severe cases, jaundice.

Which ARVs can cause it? Many drugs can affect the function of the liver. These include ARVs, especially Nevirapine and Efavirenz. The function of the liver is also affected by some natural or traditional medicines, excessive alcohol and the hepatitis viruses (A, B, C, etc).

What should a person do?

- Ensure that their doctor takes regular liver tests, usually at the start of treatment and at the same time as checking the CD4 count.
- The patient must always inform the doctor if they are taking any other medication, including traditional remedies, as these can also affect the liver.
- If the person has a hepatitis virus, regular blood tests must be done to monitor the liver.
- If the level of transaminase enzymes increases too much, the doctor may decide to halt a treatment and prescribe another.

How can a person prevent or reduce these effects? it?

Healthy eating and drinking is essential for having a healthy liver:

- Avoid too much alcohol, smoking or fatty foods
- Do not take other medications when taking ARVs unless the doctor has said it is alright

Kidney Stones - What is it?<0}

Small stones formed from crystals, which develop inside the kidneys.Symptoms can include:

- Intense pain in the base of the spine that irradiates towards the bladder.
- Blood in the urine.

Which ARVs can cause it?

Indinavir is removed from the body through the kidneys - where it sometimes forms stones.

What should a person do?

- Consult the doctor.
- The doctor might prescribe an antispasmodic drug such as Buscopan and a pain-killer, usually an anti-inflammatory.

How can a person prevent or reduce these effects?

- Drink 2-3 litres of water or other liquids per day, starting with 3-4 glasses during the half-hour following each dose of Indinavir. This can be any liquid – except alcohol, coffee, tea and milk which can cause other problems.
- Avoid drinking more than the recommended amount, because this might cause loss of nutrients from the body through the urine.

How can a person prevent or reduce these effects?

A serious disorder of the blood. Effects can include:

- Immense tiredness without any particular reason.
- Sudden loss of weight.
- Digestive problems: nausea, vomiting, loss of appetite.

- Muscular weakness or repeated cramps.
- Stomach pains.
- Breathlessness.

Which ARVs can cause it?
Stavudine, Didanosine, Combivir, Zidovudine, Lamivudine.

It can occur several months or years after first taking ARV treatment.

What should a person do?

- Consult the doctor as soon as possible, especially if treatment has been tolerated well so far.
- The doctor will order a blood test to measure the level of lactate in their blood. If it is abnormally high, it can mean lactic acidosis.
- If this is the case, the person must be admitted to hospital and ARV treatment must stop immediately. Treatment can be started with different drugs later, after the person recovers

How can a person prevent or reduce these effects?
This is an unexpected and rare side effect. There are no known methods of preventing or foreseeing it.

Pancreatitis- What is it?<0}
An inflammation of the pancreas - which is important for digesting fats and proteins. It can cause a serious infection. Symptoms can include:

- Strong pains in the stomach or back which start suddenly.
- Diarrhoea.
- Nausea.
- Vomiting

Which ARVs can cause it?
Didanosine

What should a person do?

- Inform the doctor immediately.
- The doctor will usually take a blood test to measure amylase and lipase.

These are enzymes that increase when the pancreas is infected. If there is risk of infection, antibiotics will be prescribed

How can a person prevent or reduce these effects?

When recovering from pancreatitis:

- Avoid fatty foods
- Avoid alcohol

Lipodystrophy or lipoatrophy- What is it?<0}

Lipodystrophy is excess fat, which can occur in different places on the body: chest (with women in particular), stomach and neck.Lipoatrophy is loss of fat: This can affect the limbs, buttocks and face.

Which ARVs can cause it?

Excess fat is mainly caused by protease inhibitors: Indinavir, Nelfinavir, etc.

Loss of fat: is mainly due to nucleosides (Combivir, Lamivudine, Zidovudine, Didanosine, Stavudine).

These problems can appear after several months or several years of treatment.

What should a person do?

Talk to the HIV doctor. Changing treatment can sometimes reverse the changes

How can a person prevent or reduce these effects?

- Exercise when possible.
- Maintain a balanced diet and avoid becoming overweight.
- Avoid smoking and alcohol

Muscle pains and weaknessWhat is it?<0}

Cramps or weakness in leg muscles.

Which ARVs can cause it?

Zidovudine (AZT) and Combivir which decrease the amount of fat in the blood and can damage muscle cells.

What should a person do?

- Take magnesium – to limit the effects of cramps.
- If muscle weakness progresses rapidly or cramps happen very often, along with tiredness, breathlessness or stomach pains, consult the doctor

urgently – as there is a risk of lactic acidosis.

How can a person prevent or reduce these effects?

- Take regular, gentle exercise
- If cramps happen, massage the muscle to relax it.

Peripheral NeuropathyWhat is it?<0}

These are problems of the nervous system. Symptoms can include abnormal sensations or pain in the feet, tingling, sensations of burning or strange feelings in the legs or feet.

Which ARVs can cause it?

Didanosine, Stavudine and, on rare occasions, Lamivudine.

Anti-tuberculosis drugs, the HIV virus itself, or dietary deficiencies, can cause neuropathies.

Neuropathies can appear several weeks, months or even years after first taking ARV treatment.

What should a person do?

- Consult their doctor immediately,
- For moderate pain, the doctor might prescribe anti-inflammatory drugs such as ibuprofen or indometacin.
- For serious nerve pain, the doctor might prescribe an anti-depressant or anticonvulsant which can also control pain.
- Use complementary treatments, such as: B vitamins, magnesium, calcium; massage.

How can a person prevent or reduce these effects?

- Soak the affected foot in very cold water.
- Ensure shoes are not too tight.
- Do not stand or walk for long periods - take regular rests.

TirednessWhat is it?<0}

This is a general feeling of lack of energy that can occur even after a long rest. The symptoms often include feeling 'drained' during the day. It can last several days or even longer.

Which ARVs can cause it?	ARVs can cause tiredness, particularly at the start of treatment. It takes about one month for the body to get used to the drugs.If tiredness occurs or increases during a treatment that is well tolerated, it is necessary to consult a doctor.
What should a person do?	· Inform their doctor. · In some cases, the doctor might prescribe vitamins A, B, C and E, as well as magnesium, calcium and selenium. These must never be taken in very large quantities or they will cause problems.
How can a person prevent or reduce these effects?	· Rest, but do not sleep more than normally needed. · Try to maintain a balanced diet, with enough vitamins (e.g. from fresh fruit and vegetables). · Avoid coffee and tea in large quantities, as well as alcohol. · Exercise when possible.
Sexual problemsWhat is it?	Loss of sexual desire. Failure to achieve or maintain an erection for men and difficulty in reaching orgasm for women.
Which ARVs can cause it?	Many people on triple therapy have experienced such problems, although it is not known exactly why it happens.There might also be other causes. These include: tiredness, stress, depression, alcohol, smoking and drug use.
What should a person do?	· A man with impotence might choose to take Viagra.
How can a person prevent or reduce these effects?	· Speak to a specialist in sexual issues, such as a psychologist or urologist. · Eat well and get enough rest · Reduce alcohol, tobacco or drug use

SleeplessnessWhat is it?<0}	Difficulty falling asleep, or waking in the night and failing to go back to sleep
Which ARVs can cause it?	Efavirenz, especially at the start of treatment.Sleeplessness might also be due to a many other causes: · stress or depression, · stimulants such as caffeine, tobacco or alcohol, · anxiety about living with HIV or starting or changing treatment, · other problems not linked to HIV.
What should a person do?	· Inform the doctor. · The doctor might decide to prescribe sleeping tablets (to help with sleep) or tranquillisers (drugs to combat anxiety). The choice must take into account possible interactions with ARVs.
How can a person prevent or reduce these effects?	· Do not sleep longer than needed. · Go to bed and get up at set times, because an irregular life can make insomnia worse. · Exercise every day, preferably soon after getting up from bed. · Have smaller meals in the evening so that the stomach is not full when going to bed · Reduce or cut out stimulants, such as tea, coffee, alcohol and cigarettes. For example, drink herbal tea in the evening. · Try to sit and relax before going to bed. · If possible, create an area of calm in the home.

Dark blotches, purplish marks, spots, allergic rashes on the skin - What is it?	Marks which appear on the skin after starting ARV treatment
Which ARVs can cause it?	Red blotches, purplish marks and spots: Efavirenz, Nevirapine and Delavirdine. These generally appear about two weeks after the start of treatment. Allergic reaction on the skin: Nevirapine. This usually appears two to three weeks after starting treatment.
What should a person do?	For red blotches, purplish marks and spots: Inform the doctor – this type of skin problem can be the result of many other cause as well as HIV or ARV drugs. For allergic rashes on the skin: · Inform the doctor. · This usually disappears and ARV treatment does not need to be stopped. · In some cases, the doctor might decide to stop Nevirapine and start a different ARV instead. · For the first two weeks of using Nevirapine, it is vital to take just one 200 mg dose. Then, if there are no negative reactions, the doctor will increase the dose to two tablets per day.
How can a person prevent or reduce these effects?	For dark blotches, purplish marks and spots: · It is not usually necessary to use any medication · If the doctor thinks there is infection, an antibiotic might be prescribed.

	For allergic reaction on the skin: · Itching can be relieved by using calamine or some other calming lotion on the skin
Other skin, hair or nail problemsWhat is it?	Changes in the texture and colour of the skin, hair and finger or toe nails, which can appear some time after starting ARV treatment
Which ARVs can cause it?	Indinavir can cause several problems such as: · Dry skin. · Chapped (sore) lips. · Change in the texture of head and body hair. · Loss of body hair. · Inflammation around the nails (whitlow). · In-growing nails. (whitlow).
What should a person do?	· Inform the doctor. The changes might also be caused by the HIV virus itself, or other factors. · If the problems are very significant and continue for a long time, the doctor might decide to stop prescribing Indinavir.
How can a person prevent or reduce these effects?	For dry skin and cracked or sore lips: · Keep the skin hydrated and keep the lips lubricated. · Use shea butter on the skin.

Limited Access to Sufficient Food for PLWHAs

Due to the scarcity of food in many resource limited settings, people with HIV/AIDS may be unable to manage the effects of food-medication interactions. Health workers should involve PLWHAs in identifying feasible options for the nutritional management of food and drug interactions, which may also contribute to maintaining drug adherence by generating ownership and interest in the continuation of the treatment. Food insecurity is aggravated by the economic consequences of HIV/AIDS, such as loss of earnings of a sick household member, depletion of assets and savings in order to pay for healthcare, or reduced availability of household labour to produce food.

Stigma and Discrimination Faced by PLWHAs

The stigma directed at PLWHAs can cause anxiety and depression in affected individuals, which is may cause a reduction in appetite and food intake. Stigma can also create additional obstacles and challenges for HIV-infected people trying to follow recommended feeding practices. Involving HIV-positive people in the programme design and implementation has been shown to reduce stigma and engage communities.

Impact of Antiretroviral Treatment on Wasting :

While effective antiretroviral therapy has dramatically reduced the incidence of severe wasting, moderate weight loss is still a prominent feature of HIV disease. Recent data suggest that participants taking HAART were more likely to experiencing wasting than those not receiving anti-HIV treatment (86% vs 67%).

Lipoatrophy

Research evidence suggests that fat maldistribution may be related to use of protease inhibitors, nonnucleoside reverse transcriptase inhibitors, or a combination of these two classes of drugs. To date there have been no remedies for the loss of subcutaneous fat, but recent evidence has suggested that discontinuation of Stavudine or Zidovudine therapy may be associated with limited restoration of extremity fat. For fat accumulation, a number of strategies have been attempted, including treatment with human growth hormone, androgens, or metformin, and changes in diet and exercise. It is expected that the cornerstone of management, especially in the presence of central obesity, dyslipidemia, and insulin resistance, will include a diet low in saturated fat, with low-glycemic index carbohydrates, and high in fibre.

Initial reports of fat maldistribution suggested that these changes were related to use of PIs. The use of PIs also increases the probability of intra-abdominal fat accumulation.

Cross-sectional studies also suggest that the NRTIs may be causally related to changes in body habitus, possibly by causing mutations in the mitochondrial DNA polymerase gamma gene and thus adversely affecting mitochondrial oxidative phosphorylation Length of therapy with NRTIs may also increase the risk for fat loss. Finally, dual NRTI therapy is more likely to cause fat wasting than is therapy with a single NRTI .

Combination antiretroviral therapy. It is also possible that NRTI and PIs together contribute to abnormalities in fat distribution. Indeed, PI therapy combined with dual NRTIs resulted in faster lipoatrophy than therapy with dual NRTIs, whereas PI therapy per se did not exert a strong independent risk for fat loss.

Rather than dramatic whole-body weight loss, today many HIV positive people on HAART experience lipoatrophy, or fat loss in the face, limbs, and buttocks. Paradoxically, this may coincide with fat accumulation in other areas of the body . Lipoatrophy is most strongly associated with use of nucleoside reverse transcriptase inhibitors (NRTIs), especially d4T (stavudine or Zerit).

Diet and exercise: The cornerstone of management for central fat accumulation should be diet and exercise. The goal is to decrease intake of saturated fat and excess caloric energy. Aerobic exercise is expected to augment the effects of dietary change because intra-abdominal fat (mesenteric and omental adipose tissue) is metabolically more active than peripheral fat in responding to lipolytic stimuli, such as increases in epinephrine with exercise. In persons without HIV, intensive aerobic exercise can decrease intra-abdominal adipose tissue by 17%20%. In addition, aerobic exercise increases peripheral glucose disposal in obese persons, even in the absence of weight loss, and should be beneficial for subjects with insulin resistance. A recent report suggests that an aerobic exercise programme with a moderate-fat, lowglycemic-index, high-fiber diet can reverse aspects of lipodystrophy.

Insulin and Carbohydrate Dysregulation

Patients with human immunodeficiency virus receiving highly active antiretroviral therapy (HAART) may experience abnormal body composition changes as well as metabolic abnormalities, including dyslipidemia, increases in triglycerides, low high-density lipoprotein cholesterol levels, and abnormal carbohydrate metabolism, ranging from insulin resistance(IR) with and without glucose intolerance to frank diabetes. The use of HAART with and without therapy with protease inhibitors (PIs) is related to carbohydrate abnormalities and changes in body composition. Regimens that include PIs appear to have a higher incidence of insulin resistance (up to 90%) and diabetes mellitus (up to 40%).

Existing data suggest that patients receiving therapy with PIs have a greater incidence of insulin resistance (IR) (30%-90%) than patients receiving nonPI-containing regimens (up to 20%).

Diet and exercise, mainstays of therapy for type 2 diabetes mellitus, are also appropriate for HIV-related IR and diabetes. Diet should be composed of 50%-60% carbohydrates (mostly complex carbohydrates) and protein intake of 10%20% of all calories; total fat intake should be restricted to 30% of total calories (with saturated fat limited to 10% of total calories and total cholesterol intake <300 mg/d). It may be wise to assess the cardiac status of the patient before starting an exercise programme, particularly if the patient has other risk factors for coronary artery disease.

Medical nutrition therapy is integral to total care and management. Achieving nutrition-related goals requires a coordinated team effort that includes the patient.

Lactic Acidemia in Infection with Human Immunodeficiency Virus

Lactic acidosis in patients infected with the human immunodeficiency virus was initially identified as a rare complication of therapy with nucleoside analog reverse transcriptase inhibitors (NRTIs). The only patient group that appears to be at greater risk is pregnant women. Lactic acidemia (defined by venous lactate >2.0 mmol/L) is common to several toxicities associated with nucleoside analog reverse transcriptase inhibitors (NRTIs) and nucleotide analog reverse transcriptase inhibitors that may have a mitochondrial pathogenesis. Virologically active triphosphate forms of NRTIs and nucleotide analog reverse transcriptase inhibitors can inhibit mitochondrial DNA polymerase-, which could in turn lead to impaired synthesis of mitochondrial enzymes that generate adenosine triphosphate by oxidative phosphorylation of glucose and fatty acids. Lactic acidemia with no or mild symptoms was detected in 8%21% of patients receiving at least one NRTI versus 0%-1% of patients receiving no antiretroviral therapy. Severe lactic acidemia has been described in association with all NRTIs, particularly if treatment duration is >6 months .

The primary clinical features of moderate to severe lactic acidemia are fatigue, weight loss, myalgias, nausea and vomiting, abdominal distension, and pain, dyspnoea, and preterminal cardiac dysrhythmias. The onset is acute or subacute (with symptom duration a median of 4 months in one series). Features of hepatic dysfunction are common and can include soft, tender hepatomegaly, peripheral oedema, ascites, and encephalopathy, but jaundice is rare.

Overall mortality was 80% in patients with HIV-related lactic acidemia >10 mmol/L, whereas no deaths have been reported in those with lactate <10 mmol/L. Prognosis of lactic acidemia depends on the level at the time of diagnosis. In one study, lactate levels (mean, 4.2 mmol/L) returned to normal at a mean of 3 months after NRTI cessation. Clinical features may take longer to resolve.

There is no proven intervention for lactic acidemia apart from NRTI cessation.

Bone in HIV -infected patients receiving antiretroviral therapy

Before the era of HAART, studies indicated that bone mineral metabolism was only minimally affected in HIV-infected individuals

The use of NRTIs has been associated with mitochondrial toxicity and lactic acidosis. The common risk factors for BMD loss in HIV-infected individuals include history of wasting or poor nutrition, past steroid usage (i.e., for pneumocystis carinii pneumonia or myopathy), hormonal deficiencies, or the potential contribution of HIV-related immune system activation and immune reconstitution

The recommended intake of Calcium from all sources is 1500 mg/d, and for vitamin D, the recommended intake is 4001000 IU/d. Other nutrients are also important in relation to bone health. Diets with very high protein content, excess caffeine, phosphorus, and sodium can increase calcium losses. Moderate physical activity is also recommended to help preserve bone mass.

Some ARVs have been associated with increased risk of osteoporosis and weakening of bones that may require medical and dietary responses. For osteoporosis, a balanced diet with high calcium foods, such as milk, yogurt, cheese, and vitamin D supplement, is recommended, along with medical care. Some side effects of ARVs are similar to symptoms of opportunistic infections, such as diarrhoea. Therefore, the health worker must continue to be alert to recognize symptoms of infections and treat these infections appropriately.

Lipid Abnormalities

Dyslipidemia is an important clinical problem in individuals infected with human immunodeficiency virus (HIV) who are receiving antiretroviral therapy. Abnormalities of lipid metabolism are common in HIV-infected patients and tend to be accentuated in those receiving antiretroviral therapy, particularly with protease inhibitors (PIs). During therapy with PIs, increases in serum triglycerides may be extreme, particularly with Ritonavir therapy. In addition, significant elevations of both total cholesterol and HDL-C have also occurred during therapy with the nonnucleoside reverse transcriptase inhibitors (NNRTI) Efavirenz and Nevirapine

Nondrug interventions should be the first approach for management of abnormal lipid levels. Clinicians should consult with dietary specialists as a first step, when initial attempts at dietary intervention fail to achieve the desired effects, or when intensive dietary modification becomes necessary. Other nondrug therapies are expected to be beneficial, as they are in persons without HIV. For example, structured exercise plus diet resulted in a 21% decrease in triglyceride levels in HIV-infected patients, and resistance training improved triglyceride levels Smoking cessation and weight reduction for obesity also improve the overall cardiovascular risk profile.

Diet. These diets reduce serum triglycerides. For patients with low HDL-C, reduction of dietary fat will further reduce HDL-C. Monounsaturated fats (e.g., canola and olive oil) should be substituted for saturated fats. Moreover, if carbohydrate intake is increased as ingestion of fat is reduced, this may increase triglyceride levels. The management of severe hypertriglyceridemia and hyperchylomicronemia requires a verylow-fat diet and avoidance of simple sugars (i.e., use of lowglycemic-index carbohydrates) and alcohol. Fish oils (omega-3 fatty acid supplements) variably decrease triglyceride synthesis and may be tried in patients with severe hypertriglyceridemia.

Body Shape Changes Associated with Protease Inhibitors

Although weight loss is usually seen as the primary nutritional challenge faced by HIV+ people, a new problem involving fat accumulations in specific areas of the body is now being observed. These fat accumulations seem to be associated with the use of protease inhibitors. Fat accumulations are usually seen across the belly or between the shoulder blades of HIV+ men. Women may also experience increases in breast size. Fat accumulation is often accompanied by tissue loss in the arms, legs, buttocks, and face, the pattern typical of muscle wasting. High triglycerides, which have previously been observed in people with HIV, and high cholesterol levels which were previously uncommon, have been observed in conjunction with these patterns of fat distribution in some cases.

Anecdotally, people are experimenting with a number of possible treatments, including nutritional supplements, although none of these has more than theoretical evidence to support it. Alpha lipoic acid is being used by some people with HIV. Alpha lipoic acid is naturally produced by our cells and is part of our normal cellular metabolism. Some people believe it helps compensate for both liver damage and metabolic deficiencies in HIV. Carnitine is also being used, as it has been shown to lower triglycerides in people with HIV and may also help prevent muscle wasting. People who use this often take very high doses of 3-4 grams a day. Fish oil, containing omega-three fatty acids, has also been shown to lower triglycerides in HIV+ men. Theoretically this might be useful. Finally, supplements that may help to prevent muscle wasting like l-glutamine and whey protein might be useful.

10

Drug and Food Reactions

At some point during your medical treatment you may have to take some medicines. The food we eat can effect how the medicines work. Also, the medicines we take can effect how our bodies use the food we eat.

There are new and different medicines for HIV and AIDS being tried every day. It is important that you ask your doctor about each medicine you are taking to see if there are any foods you cannot eat with them. It is also important to know that many of the physical symptoms associated with HIV can be made better or made worse by the foods you eat. The right foods to eat for one problem may be exactly the wrong foods to eat for another. If you have more than one problem, it can be difficult to know what to eat. Always try to ask your doctor for advice on what is best for your condition.

Bacteria and Food Poisoning

"It must have been something I ate!" How many times do people say this following a bout with nausea, upset stomach, cramps, diarrhoea, or vomiting?

Indeed, these can be the symptoms of food poisoning—illness caused by eating food on which harmful bacteria have grown. The bacteria that cause food poisoning are difficult to detect by a food's appearance, taste or smell. But they can cause illness ranging from mild to very severe and even life-threatening. The human body ordinarily is well-equipped to deal with these bacteria, but individuals with weakened immune systems—such as those with acquired immune deficiency syndrome (AIDS) and those infected with the human immunodefiency virus (HIV)—can be far greater risk of serious illness. Because of their weakened immune systems, these individuals are more susceptible to contracting a foodborne illness. Once contracted, these infections, with their severe vomiting and diarrhoea, can be difficult to treat and they can come back again and again. This can further weaken the immune system and hasten the progression of HIV infection and be fatal for person with AIDS.

Since most foodborne illnesses result from improper handling of food, person with AIDS or HIV infection can help themselves by following basic food safety guidelines. Applying these guidelines when buying, preparing and storing food, along with having a basic knowledge of the most common harmful bacteria and the foods on which they are found or can grow, can allow persons with AIDS to eat defensively while choosing a nutritious diet.

People cannot get AIDS from food. While many kinds of bacteria can cause food poisoning, three are the most prevalent threat to persons with AIDS and HIV infections. These are: Campylobacter, Listeria and Salmonella.

The symptoms of **Campylobacter infection** (campylobacteriosis) include acute abdominal pain, diarrhoea (which can be watery and contain blood), nausea, headache, muscle pain, and fever. Symptoms can begin 2 to 5 days after eating contaminated food and generally lasts 7 to 10 days. Campylobacter bacteria are most commonly found in raw or undercooked poultry, unpasteurized milk, and non-chlorinated water.

Listeriosis, the disease caused by Listeria, is characterized by flu-like symptoms of chills, fever and headache, sometimes accompanied by nausea and vomiting. These early symptoms can appear 2 to 30 days after exposure and can be followed by bacteremia (a bloodstream infection), meningitis (an inflammation of the membranes covering the spinal cord and brain), or encephalitis (an inflammation of the membranes of the brain itself). Foods found to contain Listeria are unpasteurized milk and cheeses, raw or undercooked meat, poultry, and fish.

Salmonellosis is the illness that can develop from eating foods containing Salmonella bacteria. It is characterized by flu-like symptoms, possibly accompanied by nausea, vomiting, abdominal cramps, and diarrhea. Symptoms can develop 6 to 48 hours after exposure and last up to a week. Foods most often associated with salmonellosis include raw or undercooked meat, poultry, fish, and eggs.

Food and drug interactions and their dietary management

The main food and drug (modern and traditional medications) interactions are listed below.

- Food effects on drug efficacy
- Drug effects on nutrient absorption, metabolism, distribution, and excretion
- Side effects of medications that affect food intake and nutrient absorption
- Drug and food interactions that cause unhealthy side effects

Types of interactions between medications and food

The side effects of drugs on food intake and the effects of drugs on nutrient absorption, metabolism, distribution and excretion may have the most negative impact on the nutritional status of people living with HIV/AIDS. The side effects of drugs and the effects of the disease are often difficult to distinguish. For example, headaches, malaise, fever, and gastrointestinal symptoms may be side effects of drugs but can also be associated with HIV and AIDS. Appropriate dietary responses may help address these.

Moreover, the effects of food on drugs' efficacy and the unhealthy side effects caused by the interaction of food and drugs also require appropriate dietary responses to maintain nutritional status and ensure the client's adherence and the effectiveness of the treatment.

Food effects on drug efficacy :

Food intake or meals can enhance or inhibit the absorption, metabolism, distribution, and excretion of medications. This type of interaction varies from one drug to another and requires appropriate dietary responses to improve the client's adherence and optimize the medication's efficacy. Dietary management to improve the efficacy of a medication includes taking the medication with food, on an empty stomach, or with or without certain types of foods. Examples of the ways food intake affects drug efficacy are listed below.

- Food reduces the rate of absorption of aspirin (acetylsalicylic acid), commonly used to treat the fever and pain that are common in people living with HIV/AIDS. Aspirin is best taken 2 hours after meals with a full glass of water.
- Food reduces the absorption of Isoniazid, a medication commonly used to treat tuberculosis. Therefore, Isoniazid has to be taken 1 hour before or 2 hours after meals.
- Rifampin is also used to treat tuberculosis. As with Isoniazid, food reduces the absorption of Rifampin. Rifampin should be taken 1 or 2 hours after meals to increase the medication's absorption.
- Food enhances the absorption or metabolism of some ARVs and inhibits the absorption or metabolism of others. For example, a high-fat meal increases the bioavailability of the nucleoside analogue.
- A high-calorie, high-fat, high-protein meal decreases absorption of the protease inhibitor Indinavir and reduces the absorption of the nucleoside reverse transcriptase inhibitor Zidovudine. It is therefore recommended not to take Zidovudine with high-fat meals (>40g of fat). As the effect of food on the efficacy of a drug is food and drug specific, the counsellor should help the client draw up a food and drug timetable. This timetable should take into account both the food and drug interactions of each drug to be taken and the client's eating habits to ensure the greatest efficacy of the treatment.

Drug effects on nutrient absorption, metabolism, distribution, and excretion

Certain modern medications affect nutrient absorption, metabolism, and excretion. Modern medications that inhibit or enhance nutrient absorption and metabolism may have negative effects on nutritional status. Dietary management may require either increasing food intake, taking a nutrient supplement to compensate for the nutrient affected, or reducing the nutrient intake if the metabolite produced can negatively affect health.

Drugs that may require increased food or nutrient intake

The medication Isoniazid, commonly taken to treat tuberculosis, inhibits the metabolism of vitamin B6. Supplementation of this vitamin is therefore recommended. The antibiotic and anti-tuberculosis medication Rifampin may increase vitamin D metabolism. Supplementation of this vitamin D may be required.

Drugs that may require reduced food or nutrient intake :

Studies have reported lipid abnormalities, including increased level of triglycerides, cholesterol, and fat maldistribution, in people who have taken protease inhibitors or non-nucleoside reverse transcriptase inhibitors.

The protease inhibitors Saquinavir and Ritonavir may cause an elevation in cholesterol and triglycerides levels, which may increase the risk of cardiovascular diseases (Pronsky, Meyer, and Fields-Gardner 2001). Most of the protease inhibitors may cause changes in lipid levels that require both dietary and medical responses. Lipid abnormalities include hypertriglyceridemia, hypercholesterolemia, and lipodystrophy syndrome.

For hypertriglyceridemia, it is important to maintain a healthy weight, eat a variety of foods, reduce the intake of refined sugar and excessive carbohydrates, increase intake of fibre , avoid alcoholic beverages, exercise daily, and take medication to lower triglycerides.

For hypercholesterolemia, it is important to maintain a healthy weight, eat a diet low in fat and limited saturated fat, increase intake of fruits and vegetables, avoid food rich in cholesterol, avoid alcohol and smoking, exercise daily, and take medication to lower the cholesterol (Pronsky, Meyer, and Fields-Gardner 2001).

The effective management of fat maldistribution or lipodystrophy syndrome has not yet been established. Diet and exercise, use of medications, and change in the ARV regimen can help.

Some antiretroviral drugs may affect glucose metabolism and cause insulin resistance(IR). Insulin resistance is associated with increased risk of diabetes (Gelato 2003). For diabetes, specific carbohydrate controlled diet, reduced intake of refined sugar and saturated fat, exercise, and anti-diabetic medications are recommended. Progressive lactic acidosis is a complication of NRTI therapy (Carr 2003). The signs of severe lactic acidemia include fatigue, weight loss, abdominal pain, dyspnoea, liver dysfunction, and cardiac dysrhythmias. In case of any of these symptoms, stopping the NRTI may help.

Management of drug and food interactions

Medications to treat HIV and opportunistic infections often require specific complementary food responses to alleviate side effects, improve efficacy, maintain nutritional status, and ensure continued adherence to the drugs. Many people living with HIV/AIDS, however, cannot follow optimal food and nutrition guidelines because they cannot access the foods required. This has serious implications both for the individual, whose health will likely decline following termination of the medication, and for others in the household and community, as poor adherence can lead to resistant strains of infections or viruses, including tuberculosis and HIV. Rapid deterioration of the individual's health can also lead to more severe declines in household food security because of lost labour and productivity.

Counsellors and service providers who offer guidance on management of drug and food interactions should help clients identify factors that might prevent them from following guidelines and help address these constraints by identifying foods and schedules suitable for the specific medications.

11

Nutrition Side Effects and Coping with the Complications of HIV/AIDS

Side effects can result from HIV, other infections or medication, and can be harmful to your nutritional health and overall well-being. Side effects left untreated can lead to decreased absorption and processing of medications and nutrients. Some side effects can cause changes in food and fluid intake, cause fatigue and generally can make you feel bad. People are not the same. Different people taking the same medication can have different side effects and those with the same side effects can have them at different levels of intensity. Mild or severe, any side effect must be addressed by you and your doctor and when needed, your dietitian.

There are other conditions or diseases that people with HIV may have and which involves nutrition. These conditions often require special nutrition information and support to help people make important diet and activity changes. You, your doctor and your dietitian must work together if you are diagnosed with any one or more of the following conditions:

The most important first step is for you to recognize any condition you are experiencing that is not "normal" and to bring it to the attention of your doctor. Your doctor can help you find out what the real reason is for the problem and to figure out how to correct it. Not all problems will "just go away" but you can learn

Side effects among people living with HIV include:

Anorexia or reduced appetite	Excessive or frequent urination	Mouth sores or pain
Bloating	Fat gain	Muscle loss
Constipation	Fat loss	Nausea
Cramps	Fatigue	Not able to eat
Diarrhoea	Feet, leg, hip, or shoulder pain	Poor fluid intake
Difficulty or pain chewing	Fever	Taste or smell changes
Dental caries	Gas or flatulence	Vision problems
Dizziness	Headache	Vomiting
Dry mouth	Heartburn	Weight gain
Excessive fluid intake	Hungry all the time	Weight loss
Anaemia	High blood sugar	Liver problems like hepatitis
Cancer	High cholesterol	Low cholesterol
Diabetes mellitus	High triglycerides	Obesity
Eating Disorder	Insulin resistance	Pre-Diabetes
High blood pressure	Kidney problems	Pregnancy

what to do to lessen or better control them. Left unchecked, these side effects or disease conditions can harm your nutritional well-being, overall health and even your life.

If you are living with HIV/AIDS, you may develop the following conditions sometime or the other.

- Dry mouth
- Mouth and throat soreness
- Loss of appetite
- Constipation
- Changes in the taste of foods
- Nausea and vomiting
- Diarrhoea
- Fatigue / Feeling tired
- Gas and bloating
- Unintentional weight loss / wasting
- Problems with fat digestion
- Skin problems
- Colds, coughs and influenza
- Fever

A person may have two or more of these conditions at the same time so will need to choose suitable foods carefully. Since people react to foods differently, they will have to select those that work for them. Normal mixed diets can be resumed as soon as the problem is resolved.

1. Oral Health Problems :

Oral conditions may have an impact on your food intake .Oral health problems (problems inside your mouth) can interfere with your ability to chew and swallow, take medications, and affect your overall health and quality of life if not treated. Mouth or throat infections like thrush, dental problems, or mouth ulcers can all be painful barriers to eating. The best way to resolve this problem is to treat the infection or have the necessary dental work.

Changes in the tissues of the mouth are associated with deficiencies in some vitamins, particularly B complex vitamins and vitamin C. Since these deficiencies have been observed in people with HIV, a B complex supplement or a vitamin C supplement (maybe one of the "stress" formulas that contain both) might help ward off oral health problems.

Oral health problems commonly diagnosed in people with HIV/AIDS

1. Candidiasis (thrush) is a fungal infection that produces cottage cheese-like bumps or red patches on the tongue, gums and inner cheeks.
2. Oral warts, caused by the Human Papilloma Virus(HPV), are little cauliflower-like bumps that appear inside your mouth on your cheeks, gums and lips.
3. Dry mouth is often caused by medications prescribed for anxiety, depression, and high blood pressure and from antihistamines as well as some protease inhibitors. Dry mouth may lead to dental caries (cavities) since there is little saliva to wash away food particles and prevent bacterial growth.

What your dentist can do for you

Regular visits to your dentist can help detect the start of dental caries, gingivitis (mild inflammation of the gums caused by plaque buildup), and periodontitis (a more severe infection leading to bone loss). Your dentist can also diagnose and prescribe treatment for oral warts, thrush, Hairy Leukoplakia, Kaposi's sarcoma, canker sores, and dry mouth. Your dentist may also be the first one to notice if a condition seen in the mouth requires medical attention and refer you to your physician for follow-up.

Food, cavities and the role of saliva

Food, if left on your teeth too long, can promote the beginning of a cavity. Bacteria in the mouth combine with food and can damage the tooth enamel making it easier to get a cavity. There may be no pain as the cavity forms until it becomes a more serious problem and more damage to the tooth structure has occurred. Saliva lowers your risk of getting a cavity. Saliva washes over your teeth and contains substances, which can reduce bacteria activity and help remove the bacteria and food particles on and between the teeth.

When these problems can not be quickly resolved, there are strategies to help you eat appropriate nutrients over the short term

Remember these 4 simple tips for a healthy mouth

1. Brush after meals and snacks. Regular brushing, flossing, proper nutrition can help prevent and detect problems. Referral

to a qualified dietitian may be necessary to assist with eating problems.

2. Floss at least once a day. Leave the floss on the bathroom counter as a reminder.
3. Drink water throughout the day to wash food from your teeth.
4. Visit your dentist twice a year.

Drink apple juice or milk (if you are not lactose intolerant).

These low-acid beverages also have significant nutrients. Choose soft moist foods like casseroles or mashed potatoes. Dunk bread or other foods in liquids including gravy or melted butter. These animal fats will not only soften foods but are also a good source of energy. Use a straw for liquids and/or liquid supplements if most of the problems are located in the mouth. Avoid heating your food too much as hot foods can cause pain, especially for those with dental problems.

2. Dry mouth

Certain medications and treatments decrease saliva production and may cause you to have a dry mouth. This makes eating and swallowing difficult, can cause dental problems, and may dull your sense of taste.

Dry mouth can occur with a number of medications, or it can be from HIV itself. Allergies can cause it, and dry mouth occurs with some infections, too. Decreased saliva can make chewing and swallowing difficult; it is also a problem because in the mouth digestion starts and saliva contains digestive enzymes. Without saliva, you can get food build-up which promotes decay and also thrush. Decreased saliva also effects the taste of food. Each time you eat you produce food acids, with normal salivary flow it returns to normal pH within two hours; this environment in your mouth can cause various oral health problems.

How to prevent dry mouth

- Quit smoking.
- Brush at least twice a day or after meals and snacks. Not only does this prevent cavities, it also stimulates saliva production. Rinse your mouth with warm, salted water.
- Moisten your mouth with fluids, frozen yoghurt, pudding or ice.

- Carry water with you at all times and drink throughout the day.
- Suck on hard candy, especially sour candy. This will help keep your mouth wet.
- Drink mild beverages such as apple juice or punch throughout the day.
- Have at least 8-10 small glasses of water a day.
- Avoid dry, rough foods like crackers, toast or cookies. you may also try soaking them in milk or other liquids before eating.
- Avoid dry foods Add gravy, creamy sauces or juice to your foods to moisten before eating.
- Avoid sweet, sticky foods. Too much sugar can dry out your mouth and damage your teeth.
- Avoid spicy, salty, or crunchy foods if they cause pain.
- Enjoy soups, casseroles and stews, oatmeal or other soft cereals, yogurt, pudding, applesauce and similar moist foods. They are all easy to follow.
- Avoid caffeinated or alcoholic drinks since they may aggravate dry mouth.
- Choose foods that are soft and easy to chew and swallow such as shakes, cream soups, hot cereals, scrambled eggs, noodle dishes, yogurt, mashed potatoes and pureed meats.
- Choose moderate-temperature foods that are not too hot or too cold. Moisten dry lips with lip balm.
- To stimulate saliva production
    - suck sugar-free sweets
    - add lemon to beverages
    - dilute juices and soups

Treatment

- Rinse your mouth often with salted warm water or mouthwash.
- Try chewing sugarless gum, which stimulates saliva and helps return acid level to normal.
- Suck on sugarless candies — making sure they are smooth and flat — lozenges or sour drops or crushed ice. Avoid sticky sweet foods and sugar containing gums and candies; they can make you even drier.

- Drink plenty of liquids at and between meals, such as water, fruit juice diluted, and also try fruit ices, popsicles, applesauce, pudding or gelatin.
- Place a pan of water near a heat source in winter to humidify room.
- Try Biotene chewing gum.
- Pilocarpine — medication prescribed by doctor to treat dry mouth.
- Herbs to try: demulcents chickweed, slippery elm, marshmallow, licorice.

3. Mouth and throat soreness

Your mouth and throat are some of the most sensitive areas of your body. . Soreness of the mouth and tongue is common in people with HIV/AIDS. A sore mouth can make it difficult to eat, thus reducing food intake. An HIV infection can allow sores to develop there. These sores can make it hurt to chew or swallow and that makes it hard to eat. Common causes of mouth and throat soreness in people with HIV/AIDS include gingivitis (gum inflammation), mouth ulcers and Candida (thrush), bacteria, herpes or other types of infection, or certain medications such as AZT or ddI, apthous ulcers. Mouth and throat soreness can lead to decreased appetite and food intake, and poor dental hygiene. It can become severe in the mouth and lower down in the oesophagus.

Here are some tips to make eating easier for you.

- Eat soft foods that are smooth in texture. Try mashed potatoes, yogurt, pudding, custards, oatmeal, cream of wheat, ice cream, applesauce, mashed banana, cream soups (Cream of Mushroom, Cream of Chicken, Cheddar Cheese).
- Put your food in a blender to make it smooth.
- Avoid spicy, salty, sticky foods that are difficult to swallow; dry, rough or hard foods like potato chips; fizzy drinks; and sour foods and juices like tomato, pineapple and citrus fruits. These may irritate mouth sores and the mouth and throat lining.
- Use more herbs and less salt and spices to season food.
- Soften toast and biscuits by dipping them in milk, tea or soup.

- Moisten cooked food with gravy, sauce and butter or margarine.
- Avoid very hot food.
- Rinse your mouth often with cool water. Avoid commercial mouthwashes that contain alcohol or other irritants.
- Try baby food. it is smooth and easy to swallow, and comes in single serving containers.
- Use a straw or drink your food from a cup instead of using a spoon. Sip soothing beverages like cold drinks and milk; try using a straw.
- Try tilting your head forward or back to make swallowing easier.
- If you are able to handle some lumps, try scrambled eggs, cottage cheese, macaroni and cheese, baked fish, tuna salad, and canned fruits. Most stews, casseroles and hearty soups would be soft enough to eat, too.
- Moisten your food to help it slide down. Cut meats up in small pieces and add gravy to them. Add gravy or cream sauces to vegetables before eating.
- Soak dry foods in milk, coffee or other warm beverage before eating. This works well with toast, crackers, and cookies.
- Do not eat spicy foods. They can sting your mouth.
- Avoid rough or crunchy foods such as raw vegetables, apples. Try cooked vegetables and soft fruits like bananas or canned pears instead.
- Stay away from oranges, grapefruit, tomatoes or their juice. They have a lot of acid and can cause your mouth to sting.
- Avoid very hot foods and beverages. Cold and room temperature foods will be more comfortable to your mouth. If really cold foods feel good, try adding ice to milk and other beverages to make them extra cold. Try eating a lot of ice cream, sherbet or popsicles to numb some of the pain.
- Rinse your mouth whenever you feel you need it. This can moisten your mouth, remove bits of food, and give it a fresher taste. Rinse your mouth with bicarbonate of soda mixed with water.

Possible medical treatments or medications:

- Aspirin, Tylenol or Motrin for pain — taken orally.

- Miracle mouthwash, which is Nystatin or tetracycline (according to if apthous ulcers are fungal or bacterial infection), Maalox, Lidocaine and Benadryl — applied topically.
- Thalidomide is also successfully being used.

Foods and drinks to avoid

- Very spicy and salty foods such as chillies and curries.
- Acidic or very sour foods such as oranges, lemons, pineapple, vinegar and tomatoes.
- Food and drinks that are too hot or too cold. Keep food and drinks at room temperature.
- Foods that need a lot of chewing such as raw vegetables, or are sticky and hard to swallow such as peanut butter.
- If candida (oral thrush) is diagnosed, cut down on sweet foods such as sugar, honey and sweet fruit and drinks because sugar may make the condition worse.

4. Thrush.

Thrush is a fungal infection caused by the Candida fungus and is common in HIV infected people. Thrush refers to whitish spots on the inside of the mouth, tongue, oesophagus, intestines, vagina, or anus. Although these sores are uncomfortable, they are not life threatening. These sores can result in difficulty in eating foods, loss of appetite, reduced food intake, and malabsorption, leading to weight loss.

Eat one to two cloves of raw garlic every three to four hours if available. If the raw garlic is too strong, crush the cloves and mix with a small amount of clean boiled water. Rinse the mouth with this mixture and then swallow the rest. Repeat every three to four hours.

- Drink sour/fermented milk. This will help to prevent yeast from growing.
- Eat green papaya as a relish or side dish.
- Gargle with slightly salty, warm, clean water.
- Avoid sweet foods and sweet drinks (e.g., carbonated soft drinks), which will increase the soreness and help the yeast to grow. Avoid sugar and honey.

4. Gas and bloating

Causes of gas and bloating include physical changes in the gut, emotional stress, and certain foods and medications.

To help manage gas and bloating:

- Don't smoke.
- Eat smaller meals more regularly.
- Avoid gas-forming foods such as beans, cabbage, broccoli, cauliflower, onion and fizzy drinks.
- Avoid spicy foods such as curry.
- Avoid fried or greasy food.
- Wait a couple of hours after a meal before lying down.
- Avoid alcohol, coffee, peppermint and chocolate.
- Try to relax, especially during meals. Eating and drinking while stressed may cause you to swallow air and may interfere with digestion.
- Eat slowly and chew well.
- Sip drinks slowly - don't gulp - especially when swallowing pills with water.
- Avoid chewing-gum, which may cause you to swallow air. Sugar-free gum containing sorbitol can cause diarrhoea and gas.
- You may be lactose intolerant, a condition which can cause gas and bloating. If you are, reducing your intake of milk products may relieve symptoms.

How to prevent a bloated feeling

- Do not drink too much with food.
- Avoid foods such as cabbage, beans, onion, broccoli, Brussels sprouts and cauliflower and cold fizzy drinks that create gas in the stomach.
- Some people find it difficult to digest wholemeal foods and foods rich in dietary fibre, particularly when the diet also contains sugar and sugary foods. Try to exclude sugar and sugary foods from the diet for a while.

Recommendations:

- Artichoke extract.
- Activated charcoal.

- Digestive enzymes with each meal.
- L-Glutamine, 30 grams (3 grams per teaspoon, so 10 teaspoons) per day; after 7 days you can cut back to 10 to 15 grams per day (1 to 2 rounded teaspoons).
- Probiotics (good bacteria in gut): acidophilus, lactobacillus, bifidum, s. Boulardii — any of these in powder form can be taken, 1/4 to 1/2 teaspoon twice a day dissolved in room temperature water. You can do a swish and swallow, this will help to control thrush also.
- Some people have had success with taking liver herbs, milk thistle and dandelion to help reduce gas.

5. Loss of Appetite

Loss of appetite or Poor appetite is one of the most common problems in people with HIV/AIDS. It can have many causes including infections, pain (particularly in the mouth or gut), depression, anxiety, tiredness or poor nutritional intake. The feeling of hunger may disappear or the person may be easily satisfied and therefore not want to eat enough. However, it is very important to continue eating to prevent weight loss and malnutrition and to maintain strength in order to speed recovery.

When not hungry ... the best way to regain appetite is to eat

- Try different foods until you find those that you like and try to have a mixed diet.
- Eat smaller meals more often. Eat whenever your appetite is good - do not be too rigid about fixed times for meals.
- Maximize caloric intake by keeping nutritional snacks around such as peanut butter and crackers, cheese, cereal, yogurt, fruit nectars and commercial or homemade breakfast drinks.
- Eat your favorite foods; you are likely to eat more of these.
- Try walking before a meal to increase appetite.
- Try to drink a lot of water, milk, yoghurt, soups, herbal teas or juices throughout the day. Drink mainly after, and in between meals - do not drink too much before or during meals.
- Add flavour to food and make it look and taste interesting. Squeeze some lemon juice over it or add spices such as cardamom, fennel, coriander and cinnamon.

- Avoid fizzy drinks, beer and foods such as cabbage, broccoliand beans that create gas in the stomach and canakefeel bloated.
- Try rinsing your mouth out before eating as this can make food taste a fresher.
- Avoid coffee, cigarettes and candy. Coffee, cigarettes, cola, chocolate and alcohol dull your appetite.
- For diarrhoea and vomiting, drink plenty of fluids to avoid dehydration, replenish sodium and potassium loss by eating bananas, potatoes, fish, meat, apricot nectar, tomato juice and sports drinks. Eat soluble fibre foods such as white rice, oatmeal, pears and mashed potatoes. Avoid insolubie high-fiber foods like wheat bran, brown rice and popcorn.
- For nausea, dry salty foods like crackers or pretzels are usually tolerable as well as simple foods like scrambled eggs, toast, noodles and bananas.
- Protein is essential for the immune system. Four small servings a day are suggested for people with HIV. Try adding diced meat, hard-boiled eggs or cheese to your diet. Protein powder can also be used and added to beverages, hot cereal or casseroles. Peanut butter is a good source of protein. However, avoid peanut butter made from raw peanuts. Instead, use one made from roasted nuts.
- Take light exercise such as walking outdoors, for example, and breathing plenty of fresh air to stimulate an appetite.
- Eat in a well-ventilated room away from cooking or unpleasant smells.
- Eat with your family or friends. If you have to stay in bed, they can join you at your bedside.
- Avoid alcohol. It reduces appetite, weakens the body and interferes with medicines.
- If the reason for lack of appetite is diarrhoea, nausea and vomiting, or a sore mouth, follow the guidelines given later in this chapter.

Anorexia is generally a loss of appetite leading to weight loss. Anorexia nervosa however, is a preoccupation with dieting and thinness that leads to excessive weight loss without loss of appetite. While anorexia nervosa generally begins to emerge in adolescence, concerns about weight usually begin earlier. Adolescence is a time of transitions, increased independence and dramatic bodily changes. Young women with low self-esteem and difficulty coping with the demands of adolescence are more at risk of developing eating disorders. Boys and girls involved in certain activities such as gymnastics, dance, wrestling or other sports where there is an emphasis on a small body frame or light weight may feel pressure to begin dieting. Young women may find their developing breasts and hips impossible to accept and the body itself becomes an enemy that they want to destroy. Obsessive preoccupation with food, weight and dieting is a way of bringing a sense of control to the adolescent who fears the rapid changes and anxiety of the increased expectations of adolescence.

Anorexia nervosa is one of the most serious eating disorders with a mortality rate as high as 15 percent. The characteristic of the disorder is excessive weight loss not caused by organic disease. In addition, it is typically associated with the loss of menstrual periods (amenorrhea) for young women and other medical abnormalities, including electrolyte imbalances.

Restricting and binge eating/purging are two subtypes of anorexia nervosa. Those with restricting anorexia nervosa do not engage in binge eating or purging behaviours. Those with binge eating/purging anorexia nervosa binge eat and then attempt to lose weight through purging behaviours.

Theories on the causes of anorexia nervosa have identified social, biological, family and personality factors.

Treatment of Anorexia Nervosa :

Anorexia nervosa is a chronic ongoing illness that may require lengthy treatment. Patients often do not view their severe weight loss as a problem and they do not want to change, therefore they do not generally seek help on their own. Parents need to be aware that teenage dieting can escalate out of control. They need to be concerned if their daughter's menstrual period has stopped or never began due to dieting and weight loss. Medical and professional mental health intervention may be required.

Depending on the severity of the weight loss, hospitalization may be necessary. The focus is on weight gain initially and gradually progresses to psychological issues. It is critical for the therapist to establish trust with the patient. Psychotropic medications are sometimes prescribed to treat underlying depression, and to lessen binging and obsessive thinking. Different behavioural techniques can be used to change behaviour such as monitoring eating behaviour and rewarding weight gain with activities that are pleasant to the patient.

Studies have shown that it is very helpful to involve the family in therapy if the patient lives at home. Relapse of anorexia nervosa may occur at times of job stress, when beginning college or graduating from college, pregnancy, illness, relationship problems including domestic violence, or environmental changes such as moving. Preparing for relapse is important for families and those suffering from anorexia nervosa. Coping skills can be taught to help deal with transitions to avoid a setback.

HIV/AIDS and Anorexia

Many people with HIV suffer from anorexia from time to time, but since not eating can reduce the absorption of medications and therefore their effectiveness, it is important to deal with this problem as soon as possible. Anorexia associated with AIDS wasting is somewhat different. The person just does not have the desire to eat. Nausea, vomiting and diarrhoea may coincide with a diminished appetite and cause a lack of intake leading to dehydration and malnutrition. You should keep in mind that taking the current HIV medications on a daily basis is something you have to do until better medications are developed. So having a diet that you can live with will make all the difference. Ask others how they are managing.

Side effects of HIV medications may also interfere with eating and general level of energy. Fatigue associated with HIV/AIDS may also be a factor. Depression, feelings of low self-esteem and other psychological problems can affect eating. Sometimes the reduced appetite and weight loss may seem welcome to someone who has been struggling to lose weight for much of their life. Unintentional weight loss, however, can lead to or be a sign that there is an opportunistic infection. It is not to be ignored.

Those with anorexic nervosa may be using amphetamines to lose weight. Using harmful substances for any reason may be an attempt to deal with inner pain and issues around being HIV-positive. It may be a way to avoid stress that has become habitual. Addictive behaviours can cause complications with interactions among substances and medications. It is likely that using substances interferes with eating healthy meals, and drinking enough fluids as well as remembering to take medications on time. An unintended weight loss in HIV patients is to be avoided. As little as a 5 percent weight loss over a four-month period is associated with increased risk of death and opportunistic complications. Determining the underlying medical cause of weight loss is important. If there is an underlying psychological reason for serious weight loss/wasting, binging, purging or obsessive thoughts about body image and weight, seek the help of a mental health specialist; the sooner the better.

6. Constipation:

Constipation occurs when you don't have regular bowel movements and you find it difficult to pass stools. Causes of constipation include:

- side-effects from certain medications
- not enough fibre in the diet
- not enough fluid intake
- lack of exercise
- stress.

Lower-gut infections can also make it uncomfortable to pass stools.

People with HIV/AIDS may have problems in digesting certain foods or may suffer from constipation. The problems may be caused by damage to the naturally occurring bacteria in the intestine, which are needed to digest food. These bacteria may be destroyed by antibiotics or other medicines.

Ho·v to deal with these problems

To help manage constipation

- Drink at least eight cups of fluid (water and other beverages) a day. Prune juice is a natural laxative that often brings relief.
- Eat foods high in insoluble fibre. Fibre, or roughage, is the part of food that doesn't get digested by the body, but which helps keep the digestive tract working properly. Insoluble fibre is a type of fibre that passes through the digestive tract

easily. It speeds up the movement of food through the gut and produces less dense stools that are easier to pass.

- Chewing food well will make it easier to digest.
- Chopped papaya added to meat acts as a tenderizer and helps digestion.
- Fermented foods such as sour cabbage water, sour porridge, yoghurt and sprouts can be easier to digest and help the digestion of other foods.
- Use recommended foods as if they were medicine, particularly during and after antibiotic treatment. Eat three times a day before or with meals and continue for two weeks.

Foods to avoid

- People can experiment by omitting a particular food and seeing if it makes them feel better. Some people find fatty foods such as fried foods, chips, hard cheese, peanut butter and cream difficult to digest. However, they can go back to a normal mixed diet once they feel better.

How to stop constipation

- Eat insoluble fibre, contained in foods such as raw vegetables and fruit, dried fruit, wholemeal dark bread, whole-grain cereals, nuts and seeds.
- Eat frequent and small meals regularly throughout the day.
- Drink plenty of fluids throughout the day.
- Be active and exercise regularly to stimulate bowel movement and improve digestion.

Tips for increasing fibre intake:

- Eat foods high in insoluble fibre, which include: nuts, seeds, fresh fruits and vegetables, fruit and vegetable peels, dried fruit, fruits with small seeds (berries, figs), prunes and prune juice, seeds, nuts, corn, whole grain breads and cereals, brown rice, bran, wheat germ, dried beans, peas and lentils.
- Add a little bran to stews, porridge or cereals.
- Eat more fruit and vegetables raw. Otherwise, steam or bake them only slightly to preserve their fibre.
- Increase fibre intake gradually over several weeks.

- Make sure you drink plenty of fluid to help the fibre pass easily through your system.
- Exercise regularly to strengthen your abdominal muscles, stimulate intestinal movement and reduce stress.
- Don't skip meals.
- Don't resist the urge to pass stools: this can worsen constipation.
- If the above measures don't provide relief, talk to your doctor about laxatives (medicines that soften the stools and stimulate bowel movements). Generally, however, it is best to avoid laxatives, as they cause loss of water and essential salts.

7. Changes in the taste of foods

Medication side-effects, poor nutrition and infections such as thrush or other infections, or possible nutritional deficiencies may affect your sense of taste, so that some familiar foods taste strange. They may develop cravings for food that they did not like in the past. However, these situations are common during illness.

How to deal with these changes

- Experiment with different foods and spices until you find foods you like. Try to have a varied diet. If red meat tastes bitter, choose other protein-rich foods such as cheese, eggs, chicken, fish, yoghurt and peanut butter.
- Try eating high-protein foods cold.
- Use lemon juice, herbs, spices, onion, garlic, vanilla or cinnamon to add flavour.
- Mint, garlic, ginger and other herbs and spices may seem to lose their taste when medicines are being taken. Try preparing food with sugar, vinegar or lemon instead.
- Brush and floss your teeth regularly.
- Increasing level of zinc supplement regimen up to 50 to 75 mg a day.
- Try rinsing your mouth with 1/2 teaspoon of baking soda in one cup of warm water before meals. This may freshen your mouth but may also change the pH.
- Use of tangy and or sour or spicy seasonings help: barbecue sauce, lemon and garlic, Italian dressing, soy sauce, fruit juices, vinegar and lemon help stimulate taste buds.

- Generally foods served at room temperature the flavour is maximized.

8. Nausea and vomiting

Nausea is the tendency to vomiting . Nausea has many causes and is a common side effect of many HIV drugs. It is important to determine what is making you nauseous. Nausea can be a sign of gastrointestinal infections or other intestinal problems. Nausea reduces the appetite and can be caused by certain foods, hunger, infections, stress and lack of water. It can also be a side-effect of medicines although certain medicines can help to relieve nausea. Nausea may be caused by the medicines you are taking or by infections in your body. Being infected with HIV can make it hard for you to eat sometimes. This is very common. You may not be able to digest certain foods that you used to eat all the time. The medicines you take may make you feel sick to your stomach. You may have infections in your mouth which hurt when you swallow. You may just feel too tired to eat. And you may worry a lot because you know you should eat, no matter how you feel. If nausea or vomiting last more than 2-3 days you should call your doctor. Call within 48 hours if you can't eat solid foods at all. There are some anti-nausea medications that you may be able to purchase over the counter. Your doctor can also prescribe some. Some PLWHAs have found that smoking marijuana helps them deal with nausea. Ginger, as in ginger ale, has been shown to decrease nausea.

The good news is that there are certain foods that can help you feel better when you are having these problems.

Cause of nausea:

Nausea can have many causes, such as HIV or other infections, some medications, toxicities to medication, not eating, dehydration, overeating, certain foods and odours, migraine headaches, food poisoning, and food allergies.

Consequences of nausea:

Nausea can result in loss of appetite, reduced food intake, weight loss, and interfere with doing daily activities. It can be serious. Make sure your doctor knows you have nausea. In the meantime, try the following to control nausea.

Try these tips:

- Eat small frequent meals. Do not skip meals and do not go hungry.
- Eat more during the times you are feeling better but do not overeat.
- Don't eat your favorite foods when you are nauseated. This could cause you to be "turned off" by them later.
- Eat salty foods, avoid very sweet foods.
- Plain, simple foods are best to eat now. Try these: soups, puddings and custards, ice cream, rice, macaroni, noodles, toast, yogurt, soft-cooked eggs, cream of wheat, farina, oatmeal, bananas, canned fruit, mashed potatoes, crackers, cottage cheese and fruit, eggs.
- Stay away from fried and greasy foods. Use only small amounts of margarine, butter, cream or oil in your food.
- Eat and drink slowly. Drink small frequent sips, rather than large amounts at a time.
- Check with your doctor about the amount of fluids you should be drinking if you have stomach or leg swelling.
- Drinking large amounts of sugary beverages quickly can cause nausea. This includes juices, soda, and supplement drinks.
- Drink fluids, including soups, between meals rather than with the meal.
- Eat dry toast, crackers, or melba toast when first getting up in the morning.
- Avoid overly sweet, greasy, hot, or spicy foods. Salty foods may be well tolerated.
- Avoid strong smelling foods and cooking odours. If strong odours make you feel nauseous, cooler foods have less of an odour and may be better tolerated. Try sandwiches, fruit, and cottage cheese. Eat in a well-ventilated area. Open the windows or eat outside.
- Prepare and freeze foods when you feel good to eat when you are not feeling well.
- Avoid getting overtired.
- If taking any dietary supplements (ex. multi-vitamins, minerals, herbs, etc.), take with food.
- Try ginger (tea, ale, grated root or powder), club soda, smelling the rind of citrus fruits.

- Do not lie down flat for at least 2 hours after eating. If you wish to rest, sit down. If you must lay down after eating, prop your head up at least 4 inches higher than your feet.
- Some medicines cause nausea. If possible, take them at a time of day when nausea will not interfere with meals.
- Sometimes just the smell of food can make you feel sick. Open the windows for some fresh air. Avoid making foods that will produce a strong smell in your home, like brewing coffee, frying meats or fish, or cooking spaghetti sauce or chili.
- If medications have been prescribed for your nausea and vomiting, take as directed by your doctor and pharmacist. If vomiting occurs, the body will lose water and will dehydrate even more quickly. If a person is too sick to eat, small and frequent drinks of water, fruit juice and vegetable soups may help.

How to deal with nausea and vomiting

General recommendations

- Sit up when eating. Try not to lie down until one or two hours after eating.
- Drink plenty of fluids after meals.
- Try not to prepare food yourself. The smell of preparing or cooking food may worsen the feeling of nausea. Ask somebody else to prepare food or eat foods that require little preparation.

Recommended foods to eat and drink

- If vomiting occurs, keep drinking small amounts of water, soups and spice teas. Eat soft foods and go back to solid foods when the vomiting stops.
- You may be able to relieve the feeling of nausea by smelling fresh orange or lemon peel, or by drinking lemon juice in hot water or a herbal or ginger tea
- Eat dry and salty foods such as toast, crackers and cereal.

Foods to avoid

- Fatty, greasy and very sweet foods can make nausea worse. Try to remove one food at a time from the diet to see if it makes a difference. If so, avoid that food. What affects one person may not affect others. People need to find out what suits them best.

- There are medicines that can reduce nausea.
- Even if you are not eating you need to replace your body fluids. You can also try sipping liquid supplements. Again, don't go without solid foods for two days without calling your doctor. When you are ready to try and eat start with bland, dry foods like toast or crackers. Generally, cold foods without much of an odour are easier to take when you are feeling nauseous. Don't push it. Several small meals will be easier to take than one large one. Eat slowly and don't lie down immediately. If you are feeling nauseous it is probably easier to let someone else prepare the food for you, if possible.

9. Diarrhoea

Diarrhoea is a common side effect of HIV-related infections and HIV-related medications. Everybody ends up coping with it at one time or another but that doesn't mean that it is unimportant. You should tell your doctor when you have had diarrhoea and call her/him if unexplained diarrhoea lasts for more than three days. Diarrhoea can be a sign of an infection in your intestine. Intestinal infections are often caused by the same bacteria and parasites that cause food poisoning. They can be serious for people with HIV and need to be treated.

Definition: Diarrhoea can be defined as bowel movements that occur too often and that are too loose. The average number of regular bowel movements varies greatly from 3-21 times per week. What is your normal bowel habit? Infections, medicines and emotional stress can all cause diarrhoea. it can make you feel weak and become dehydrated

Consequences: Decreased appetite, malabsorption of nutrients and drugs, contributing to malnutrition, weight loss, wasting and possible drug failure. Persistent diarrhoea may lead to dehydration, electrolyte imbalance, hospitalization and death. Until diarrhoea is controlled, good nutrition and hydration is absolutely necessary.

Causes of diarrhoea could be from:

- Changes in the gastrointestinal tract from HIV infection

- Infections that injure the bowel (parasitic, bacterial, viral)
- A number of drugs
- Difficulty in absorbing fats
- Lactose intolerance
- Mega dose of vitamin C
- Food sensitivity (ex: raw fruits or vegetables, fatty foods: bacon, fried foods, gravies, sauces)
- Stress
- Drinking supplements or other concentrated beverages too fast

Let your doctor know about the state of your bowel movements and when they changed. Call your doctor if you have diarrhoea that persists for three days. A doctor should be notified when diarrhoea persists two days for a baby under twelve months old. Diarrhoea always has an underlying cause. The first step is to find out what that cause is and to resolve it by treating the infection or adjusting current medications.

Tips to control diarrhoea

Allow your bowel to rest for 24 hours and only have clear fluids that have some calories. Avoid foods that can increase diarrhoea. Problem foods can include the following:

- Fatty, greasy and fried foods. Choose a baked potato over French fries, hard-boiled egg over scrambled, and broiled chicken over fried chicken. Reducing the amount of fat eaten at one time can make a big difference.
- Spicy or overly sweet foods: Cajun, curries, chili peppers, or candy bars, glazed donuts, etc.
- Caffeinated foods and drinks: chocolate, coffee, strong teas, colas and others containing caffeine
- Foods high in bulk and roughage, such as bran, whole grain cereals and breads, popcorn, nuts, seeds and skins, raw vegetables and fruits, and gas producing foods: cauliflower, beans, bell peppers, onions and cabbage. Beano, an over the counter enzyme product, might help.
- Watch out for milk products – you may have developed an inability to digest the sugar in milk called lactose. This condition is called lactose intolerance. Symptoms of lactose

intolerance are stomach distention, bloating, gas and diarrhoea.

- Drinking liquid nutritional supplements, especially quickly and on an empty stomach, can cause diarrhoea and nausea.
- Cigarette smoking and alcoholic beverages may also make diarrhoea worse.

Keep trying to adjust your diet to reduce your diarrhoea. Consider these recommendations:

What to do if you have diarrhoea :-

- Replace fluids lost to your body in the diarrhoea. Drink 10–12 eight ounce glasses per day.
- Drink between meals. Try mild liquids like diluted fruit juices or fruit drinks or defizzed fruit flavored sodas, sports drinks, rice water, weak tea, soups and broth.
- Rice drinks can be made easily: 1 cup white rice into 6 cups of boiling water, reduce to a simmer until rice is cooked. Blend the rice and add flavorings, like sugar, cinnamon, and lemon rind, to taste.
- Rice soups, like congee, a classic Chinese dish, are easy to make and serves the same purpose as horchata. Combine 1 cup of washed short grain rice and 8 cups of water in a large saucepan with a tight-fitting lid. Bring to a boil, cover, and reduce heat to simmer. Cook for 1 1/2 hours. Serve hot.
- You can add salt and pepper to taste. Also as tolerated, you can add and cook till hot vegetables like spinach, tomatoes, or scallion, and tofu or an egg, slightly beaten then thoroughly cooked.
- Electrolyte solutions and drinks. Oral rehydration therapy (ORT) drink can be easily made and taken: 1 quart of water, 1 teaspoon salt, 4 teaspoons sugar, and 1 heaping teaspoon of baking soda, boiled for 3–5 minutes, refrigerated and then flavored with lemon, lime or fruit juice. It is also available in most pharmacies/ chemists .
- Purchase commercial electrolyte replacement
- Replace the potassium lost to your body in diarrhoea. If you do not have enough potassium you can feel very weak. These foods are high in potassium: bananas, potatoes, fish and meat.

- Some food can actually help stop the diarrhoea. It would be good for you to eat plain white rice, cream of wheat or farina cereal, toasted white bread, plain macaroni or noodles, boiled eggs, oatmeal, ice cream, jello, applesauce, bananas, canned fruit, mashed potatoes, yogurt, and plain crackers.
- Don't skip meals , even though you don't feel like eating. Eat small amounts of food every couple of hours.
- Try eating foods at room temperature rather than very hot or cold.
- Every 1/2 hour or so eat small servings of bananas, ½ cup boiled white rice, 1/2 cup applesauce, 1 slice of dry white toasted bread, or caffeine-free tea.
- Add other easy to digest foods: mashed potatoes, cream of rice or wheat, dry crackers, flavored gelatin, broth, cooked carrots, or yogurt with live cultures.
- Add other low fibre foods that are soft and easy to digest: noodles, hard boiled eggs, saltine crackers, rice–cakes, etc.
- Foods with soluble fibre can actually help: white rice, oatmeal, apple sauce, fruits and vegetables without skin, like apples, grapes, apricots, pears, and peaches, potato, sweet potato, carrots, unseasoned split pea soup, etc. Psyllium, Metamucil, Fibercon and other bulking agents are formulated in powders or bars and can be purchased over the counter.
- Try enteric-coated Lactobacillus acidophilus tablets.
- Slowly return to your normal diet.
- Stay away from fatty, greasy foods and fried foods. Do not eat doughnuts, chips, fried potatoes or french fries, bacon, sausages, gravy, bologna, hot dogs, fried chicken, fried fish, or other fried meats. Use only small amounts of margarine, butter, cream or oil in your food.
- Stay away from spicy foods. Do not eat chili, pizza, hot sauce or tacos.
- Avoid foods with a lot of crunchy fibre. They can irritate your intestines. Do not eat raw fruits or raw vegetables or the skins or seeds of any fruit or vegetable. Do not eat corn. Do not eat whole wheat breads. Do not eat nuts.
- If you have cramps, stay away from foods that can cause gas. Do not eat dried beans, canned beans, cabbage, broccoli, cauliflower, carbonated drinks, or beer. No chewing gum.

Food and Water Safety First!

Make sure you are following sanitation guidelines:

- Don't eat raw or undercooked meats, fish, poultry or eggs. Use only pasteurized milk and cheese products. Avoid hard to clean raw vegetables, like lettuce or broccoli and sprouts.
- Wash your hands after you use the bathroom, and before and after you prepare foods or eat.
- Wash all kitchen surfaces and utensils with hot, soapy water, then apply a cleaning solution of 3 tablespoons of bleach to 1 quart of water, let stand for 5–10 minutes, rinse thoroughly and air dry.

Drink water that is considered safer, i.e. water that is:

1. Brought to a rolling boil for at least 1 minute (may then be refrigerated)
2. Distilled
3. Processed via reverse osmosis.
4. Filtered at or less than 1 absolute micron through a filter
5. Bottled mineral water that meets these guidelines
    - Water from a water- dispensing machine is not guaranteed to be safe.
    - Do not drink water from lakes, ponds, river , streams or springs.

Consider with your doctor medications to control diarrhoea:

- Antidiarrhoeal Combination Products (Diasorb, Donnagel, Kao–Spen, Kaolin w/Pectin, Kepectolin, Kaopectate Advanced formula, Parepectolin, K–Pek, K–C, Kaodene, Rheaban) (contains salicylate, which is also found in aspirin; therefore, use with caution in patients with bleeding disorders or salicylate sensitivity)
- Bismuth Subsalicylate (Pepto–Bismol and Maximum Strength, Bismatrol and Extra Strength, Pink Bismuth) (may reduce absorption of tetracyclines)
- Difenoxin HCI with Atropine Sulfate (Motofen) (do not use concurrently with MAO inhibitors)

- Diphenoxylate HCI with Atropine Sulfate (Logen, Lomotil, Lonox, Lamanate) (do not use at the same time with MAO inhibitors, Barbiturates, tranquilizers, and alcohol)
- Loperamide HCI (Imodium A–D, Kaopectate II, Maalox, Loperamide, Pepto Diarrhea Control) (may cause drowsiness)

Other treatments that might lessen diarrhoea:

- Pancreolytic Enzymes: Sometimes diarrhoea is due to an absorption problem, sometimes due to enzyme deficiencies. Pancreolytic enzymes are available through prescription, buyers clubs, or health food stores.
- L–glutamine: Typical recommendations for glutamine may be 0.4g/kg up to 30g/day for about 5–14 days, followed by 5–10g/day. (Do not use with endstage liver or kidney disease).
- Total parenteral nutrition (TPN): Intravenous feeding for people with severe malnutrition.
- Probiotic preparations: Live bacteria to supplement the microbes in the GI tract. Usually contain strains of Lactobacilli, bifidobacteria, saccharomycis, etc. Not for long term use.
- FOS: fructo-oligosaccharides. Prebiotics that mainly stimulate the activity of bifidobacteria.
- Florastor™ contains Saccharomyces boulardii, a yeast, that is to help protect your intestinal tract and keep your intestines functioning well. Often considered a probiotic. See www.florastor.com

Drugs that are known to cause diarrhoea:

- **Antibacterials:** Ampicillin, Amoxicillin, Cefamandole, Cefnaxone, Ciprofloxacin, Clarithromycin, Clindamycin, Clofazimine, Doxycycline, Erythromycin, Ethionamide, Flagyl, Imipenim–cilastin, Para– aminosalicylic acid (PAS), Paromomyncin sulfate, Rifabutin, Rifampin, Tetracycline
- **Antifungals:** Amphotericin B, Fluconazole, Flucytosine, Foscarnet, Ketoconazole, Miconazole, Nystatin
- **Antineoplastics:** Adriamycin, Bleomycin sulfate, Etopside, Vinblastine sulfate
- **Antiprotozoals:** Atovaquone, Azithromycin, lodoquinol, Metronidazole, Thiabendazole, Trimetrexate

- **Antiretrovirals:** Epivir (3TC), Zalcitabine (ddc), Zidovudine (AZT), Videx (ddI), Zerit (d4t), Norvir (ritonovir), Kaletra (lipinavir/ritonavir),any drug boosted with Norvir, Viracept (nelfinavir), Crixivan (indinavir)
- **Chemotherapeutic Agents:** Adriamycin, Bleomycin sulfate, Etoposide, Vinblastine sulfate
- **Immune Based Therapies:** (Epogen), Granulocyte macrophage colony stimulating factor (GMCSF), Interleukin2
- **Miscellaneous:** Buspirone HCl, Chloral hydrate, Amitryptoline, Paroxetine, Sertraline,
- Metoclopramide, Sargramostin, Anadrol, Megace, Diphenoxylate

If diarrhoea persists longer than a few days, seek medical advice: you might have an infection. Your doctor may think it is necessary to prescribe anti-diarrhoeal medication.

10. Malnutrition

Malnutrition is a common complication of HIV infection and AIDS. Malnutrition is a major and early problem in HIV infection. While some people may be undernourished before becoming HIV+, in other cases HIV results in undernourishment (Beach, Baum and co-workers). In addition to malabsorption problems, nutrients such as zinc, selenium and vitamins B_6, B_{12}, E and folic acid are likely used faster than others. Deterioration of the small intestine lining may be the earliest result of HIV infection and it often becomes a dominant feature in advanced HIV disease (Batman et al, 1989; Ehrenpreis, 1992; Gazzard, 1992; Grunfeld, Kotler & coworkers; La Brooy, 1993; Laine et al, 1993; Lim et al, 1993; Ott et al, 1993; Schwarz & Greene, 1992; Smith & Mai, 1992; Ullrich et al, 1989; Zangerle et al, 1993). Even if proper digestion has begun in your mouth and stomach, nutrients still may not be fully absorbed from the intestines. Thus diet needs to be adjusted accordingly.

Malnutrition places added stress on an already weakened immune system and may complicate the treatment of the disease by affecting the intestinal tracts ability to absorb drugs, not to mention its inability to absorb proteins, carbohydrates and fats.

Malnutrition in children is particularly devastating because children are still growing and developing, placing even higher energy demands on their bodies and immune systems.

Reasons for Malnutrition:

- Changes in Metabolism
    - alterations in the function of the gastrointestinal tract and the ability to use food in an efficient way
    - increased use of body fat stores
    - recurrent fevers and infections causing a rise in metabolic rates
    - depletion of vitamin and mineral stores
- Changes in Oral Intake
    - decreased intake due to medication schedules that require the child to be without food (NPO) for a period of time before and after the medications are given, as well as potential
    - problems with nausea, vomiting and mouth sores
    - altered intake due to oral infection with *Candida* (thrush.) Bear in mind that *Candida* can invade the oesophagus (throat), as well as the small intestine without being present in the mouth
    - lack of adequate food supply in the home
    - caregivers that may be infected as well and not able to care for the child properly
    - inability to tolerate fats and lactose (milk sugars)
    - diarrhoea, the cause of which may or may not be known
- Functional Impairment
    - chewing and swallowing may be greatly affected in children with HIV involvement of the nervous system. An evaluation by a speech pathologist can be very beneficial.

A good multivitamin should be considered. A minimum of 25 mg of vitamin B_6, 50 mcg each of selenium and chromium, and no more than 10,000 i.u. of vitamin A could be a rule of thumb in choosing this multivitamin with minerals. In addition, another 50-75 mg of zinc, 400-800 i.u. of vitamin E from a natural source, vitamin B_{12} by a **non**-stomach route, and 600-1500 mg of N-acetyl cysteine (NAC) may be useful.

A preventive approach is better than a treatment approach; i.e., establish and keep adequate nourishment in the earliest stage of HIV infection as possible. Wasting, an internal deterioration of body chemistries that ultimately results in a persistent weight loss that occurs even in the absence of opportunistic infection, seems to result from problems in the body's metabolism. While protein, fat and carbohydrate in your food provide building blocks and fuel for your body, vitamins and minerals are tools that are necessary for your body to **use** those building blocks. Making sure you are not deficient in these tools should help your body use the building blocks better, and give better resilience if you get an opportunistic infection.

11. Fatigue / Feeling tired

Feeling tired is normal when you are sick. It is a sign that your body is working hard to fight off germs. Your body needs rest, but it also needs good food.

Fatigue can interfere with nutrition in that sometimes you may feel too tired to cook, or even to eat proper meals. Try these simple ideas.

Definition: A state of increased discomfort and decreased efficiency resulting from prolonged or excessive exertion; a loss of power or capacity to respond to stimulation.

Consequences: Fatigue can be a barrier to buying food, cooking meals, and even eating. When you do not eat because you are too tired to buy or make food, your body does not get the energy it needs to keep you going and to keep your immune strong.

First: Speak to your doctor immediately so you can work together to solve the problem that is causing fatigue. Be informed about your treatment. Meet regularly with a registered dietitian who can address any nutrition related concerns you may be experiencing.

Causes of Fatigue

- HIV itself because the body uses a lot of energy to fight the virus
- Some anti-HIV drugs, including AZT, which slow the production of red blood cells (which are responsible for carrying oxygen around the body)
- Decreased food intake or poor absorption in the gut may cause low levels of vitamins and minerals in the blood
- Stress, depression, and/or disrupted sleep patterns

- Low levels of testosterone
- Lactic acidosis, a side-effect of the nucleoside analogue class of anti-HIV drugs (AZT, d4T, etc)
- Anaemia (decreased production of red blood cells) caused by the HIV virus, certain medications or chemotherapy
- Other infections that you may get as a result of your decreased immune system function

Nutrition Tips to Help You Deal with Fatigue

- Rest as much as possible, and don't tire yourself with food preparation. Ask for help from family and friends to assist you with cooking or buying groceries. HIV/AIDS Positive Network or support groups can sometimes help with home care and food parcels. Don't be embarrassed to ask for their help. People like doing things for others.
- Shop by phone and have your groceries delivered or ask a friend to shop for you
- Order take-out restaurant food or have a friend or relative to bring you food
- Eat small, frequent meals packed with nutrients, for example: ½ roast beef sandwich with cheese
- Fix simple snacks, rather than meals, for yourself
- Eat canned foods. Try creamed soups, spaghetti, chili, chow-mein and other things. They may not taste the greatest, but they'll get some food in your stomach. And if you eat a piece of fruit for dessert and drink a glass of milk or juice, you've got a balanced meal!
- Eat frozen foods. Frozen dinners, pizza, egg rolls, macaroni and cheese, fried chicken and fish. Just pop them in the oven, and set a timer. Come back after a little nap, and you're ready to eat. Drink a glass of milk or juice, add a piece of toast or fruit.
- Freeze extra portions and leftovers for when you're too tired to cook. Keep stores of canned and frozen foods, which need little preparation.
- Choose high-energy, easy-to-eat foods that require no preparation, such as bananas, avocado, yoghurt and nuts.

- Convenience foods, take-aways and food delivery services may be quite expensive, but can be a help during times of fatigue.
- If you are going to spend the day in bed, put some favourite foods and drinks in a cooler with ice beside you. Then you can get your rest but not be without food. A food warmer or crock pot could be used in the same way to keep hot food hot at your bedside.
- On days that you feel well cook extra food and freeze it in little plastic containers. You'll be grateful to have these to heat up on days that you are tired.
- Decrease your consumption of coffee—it may actually add to the problem of fatigue
- Eat with nice people in a soothing and supportive atmosphere.
- Make as few dirty dishes as possible. Use paper cups and dishes, cook in the foil pans that food comes in.
- Tell your doctor if fatigue persists; it may be related to a treatable underlying condition, such as anaemia.

12. Heartburn

Heartburn, also known as acid indigestion, is a burning sensation in the chest or throat. The pain associated with heartburn occurs when stomach acid comes into contact with and irritates the lining of the oesophagus. It has NOTHING to do with the heart – it is a digestive problem. It is a common symptom of Gastroesophageal Reflux Disease (GERD). Heartburn occurring more than twice a week may be considered GERD, and it can lead to more serious health problems. You may experience one or more of the follow symptoms:

- A burning chest pain that starts from the heart area and moves up toward the throat
- A feeling that food is coming back into the mouth
- An acid or bitter taste at the back of the throat
- An increase in pain severity when lying down or bending over

Cause of heartburn

The lower oesophageal sphincter (LES) is a muscle located at the bottom of the oesophagus and acts as a valve. The LES opens to let food enter the stomach and then closes to keep the stomach contents from returning up to the esophagus. When the LES weakens, stomach acid flows backward into the oesophagus and causes heartburn.

Common factors that may cause heartburn

- Citrus fruits and their juices, chocolate, peppermint, spearmint, tomatoes or tomato products, raw onions, garlic, black pepper, vinegar, and fatty or spicy foods.
- Beverages that are caffeinated &/or carbonated and alcoholic beverages. This includes coffee and soda.
- Eating large portions of food at one time.
- Eating late night snacks shortly before going to bed.
- Being overweight.
- Stress
- Pregnancy
- Hiatal Hernia- a condition in which a portion of the stomach protrudes upward into the chest through an opening in the diaphragm.
- Certain medications: Non-nucleoside analogs (non-nukes) and protease inhibitors (PIs) for HIV treatment are noted to have caused intestinal discomfort and/or vomiting. Recurrent vomiting may loosen the muscle valve and increase the likelihood of heartburn.
- Some medications to treat high blood pressure, heart disease, depression, insomnia or anxiety, and asthma
- Smoking. Tobacco may stimulate stomach acid production.

Complications of Long-Term Heartburn: Heartburn can disrupt sleep and make eating difficult. Chronic acid injury can lead to respiratory infections, scarring of the lower oesophagus, ulcers, and even oesophageal cancer.

Preventing heartburn: All treatments are offered to decrease the amount of acid backflow or to make the stomach content less irritating to the lining of the oesophagus. Treatment options include:

Lifestyle and Dietary Modifications (Preferred Approaches)

Avoid foods and beverages that may induce heartburn

Avoid tight fitting clothes

Avoiding eating 2-3 hours before sleep

Do not over eat – stop before you are full

Keep your upper body up-right 1-2 hours after eating
Stop smoking
Raise the head of your bed 6-8 inches when sleeping
Lose weight if overweight

Medications of Heartburn :

Over-the-counter (OTC) medications are available to treat heartburn. However, many of them have been found to interact with HIV medications, in most cases decreasing their effect. Below is a brief reminder of how to prevent adverse interactions.

- Lexiva, Crixivan, and Rescriptor should be taken at least 1 hour apart from antacids such as Maalox and Tums. Reyataz should be taken 2 hours before or 1 hour after antacids.
- Crixivan and Rescriptor should not be taken with acid suppression agents (H2 blockers) such as Pepcid, Tagamet, and Zantac. They can be taken 12 hours after taking Reyataz and use with caution when taking Lexiva.
- Crixivan, Rescriptor, and Reyataz, should not be taken with proton pump inhibitors such as Nexium, Prevacid, and Prilosec. Use with caution when taking Lexiva.

If you are taking any medications for heartburn, either prescription or over-the-counter, notify your doctor before starting any HIV medication regimen or changing regimens.

Key Points to Remember

- Don't ignore frequent heartburn — instead consult with your physician.
- Heartburn is a common condition. Timely treatment is recommended to achieve early symptom resolution.
- If you are self-medicating for heartburn two or more times a week, or if symptoms remain with the use of OTC or prescription medication, you need to see a doctor and perhaps be referred to a gastroenterologist.

How Heart Attack Differs From Heartburn?

A heart attack occurs when the blood supply to part of the heart muscle is restricted or stopped, usually by blocked or narrowed arteries. Get help fast if you experience any of these signs:

- intense pressure or crushing pain in the chest that may extend into the arms, neck or back
- moderate chest pain, tightness, pressure or vague discomfort
- feeling faint, dizzy or weak
- difficulty in breathing or swallowing
- a feeling of severe indigestion that doesn't go away after taking an antacid

13. Unintentional Weight Loss / Wasting

Research has demonstrated that there is a correlation between nutrition, quality of life and managing disease progression. Malnutrition, weight loss, and lost lean body mass have been associated with poor patient prognosis and should be aggressively managed. Once lost, it can take 10 times longer to gain back lost weight and lost body cell mass.

"Wasting ... has been associated with increased mortality, accelerated disease progression, loss of muscle protein mass, and impairment of strength and functional status." Even a 5% loss has been linked to increased illness and death. Different factors contribute to unintentional weight loss and malnutrition. Unintentional weight loss can result from starvation, a condition called cachexia, or a combination of the two.

Starvation is a form of weight loss that occurs because of decreased intake of calories and protein. It can also occur in an individual who is eating enough, but who is losing many calories because of altered bowel function and diarrhoea, more commonly referred to as malabsorption. Starvation can result from a combination of both decreased intake of food and increased calorie losses. If the bowel can absorb normally, starvation can be corrected by increased intake of calories and protein. If the bowel cannot absorb normally, then the reason for the bowel problem needs to be identified and the problem corrected, so the individual can eat and absorb nutrients. Initially, starvation mainly causes a decrease in body fat, rather than skeletal muscle. If starvation progresses over a long period of time, more muscle tissue will be lost and the individual will begin to experience loss of body muscle or "wasting."

Cachexia differs from starvation. The loss of weight is mostly from loss of muscle tissue, known as a loss of "Lean Body Mass"

(LBM) or "Body Cell Mass" (BCM). Both the muscle and protein tissues in our body are the tissues in which most of our metabolic function occurs, including immune tissue, organ tissue, tissue that produces energy and support movement, and tissue that supports body functions. No protein tissue can be considered storage tissue. All protein tissues have a role and are part of body function homeostasis or balance. Loss of LBM alters the balance and can affect the body functions that support maintenance of optimal health. Cachexia is caused by metabolic alterations. These metabolic alterations affect how the body uses the nutrients that come from food. The end result of cachexia is that the body uses protein tissues for energy. When an individual suffers from cachexia simply eating adequate protein, calories and micronutrients may not reverse this form of unintentional weight loss. This is defined as "wasting syndrome."

HIV infection often causes problems with weight loss.

- Increase the number of times you eat each day. If you usually have 2 meals per day, start having 3 meals per day. if you usually have 3 meals per day, start eating 4 or 5 times per day. You may have to plan your meals something like this: Breakfast — Snack — Lunch — Snack — Supper — Snack
- Don't count on your appetite. Eat even if you aren't hungry. Watch the clock and eat something every 2 to 3 hours, whether you feel like it or not.
- Eat more foods that are high in calories and protein, such as milk, cheese, meats, and peanut butter. Make your snacks count! Eat healthy foods high in calories and protein between meals. See the list of healthy snacks in the section, "Snacking On Healthy Foods Makes A Difference."
- Add extra fat to your food. It can increase calories a lot without your having to eat a larger amount of food. Ideas for adding fat to your food are in the section, "Gaining Weight With Extra Fat."
- Add sugar, honey, syrup, brown sugar and other sweet things to your food. Put jams and jellies on breads, toast, rolls, pancakes and waffles. Put sugar or honey in your coffee and tea. Add it to your cereal.

- Eat dried fruit such as raisins, prunes, dried apricots, dried apples, dried peaches, figs and dates. These are good by themselves or mixed with nuts for a snack. Add them to hot cereal such as oatmeal and cream of wheat.

Gaining Weight With Extra Milk and Dairy Products

- Drink milk as your beverage with meals. It has more calories and protein than juice, tea, water, or soft drinks. If you don't care for regular milk, try chocolate milk, buttermilk, egg nog, hot cocoa or milkshakes.
- Use milk instead of water to make soups and hot cereals.
- Make extra-strength milk by mixing 2 heaping tablespoons of dry powdered milk into every cup of milk that you use.
- Regular milk has more calories than low-fat milk or sweet acidophilus milk. Half and Half has the most calories of them all! It can be used in place of milk for drinking and in any recipe.
- Nonfat dry milk powder can be added to a lot of foods to give them more protein. You'll never taste it in there. Try adding it to raw ground beef before making it into hamburger patties, meatballs or meatloaf. You can also add it to any casserole, macaroni and cheese, tuna or egg salad, hot or cold cereal, scrambled eggs, mashed potatoes, milkshakes and puddings.
- Have ice cream as your desert often. It also makes a great snack in a bowl or a cone. You might also try adding it to breakfast cereal in the morning. Top your waffles or pancake with ice cream.

Gaining Weight With Extra Cheese

- Mix cheese into your scrambled eggs. Melt it onto fried eggs.
- Have cheeseburgers instead of plain hamburgers. Put cheese into all your meat sandwiches.
- Melt cheese onto your meatloaf and spaghetti.
- Put extra cheese on pizza.
- Put extra cheese in macaroni and cheese and any other type of casserole.
- Put cheese into your mashed potatoes, and on your baked potato. Melt cheese onto other vegetables too.

- Put cheese on top of salads, soups and chili.
- Make melted cheese toast instead of plain buttered toast. Put a piece of cheese inside of hot biscuits, rolls and corn bread.

Gaining Weight With Extra Meat

- Double the amount of meat you usually put on sandwiches. Put two hamburger patties on your hamburger bun.
- Have two or three helpings of meat at meals. Eat less of other foods at that meal if you are feeling full.
- Put chopped, cooked meats into soups and salads, and on top of pizza.

Gaining Weight With Peanut Butter

- Spread peanut butter **thickly** on your sandwiches or crackers
- Put peanut butter on pancakes and waffles before you pour on the syrup.
- Spread peanut butter on apples, bananas or pears at snack time.
- Blend peanut butter into milkshakes.
- Put peanut butter on hot toast, hot biscuits. It tastes great melted!
- Fill the dent in sticks of raw celery with peanut butter. Makes a good snack.
- Spread peanut butter on cookies, vanilla wafers, and graham crackers before eating.

Gaining Weight With Extra Fat

Adding fat to your food can increase calories a lot! It can be hard to digest sometimes, though. Use these tips when you feel well. If you begin to have diarrhoea or nausea stop adding so much fat.

- A teaspoon of butter or margarine will add 45 calories. Mix it into hot foods such as soups, vegetables, mashed potatoes, cooked cereal, rice, and casseroles. Spread it on bread, rolls, corn bread and biscuits. You'll use more if these breads are hot when you spread on the butter or margarine.
- Salad dressings are a very tasty way to add fat to your food. Try Ranch, Blue Cheese or Buttermilk dressing on sandwiches. Pour it over baked potatoes, or use it as a dip for vegetables.

- A tablespoon of mayonnaise has 100 calories. Salad dressing looks like mayonnaise, but has only half the calories. Put mayonnaise on your sandwiches. Put a lot of mayonnaise in tuna salad, egg salad, chicken salad, ham salad. Try it on a peanut butter sandwich.
- Sour cream has a lot of calories, too. Put sour cream on cooked vegetables such as potatoes, beans, carrots and squash. Top your bowl of chili, salad and soups with it. Add sour cream to casseroles. Dip raw vegetables into sour cream. Put it on top of fresh fruit with some sugar for dessert.
- Whipping cream has 60 calories in each tablespoon. Add it to pies, fruit, puddings and other desserts. Top your hot chocolate or cocoa with whipped cream.
- Frosting is made of fat and sugar. You can buy it already-made in cans. Top fruits, cookies, pudding, cakes, and other desserts with frosting.
- Fry your foods rather than baking or roasting them. If you roll your meats and vegetables in flour or crumbs before frying them, they will hold onto more of the fat and calories.
- Put gravy and cream sauces on your meats and vegetables.

Foods Which Will Not Help You Gain Weight

When you are trying to gain weight you must think about eating a lot of calories. The more calories you eat, the more weight you can gain. You should realize that your goal of eating more calories and gaining weight is exactly the opposite of what many people are trying to do.

When people become infected with HIV they often decide to make the most of their health. They may begin to pay more attention to nutrition. But if they follow what friends and family and the media say is good nutrition, they may lose weight. And that's not what they need!

Treating Unintentional Weight Loss:

Because the causes of unintentional weight loss are so variable, treatment plans should be individualized and based on the cause of the lost weight, as well as goals for regaining both lost weight and lost lean body mass. Addressing unintentional weight loss proactively and vigorously can improve the overall health and outcomes for people living with HIV/AIDS.

Wasting or Unintentional weight loss was an important feature of AIDS in the early years of the epidemic. Even today, AIDS is referred to as "slim disease" in Africa. Experts define wasting as involuntary or unintentional loss of 10% or more of body weight.

Designing a Treatment Plan:

Weight loss can be caused by a number of factors including:

- decreased intake of food, medication side effects
- decreased absorption of nutrients
- untreated secondary infection
- alterations in metabolism

Identifying the cause of the weight loss is the first step in developing an appropriate treatment plan. Whether the cause is related to decreased intake, increased nutrient losses or changes in metabolic function, nutrition plays an important role in stopping the weight loss, and in regaining lost weight and lost LBM.

Both food and food supplements can play a valuable role in developing a successful treatment plan. The use of oral supplements can be particularly useful when an individual is unable to take in food as a source of calories and protein because of difficulty with chewing, swallowing and fatigue. People may not find time to prepare meals properly and in these situations, food supplements can also be helpful. Second line nutrition supplements, which include micronutrient supplements or amino acid supplements, can also be useful in specific situations to support the treatment of weight loss. Specific foods and nutrition supplements are helpful to specific symptom management such as diarrhoea, decreased intake, or when a patient is wasting secondary to metabolic changes.

Adequate Calories, Protein and Micronutrients

When using supplements, do not take more than the recommended dose on the label unless advised to do so by a knowledgeable doctor / dietician / nutritionist . The more is not necessarily the better. A recent case underscores this warning. As reported in the September 2005 *International Journal of STD and AIDS*, an HIV positive man in London developed severe liver inflammation with skyrocketing ALT levels after taking more than a dozen dietary supplements, many at high doses — as much as 67 times the recommended daily value; fortunately, once he stopped taking the supplements, his liver function returned to normal.

Certain vitamins and minerals (including the fat-soluble vitamins A, D, and E) can be toxic at high doses, and they may cause deleterious effects even at lower doses beyond what is provided in a typical multivitamin pill. Remember that "natural" does not necessarily mean "safe." Seek medical advice before starting a new supplement or beginning any unusual diet. Tell the doctor about any use of supplements (as well as over-the-counter medications, recreational drugs, and herbal remedies), since these can potentially interact with antiretroviral drugs.

The first line in nutrition treatment for unintentional weight loss is assuring the intake of adequate calories, protein and micronutrients, preferably from food. However, both medical symptoms and social conditions can affect an individual's ability to eat enough food to meet optimal energy and nutrient needs. Side effects of HIV/AIDS and/or medications can cause symptoms such as nausea, vomiting, and diarrhea, thereby also making the consumption of adequate nutrients difficult. In addition, alterations in metabolism can cause increased energy needs. Other issues such as economic and social conditions, including a physical inability to prepare meals can also affect the ability to eat properly. All of these symptoms and conditions can affect intake, in addition to making one feel overwhelmed by attempting to eat what appears to be so much.

- Depending on the specific symptom(s), dietary intakes can be adjusted to help manage the symptoms.

If an individual needs to add calories and protein, other strategies can come into play. Altering your meal plan to include 6 small meals per day can be helpful, as well as the inclusion of high calorie, high protein nutrient dense snacks.

Commercial Nutrition Supplements

A number of commercial nutritional supplements are also available and can help a person living with HIV/AIDS (PLWHA) gain back lost weight. In choosing a nutritional supplement consideration should be given to a number of things, including presence of diarrhoea, lactose intolerance, individual nutrient requirements, and taste, as well as weight gain and body cell mass goals.

Impact of Antiretroviral Treatment

While effective antiretroviral therapy has dramatically reduced the incidence of severe wasting, moderate weight loss is still a prominent feature of HIV disease. Weight loss was significantly associated with nausea, diarrhoea, thrush, poverty, history of drug use, CD4 cell count below 200 cells/mm^3, and HIV viral load above 100,000 copies/mL.

Rather than dramatic whole-body weight loss, today many HIV positive people on HAART experience lipoatrophy, or fat loss in the face, limbs, and buttocks. Paradoxically, this may coincide with fat accumulation in other areas of the body . Lipoatrophy is most strongly associated with use of nucleoside reverse transcriptase inhibitors (NRTIs), especially d4T (stavudine or Zerit). For this reason, U.S. government treatment guidelines no longer recommend d4T as part of a first-line regimen for people starting HAART.

Since HIV positive people and their clinicians may not recognize the early signs of wasting, it is important to monitor weight regularly to detect subtle changes. Underlying factors contributing to weight loss — such as OIs or hormone imbalances — should be promptly addressed. When it comes to weight loss, prevention is often easier than cure. While recombinant human growth hormone (HGH, Serostim) is FDA-approved for the treatment of HIV-related wasting, it is extremely expensive and is beyond the reach of the common men in developing countries and also can cause side effects including carpal tunnel syndrome, joint pain, and insulin resistance. Anabolic (muscle-building) steroids such as testosterone and oxandrolone (Oxandrin) help some patients gain weight, but can also cause adverse effects.

14. Malnutrition and Weight Loss/Wasting in Patients Infected with Human Immunodeficiency Virus

Weight loss and muscle wasting remain significant clinical problems, even in the era of potent antiretroviral therapy. In patients infected with human immunodeficiency virus (HIV), wasting, particularly loss of metabolically active lean tissue, has been associated with increased mortality, accelerated disease progression, loss of muscle protein mass, and impairment of strength and functional status. Factors that may contribute to wasting include inadequate intake, malabsorptive disorders, metabolic alterations, hypogonadism, and excessive cytokine production.

Malnutrition and wasting can be caused by four general factors. Any of these problems should be addressed with your doctor, who should also refer you to a dietitian.

1. **Low intake of calories and nutrients:** There are many causes for low intake. Some people suffer loss of appetite from depression, infection, fever, medications, treatment with chemotherapy or radiation, fatigue, diarrhoea, or nausea or have fear of eating. Other reasons are due to pain or difficulty chewing, tasting, or swallowing. Some people have financial problems or cannot get around easily and do not have access to food. The result is the protein break down.
2. **Malabsorption:** This occurs when foods are not getting broken down into nutrients, or if they are, cannot be carried out of the gut into the circulation system. If you have diarrhea or vomiting, food and liquid is not completely being absorbed. Problems causing the malabsorption can be due to medication, malnutrition, or infection. Diarrhoea or vomiting may be made worse when there is lactose intolerance or fat malabsorption.
3. **Abnormalities in metabolism:** Metabolism is the process of using nutrients to run the body. There may be an increased demand for calories protein, and nutrients.
4. **The wasting of muscles from not being used:** The "use it or lose it" concept is true. Changes in activity can occur when there are changes in work or social routines, or you just don't feel mentally or physically well enough to keep up your usual physical activity or exercise.

Protein Breakdown

Without enough calories and nutrients from foods vital body tissue protein may be used for fuel. This protein breakdown process is called catabolism. The result is called wasting or cachexia with muscle "atrophy," a decrease in the size of cells, tissues, and organs. Skeletal muscle loss may be visibly noticed and sometimes not. Weight may not change even though muscle mass has changed. Other body systems can be negatively affected, too. Other problems caused as a result of using protein for fuel include:

- A decreased in immune system competence,
- ncreased risk of infections, like PCP,
- Atrophy of the small intestine villi, resulting in difficulty digesting, absorbing, and using nutrients.

Diagnosis

- Monitor weight every 6 months in HIV-infected patients and every 3 months in patients with weight loss. Keep a weight chart in the patient's medical record.
- Assess adequacy and quality (protein, micronutrients) of dietary intake and malabsorption in all patients with weight loss.
- Distinguish between classic wasting (generalized weight loss) and lipoatrophy (disproportionate loss of fat in the limbs, face, or buttocks), considering immunologic and virologic status and medications.
- Assess potential underlying mechanisms of wasting, as follows:
- Inadequate food intake due to anorexia, gastrointestinal disturbances, or oral or oesophageal lesions.
- Active secondary infection.
- Hypogonadism and other endocrine abnormalities.
- Malabsorption and diarrhea.
- Hyperlactatemia or lactic acidosis in patients with rapid weight loss, anorexia, gastrointestinal disturbances, dyspnea, or fatigue.
- Determine impact of psychosocial factors (e.g.. access to food, depression) on food intake.

Treatment

- Provide nutrition counseling to increase caloric intake in patients with inadequate intake; maintain or increase intake in patients whose intake supports their current weight but is not sufficient to increase weight. Ensure adequate balance of protein, fat, and carbohydrate and micronutrient intake.
- Optimize antiretroviral therapy.

- Consider Resistance Exercise Training (RET) in stable, ambulatory patients with wasting. RET may be used in conjunction with other therapies.
- Administer testosterone replacement in HIV-infected men with significant weight loss and low testosterone levels.
- Consider stimulating the appetite with megestrol acetate for patients who are unable to voluntarily increase or maintain total energy intake.
- Consider other pharmacologic interventions, such as GH and anabolic steroids, for rapid weight loss associated with acute infection and in severe cases of continued weight loss refractory to nonpharmacologic therapies. Ensure adequate caloric intake during pharmacologic interventions.
- Reassess need for continued anabolic therapies in the context of the patient's overall health every 3.6 months.

Get Your Nutrition Trip Together: A Five-Point Plan

1. **The Diet**

   In general, practice eating high protein, high complex carbohydrates, and moderate fat foods, and drink plenty of fluids, 8-12 cups a day. Eat on a regular basis every few hours and whenever you are hungry. Take a general multiple-vitamin and mineral supplement daily and B complex daily. Attend to any nutrition concern. Individually, adjust this plan as conditions warrant.

2. **Physical Activity**

   Practice getting some physical activity on a routine basis. Activity can make a physical and psychological difference. It can make you stronger, more alert and relieve stress.

3. **Sleep**

   Set up a routine so that your sleep is steady and uninterrupted. Try not to sleep too few or too many hours each night. Get attention if there is a problem.

4. **Stress Management**

   Do things that make sense and support your self-esteem. Correct the tasks or situations that hurt your self-esteem. Include ways to release stress and ways to relax.

5. Unconditional Love

Make decisions and do things for you out of self-love and self-respect. This is really the key point. When you are paying attention to loving yourself, everything else is easier.

Evidence now demonstrates that nutritional counseling and support, appetite stimulants, progressive resistance training, and anabolic hormones can reverse weight loss and increase lean body mass in HIV-infected patients.

Prevention of weight loss

The significant impact of wasting on survival, disease progression, and functional status highlights the need to prevent muscle wasting and weight loss in HIV-infected patients. To prevent loss of weight and LBM, all HIV-infected patients should be encouraged to maintain adequate energy intake and engage in moderate exercise.

The following points needs to be considered :-

- Evaluation of weight and nutritional status of the HIV-infected patient. Weight history is important
- Potential risk factors for wasting before weight loss should be evaluated. Minimum basic investigation of risk factors for weight loss include history of reduced caloric intake due to anorexia or multiple factors leading to inaccessibility of food, opportunistic infections, gastrointestinal disease, malignancies, and other endocrine or metabolic conditions,
- Education on appropriate nutritional practices, exercise, and the importance of maintaining energy balance should be emphasized.
- For many patients, especially children, nutritional status is often related directly to the socioeconomic considerations that need to be recognized as an important determinant of overall nutritional status and growth.
- Recommendations on the appropriate monitoring of weight and growth in children will include consideration of increased energy requirements required for normal growth.

Treatment of active wasting

In contrast to the treatment of other HIV-related complications, a standardized approach to the management of active weight loss has not been established.

Restoration of healthy weight in stable patients with a history of weight loss

Early nutritional intervention is important in such patients to maximize gain of LBM and minimize gain of visceral fat.

Potential therapeutic interventions

A significant body of evidence now demonstrates that use of nutritional counseling and support, appetite stimulants, progressive resistance training (PRT), and anabolic hormones can reverse weight loss and increase LBM in HIV-infected patients. Treatment of associated opportunistic infections and optimization of antiretroviral therapy should be the first goal in patients with wasting, followed by an assessment for adequate caloric intake and food absorption.

Nutritional supplementation

Children and adults receiving enteral or parenteral feeding or oral nutritional supplements have commonly been reported to gain weight and in some cases body cell mass . Other forms of nutritional supplementation, including total parenteral nutrition (TPN), -hydoxy -methylbutyrate (-HMB), and high-quality oral protein have been assessed. Overall, studies suggest that increases in net daily energy and macronutrient intake can be achieved with the oral supplements, and their use may be an effective means of maintaining or increasing intake for some patients. A variety of conventional preparations are available, as well as specialized formulas for patients with specific intolerances.

Resistance exercise training

Resistance exercise can increase lean tissue in HIV-infected patients. In a recent study in asymptomatic HIV-infected men, almost all of whom were receiving HAART, a supervised 16-week weight-lifting programme was associated with a 1.4-kg increase in LBM) and significant increases in thigh muscle area.

Nonpharmacologic measures such as nutritional supplementation and exercise should always be considered and encouraged before pharmacologic interventions are instituted.

Appetite stimulation

Megestrol acetate, a synthetic progestational agent, is a potent appetite stimulant and effectively increases weight, although the weight gain is predominantly or exclusively fat.

Dronabinol ([9]-tetrahydrocannabinol), the primary active compound in marijuana, is approved by the US Food and Drug Administration for HIV-associated anorexia.

Significant weight gain was reported in a study of HIV-infected subjects receiving protease inhibitors who were randomized either to receive dronabinol or to smoke marijuana in a 3-week metabolic ward study of the safety of cannabinoids compared with oral placebo.

Anabolic androgenic steroids

Use of testosterone has been shown to increase LBM among hypogonadal men with AIDS wasting. Natural testosterone esters, rather than synthetic anabolic steroids, should be used as androgen replacement in hypogonadal men. Men receiving natural testosterone esters or synthetic testosterone derivatives should undergo a yearly prostate examination and prostate-specific antigen monitoring during long-term therapy. In addition, hematocrit and lipid levels should also be monitored. Use of physiologic testosterone replacement in hypogonadal men is unlikely to result in dyslipidemia, liver dysfunction, or insulin resistance.

The combination of testosterone analogs and exercise has also been shown to increase LBM

Growth hormone

Pharmacologic use of growth hormone (GH) has been shown to improve nitrogen balance and increase LBM in HIV-infected patients with wasting and to promote lean tissue retention in those with secondary infections.

Cytokine suppression

Several weak cytokine suppressors have been evaluated as potential treatments for wasting. For example, thalidomide suppresses TNF- production in vitro and has been shown to promote nitrogen retention in a metabolic ward study and weight gain in 3 placebo-controlled studies in patients with HIV infection

A large body of evidence demonstrates that weight loss and decreased LBM are common in HIV-infected patients, even in the era of HAART. A number of studies suggest that loss of weight and

LBM are independent predictors of increased morbidity and mortality in HIV-infected patients. Furthermore, data from randomized, placebo-controlled studies suggest that treatment strategies for weight loss, including Resistance Exercise Training, testosterone, megestrol acetate, Growth Hormone, anabolic steroids, and combination therapies, can increase weight and, in many cases, LBM, although the long-term effects of such interventions on survival and disease progression have not been determined.

15. Problems with fat digestion

People with HIV infection sometimes have problems with fat digestion, most often in the case of severe gut infection in late-stage AIDS. To cut down on dietary fat:

- Avoid fried foods, bacon, sausage, fatty cold meats, butter, margarine, mayonnaise, oil, peanut butter, cream, creamy sauces and cheese.
- Use low-fat or fat-free milk and milk products
- Choose lean meat, tuna canned in water, cut visible fat off meat and remove chicken skin.
- Bake, boil or steam instead of frying.

Decreased fat intake reduces calories, so you may need to eat more of the other food types to maintain your weight.

16. Neuropathy

Neuropathy is another common symptom of HIV disease. It is usually experienced as a numbness or tingling in the hands and feet and can be very painful. Neuropathy is also a side effect of drugs such as ddC, ddI and d4T. The simplest solution to drug related neuropathy is to avoid drugs known to cause it. However, this is not always an option. Drug treatments for peripheral neuropathy include the epilepsy drugs carbamazepine and phenytoin and the anti-depressant amitriptyline. These successfully treat the symptoms of neuropathy for some people to varying degrees.

The use of nutritional therapies for neuropathy in HIV, particularly the use of B vitamins, has not been studied extensively. Small preliminary studies have produced mixed results with some studies showing no response to B vitamin supplementation. There are some similarities between the neuropathy seen in HIV and that seen in diabetes. Confusingly, the use of B vitamins and other nutrients has been widely studied in diabetic neuropathy and has been successful, (40) particularly supplementation with the B vitamins biotin, B_6 and B_{12}. Promising results have also been shown with some of the other B vitamins including thiamine, niacin and folic acid. People with HIV who experience neuropathy might want to consider taking a B-50 complex vitamin once a day to reach the levels studied. You may also wish to approach your doctor about regular injections (at least weekly; 2-3 times weekly was most often studied) of B_{12}. Other nutrients which have seemed helpful in diabetic neuropathy included choline, inositol, caritine, magnesium, and chromium. All of these would be contained in a good quality multi-vitamin with minerals. Finally, linolenic acid found in evening primrose oil was found in at least one study to improve the symptoms of diabetic neuropathy.

17. Neurological disorders

Neurological problems such as memory loss and more serious problems like dementia occur in HIV. Although dementia is not that common, lesser problems like forgetting faces and names can be annoying irritants for people with HIV. At least one study has connected these type of memory problems in HIV to deficiencies in vitamin B_{12}. Although some studies have questioned the usefulness of B_{12} supplements in outright neurological disease like dementia, case studies have been reported of improvements in dementia when injections of B_{12} are given. Nutrition scientists like Lark Lands and Chester Meyers (USA) have suggested that 1 cc shots of B_{12} given 1-3 times a week, may help prevent some memory problems and even improve symptoms of dementia in some cases.

18. Peripheral Neuropathy

Peripheral Neuropathy can be caused by many medications such as: ddI, ddC, D4T, Vincristine, INH, Dapsone and others. It can also occur with nutritional deficiencies and overdoses, with diabetes and miscellaneous conditions. Peripheral neuropathies can vary from slight tingling and numbness to extreme discomfort, and this is why the treatments also vary.

Nutritional supplements associated with peripheral neuropathies:

- Choline.
- Inositol, 2-6 grams per day, or rich in cantaloupe, peanuts, grapefruit and whole grains.
- Vitamin B6 up to, but no more than, 200 mg./day.
- Vitamin B12, either weekly intramuscular injections, or 1000-5000 mcg. orally taken in the sublingual or nasal form.
- Acetyl-L-carnitine helps to raise inositol levels.
- Biotin, 10-15 mg./day.
- Thiamine, 50-100 mg./day.
- Gamma Linolenic Acid, 500 mg./day.
- Alpha Lipoic Acid, up to 600 mg./day.
- Magnesium.
- Chromium, 200 to 400 mcg./day.

Medical management of peripheral neuropathies:

- Elavil, 50-75 mg. taken before bed each night.
- Neurontin (gabapentin) 200-400 mg. three times per day.

Others

- Capsaicin cream (Zostrix) rubbed in to affected area, or cayenne pepper soaks. Remember, don't rub eyes afterwards!
- Manual massage to affected areas, if not too painful.

19. Colds, coughs and influenza

Colds and influenza (flu) are common virus infections that can cause a runny nose, sore throat, cough and sometimes fever. However, these infections almost always disappear without medicine.

How to deal with colds and flu

- Drink plenty of water or other fluids and have plenty of rest.
- Prepare special teas for colds and drink them for as long as symptoms last.
- A cold normally lasts about a week. If it lasts longer, or other symptoms are present such as a high fever or a cough with a lot of mucus, blood or odorous discharge, see a doctor because there may be an underlying infection.

Coughs

Coughing is how the body cleans the lungs and throat by getting rid of mucus and germs. Therefore, do not take any medicines to stop coughing but try to loosen the mucus.

- Breathe in hot vapours. Take a bowl or pot filled with very hot water and cover the head with a towel. Breathe in the vapours deeply for ten minutes, twice a day. Eucalyptus, mint or thyme leaves can be added, but hot water works just as well on its own.
- Try onion tea or cough syrup to ease the symptoms .
- Drink lots of water or other fluids.

20. Fever

Fever is a body temperature above 37 degrees Celsius. People with acute or chronic fever may have chills, sweat excessively, have muscle and joint aches, or be fatigued. Fever is common in PLWHAs and does not necessarily indicate a serious illness. The reasons for fever vary, and it is often hard to determine whether fever is due to HIV or another illness, such as malaria or untreated opportunistic infections. The body's energy expenditure increases with fever, causing increased energy requirements.

Some days you just may not feel like eating. It can be caused by many different things — pain, illness, tiredness, worry. It is important to eat well even on days like this. You'll find it helps your mood as well as your body. These ideas should help.

Drink plenty of fluids throughout the day.

- Cool down by sponging your body with a wet cloth.
- Eat food that you really love at this time. If you can find one thing you enjoy eating, just eat it all day.
- Eat smaller, more frequent meals at regularly scheduled intervals.
- Sometimes you can't eat solid food but you'll be able to drink things. Try milkshakes. Try ice cream floats — mix ice cream with your favorite juice or soft drink in a tall glass. You might also try chocolate milk, egg nog or hot cocoa. Creamy soups might go down easily, too.
- Keep snacks right beside you in your home. You might be able to nibble enough to finish quite a bit of food.

- Add high-protein snacks between meals.
- Try traditional remedies for reducing fever, such as neem tea. Aspirin or paracetamol can also be taken but read the instructions carefully about safe doses first - especially when giving to children.
- Do not give aspirin to children or people with stomach and kidney problems.
- Watch the clock. Eat something every hour or two whether you feel like it or not.
- Eliminate oils, butter, ghee, margarine, and foods that contain or are prepared with these
- Trim all visible fat from meat and remove the skin from chicken.
- Avoid deep fried, greasy, or high fat foods.
- Eat smaller, more frequent meals spaced out evenly throughout the day.
- Take a daily multivitamin, if available.
- Eat soups rich in foods that give energyand nutrients, such as maize, potatoes, and carrots.
- Drink teas from lemon, guava, and gum tree.
- Drink more than usual, beyond thirst.
- Continue to eat small, frequent meals as tolerated.
- Drink fluids to prevent dehydration, particularly clean boiled water.
- Bath in cool water.
- Rest.
- Take two aspirin or Panadol, if available, with a meal three times a day (morning, afternoon, and evening).
- Go to the health centre/ hospital in case of:
- Fever that last several days and is not relieved with aspirin
- Loss of consciousness
- Severe body pain
- Yellow eyes
- Severe diarrhoea
- Convulsion seizure

21. Lactose intolerance

Some people with HIV infection are partially or totally lactose intolerant i.e. the gut has difficulty digesting lactose, the sugar in milk. This is because of a deficiency in the enzyme lactase, which is needed to break down lactose. Symptoms include diarrhoea, gas and bloating.

If you're not sure whether or not you are lactose intolerant, try cutting out milk products (including low-fat dairy products; milk powder; ice-cream; and drinks, soups or desserts containing milk) from your diet to see if symptoms improve.

To help manage lactose intolerance:

- Lactase-treated milk, or lactase supplements, can help milk digestion. Ask your pharmacist, doctor or nutritionist where you can get these products.
- Sour or fermented milk products such as yoghurt and buttermilk are often better tolerated, since some of the lactose is already broken down in these foods.
- Hard cheeses such as parmesan may be better tolerated than soft ones.
- Read labels on foods, supplements and medicines if you are extremely lactose intolerant, to make sure they don't contain milk or lactose.
- Combining milk with other foods can improve tolerance.

22. Anaemia

Anaemia is a medical condition when the number of red blood cells is below normal. When this happens, not enough oxygen is going to body tissues. There are many reasons for anaemia and the treatment will depend upon the cause.

Two laboratory values that come from blood tests measure red blood cells. One Laboratory test is the haemoglobin (Hb or Hgb) or haematocrit (Hct or Hcrt). Normal haemoglobin levels are for adult men: 14-18 g/dL and for adult women 12-16 g/dL. Normal haematocrit levels are 42%-52% for adult men and 37%-48% for adult women. Anaemia is often defined as when there is a haemoglobin level below 12g/dL. "Normal" levels can vary. Reticulocytes are slightly immature red blood cells. If your haemoglobin is low, a "reticulocyte count" is done. This test shows whether the bone marrow is producing red blood cells at the right rate.

The other lab tests that can help identify the type of anaemia are: serum iron, total iron binding capacity (TIBC), iron/TIBC ratio, serum ferritin, serum erythropoietin, vitamin B12 and folate. Whether there is blood loss internal or external bleeding, menstruation, etc. is an important factor, too.

Consequences of Anaemia

Anaemia can affect the quality of your life by lowering your energy level, making you feel tired and making it difficult to go about your daily activities. Anaemia is a common problem for people with HIV infection. Today with highly active anti-retroviral treatments almost 50% of HIV-infected people have anaemia. Before HAART 90% had anaemia. It can occur at any stage of HIV infection, may become more severe with disease progression and has been associated with shorter survival times.

Common symptoms of anaemia

- Tiredness , low energy , fatigue
- Shortness of breath
- Pale conjunctiva or skin
- Dizziness
- Headach
- Anxiety
- Sleeping poorly
- Nausea
- Sadness
- Irritable
- Abdominal or chest pain

Causes of Anaemia

Anaemia can be due to a problem in red blood cell production, increased red blood cell destruction and increased red blood cell loss. There may be a lower than normal number, altered size or function of red blood cells. The most common type of anaemia in HIV disease is called "anaemia of chronic illness." There are many different causes and types of anaemia that can affect people with HIV and sometimes people with HIV have no specific cause of anaemia found.

Possible underlying causes for anaemia

HIV infection and other chronic illnesses	*Iron, B6, Folate and B12 deficiency*
Medications to treat HIV	Malnutrition
Opportunistic infection	Tumour or abnormal cell growth
Bone marrow disorders	Kidney disease

HIV-related drugs that can cause anaemia

Zidovudine (Retrovir, AZT)	Ribavirin (Rebetol)
Bactrim (Septra)	Interferon
Cidofovir (Vistide)	Amphotericin B
Foscarnet (Foscavir)	Flucytosine (Ancobon)
Ganciclovir (Cytovine)	Sulfonamides

Trimethoprim

Pyrimethamine

Pentamidine

Antineoplastic (anti-cancer) agent

Dapsone

Factors that make you more likely to develop anaemia

- Clinical progression from HIV to an AIDS
- CD4 count less than 200 cells/mm^3
- Viral load increase
- Being African American
- Being female
- Taking Retrovir (AZT)
- Taking Videx (ddI) or Zerit (d4T) but to a lesser degree than AZT.
- Hepatitis C infection and taking medication to treat it .

Management of Anaemia.

Management of anaemia has been shown to improve survival and quality of life. Getting treatment for anaemia is very important and the type of treatment will depend on the cause or type of anaemia. Your doctor needs to diagnose the underlying cause of your anaemia. Ask your doctor to clearly explain to you what kind of anaemia you have, its cause and its treatments. Your doctor may ask that you make changes in your diet and/or take iron supplements and/or prescribe a medication to increase red blood cell production.

Nutrition related anaemia

If your anaemia is due to low levels of a certain vitamin or mineral, treatment may include adding specific foods and/or vitamin and mineral supplements to your diet. After doing the appropriate laboratory tests, your doctor may diagnose a nutritional deficiency and prescribe single vitamin or mineral supplements if you need them. It is not a good idea to take single vitamin or mineral supplements without first speaking to your doctor. Taking too much of a vitamin or mineral can be as harmful as not having enough. Taking a daily low level general multiple vitamin and mineral supplement however has been recommended.

Iron-deficiency anaemia is the most common nutritional related anaemia worldwide, affecting about 40% of the world's population. Anaemia from an iron deficiency can be due to lack of iron in the diet, blood loss, or intestinal parasites. Iron is found in red blood cells, and its main role is to carry oxygen from the lungs to the rest of the body. Infants, adolescent girls, pregnant women, and the elderly are those at highest risk. Symptoms can include oral lesions, angular stomatitis (lesion in corner of mouth), gastrointestinal problems, thinning and brittle nails and nails that are concave, resembling a spoon. Your doctor may prescribe an iron supplement depending on the severity of your anaemia. It may take several months for your body's iron stores to increase, so it is very important that you take your medication as prescribed by your doctor.

Iron in general, meat, fish, and poultry are excellent sources. Other sources of iron include beans, dried fruits, whole grains, fortified cereals, and enriched breads. Iron supplements can cause constipation so include high fibre foods in your diet such as fruits, vegetables, and whole grains and drink plenty of fluids. Eat foods high in iron or fortified with iron. Iron from an animal source food is easier for the body to absorb and use than iron from a plant source.

Vitamin C foods included in meals or supplements will help your body absorb and use the iron from plant foods. Foods that have been cooked in a cast iron skillet are a source of iron, too.

Calcium may interfere with iron absorption, so to minimize this, do not drink milk or take a calcium supplement with your meals or at the same time you take your iron supplement (if your doctor has prescribed one).

Iron - food sources	*Protein Rich*	*Vegetables*	*Fruits*
Beef, lean		Dried peas	Dried Fruit
Calf liver		Green beans	Prunes
Chicken, dark		Spinach canned	Watermelon
Sardines		Turnip greens	Strawberries
Turkey, dark		Mustard greens	Tomato juice
Dried beans		Broccoli	Oranges
Prunes			
Grains			
Fortified cereals			
Bran Muffin			
Wheat Bread			
Oatmeal			
Cream of Wheat			
Corn tortillas			

Megaloblastic Anaemia

Megaloblastic anaemia can be caused by a deficiency in folic acid or a deficiency in vitamin B12 and occurs often in HIV infection by AZT. With megaloblastic anaemia your laboratory test would show Mean Cell Volume (MCV) above normal and your doctor must further determine the exact cause and type.

Folic acid is a B vitamin sometimes called folate or folacin. Folic acid is found in many vegetables, beans, fruits, whole grains, and fortified breakfast cereals. A deficiency in folic acid affects the synthesis of DNA and growth of red blood cells. Pregnant women, alcoholics, and vegetarians are usually at highest risk for folic acid deficiency. Folic acid is especially needed during human growth, and with alcoholism, hepatitis, infection, inflammatory diseases, use of some birth control medications, cancers and poor eating habits. Your doctor may prescribe a folic acid supplement if you need one. Be cautious, as excessive folic acid supplementation will hide a B12 deficiency if there is one. Eat at least 3 fruits a day and 2 cups of vegetables a day. Do not overcook your fruits and vegetables — heat can destroy folic acid in foods.

Protein Rich	*Vegetables*	*Fruits*	*Grains*
Tenderloin Steak	Baked Potato	Apricots	Fortified cereals
Chicken, dark	Sweet Potato	Strawberries	Wheat Bread
Turkey, dark	Asparagus	Bananas	Barley
Beans: Pinto, Black, Navy, Lima, Kidney , others	Beets	Strawberries	Wheat germm
Turnip & mustard greens, cooked		Oranges Orange Juice	
Lentils Sardines Spinach		Romaine lettuce Broccoli	

Folate – food sources , Dairy- Milk , Yogurt -Cheese

Megaloblastic and Pernicious Anaemia

Vitamin B12 deficiency can cause megaloblastic, macrocytic, and pernicious anaemia. B12 deficiency usually occurs due to poor absorption of the vitamin rather than inadequate intake, though strict vegetarians can become deficient. People at risk include the elderly, strict vegetarians or vegans, people with deficient intrinsic factor (component that aids vitamin B12 absorption) chronic small intestinal problems, partial or full stomach removal, long term use of certain medications such as Glucophage (metformin), acid-lowering agents, and cholestyramine. As with folate deficiency anaemia, B12 deficiency anaemia leads to large immature red blood cells. Your doctor may recommend an oral supplement or a subcutaneous injection of vitamin B12.

Vitamin B12 – food sources

Meat Chicken
Fish Eggs Milk

Cheese
Soymilk fortified with B12

Less common types of anaemia

- Aplastic anaemia: is a serious disease in which normal bone marrow is replaced with fat. Drug toxicity, toxic chemicals, radiation exposure, medications, and diseases can cause it.
- Hemolytic anaemia: occurs when mature red blood cells are destroyed too early. It may be caused by vitamin E deficiency.
- Sickle cell anaemia: is a hereditary disorder most common in the African American population and is usually diagnosed during infancy.

Anaemia of chronic disease: occurs in inflammation, infection, and neoplastic disorders.

23. Skin problems

Skin problems such as rashes and sores are common in people suffering from HIV/AIDS. Other problems such as dry patches or poor healing of wounds may be related to malnutrition or specific micronutrient deficiencies.

Poor skin conditions can be caused by lack of vitamin A or vitamin B6. Although many skin problems may need specific medical treatment, the addition of foods rich in vitamin A and/or B6 to the diet may help to prevent skin problems or improve the condition over time. Good sources of vitamin A are yellow, orange and green vegetables and liver. Good sources of vitamin B6 are cereals, kernels, whole grains, seeds and nuts as well as figs and green leafy vegetables.

24. Lipodystrophy

Changes in body fat in persons infected with the human immunodeficiency virus have been associated with deleterious changes in blood lipids and insulin resistance, raising concern that these changes will increase the risk for accelerated atherosclerosis.

Changes in body fat are often identified in advanced disease but may also occur early after HIV infection is detected. Research evidence suggests that fat maldistribution may be related to use of protease inhibitors, nonnucleoside reverse transcriptase inhibitors, or a combination of these two classes of drugs, but the etiologies of the various changes in body fat remain uncertain.

From early in the era of HAART, a spectrum of changes in body fat have been reported to occur in 20%80% of subjects receiving these therapies

Incidence and prevalence

There are few data on the incidence of clinical fat maldistribution. One report describing 84 subjects from the French PRIMO cohort and who were initiating HAART (88% received at least one protease inhibitor [PI]) shortly after acute HIV infection indicated that the incidence of lipodystrophy was 5% at 6 months, 9% at 12 months, and 26% at 24 months.

Pathogenesis and associated risk factors

Female sex. Women may be at greater risk for accumulation of fat. Trunk obesity rather than subcutaneous fat wasting appears to occur more often in women than in men.

Initial reports of fat maldistribution suggested that these changes were related to use of PIs. Indirect evidence did suggest that PIs were involved because the odds of fat wasting were shown to increase with the duration of therapy. The use of PIs also increases the probability of intra-abdominal fat accumulation.

Cross-sectional studies also suggest that the NRTIs may be causally related to changes in body habitus, possibly by causing mutations in the mitochondrial DNA polymerase gamma gene and thus adversely affecting mitochondrial oxidative phosphorylation Dual NRTI therapy is more likely to cause fat wasting than is therapy with a single NRTI

Combination antiretroviral therapy. It is also possible that NRTI and PIs together contribute to abnormalities in fat distribution. Indeed, PI therapy combined with dual NRTIs resulted in faster lipoatrophy than therapy with dual NRTIs, whereas PI therapy per se did not exert a strong independent risk for fat loss.

Management of lipoatrophy

Little is known about options for management of lipoatrophy

Insulin sensitizing agents. Because both fat atrophy and fat accumulation are associated with insulin resistance.

Treatment switching strategies. Although a number of switch studies in which PIs were changed to regimens without this class of drugs failed to demonstrate consistent, objective improvements in body composition.

Management of fat accumulation

Human growth hormone. Human growth hormone has potent fat-oxidizing properties and has decreased dorso-cervical fat in persons with HIV and reduced abdominal fat in HIV-negative men with abdominal obesity.

Androgens. The greatest beneficial effects occurred in men with lower levels of serum testosterone, as often occurs in men with HIV.

Metformin. Metformin is an insulin-sensitizing agent that reduces hepatic glucose production. In an open-label study in which metformin (850 mg) was administered 3 times a day to HIV-infected subjects with central obesity, fasting insulin levels and insulin response to oral glucose tolerance testing improved and visceral adipose tissue decreased.

Diet and exercise. The cornerstone of management for central fat accumulation should be diet and exercise, as extrapolated from populations not infected with HIV. For central fat accumulation, the goal should be to decrease intake of saturated fat and excess caloric energy. Aerobic exercise is expected to augment the effects of dietary change because intra-abdominal fat (mesenteric and omental adipose tissue) is metabolically more active than peripheral fat in responding to lipolytic stimuli, such as increases in epinephrine with exercise. In addition, aerobic exercise increases peripheral glucose disposal in obese persons, even in the absence of weight loss, and should be beneficial for subjects with insulin resistance. A recent report suggests that an aerobic exercise programme with a moderate-fat, lowglycemic-index, high-fibre diet can reverse aspects of lipodystrophy. Supervised resistance (strength) training modestly decreased truncal fat as assessed by DXA scanning in 2 preliminary studies, but resistance exercise is not expected to be as efficient in reducing fat as aerobic exercise.

25. Insulin and Carbohydrate Dysregulation

Patients with human immunodeficiency virus receiving highly active antiretroviral therapy (HAART) may experience abnormal body composition changes as well as metabolic abnormalities, including dyslipidemia, increases in triglycerides, low high-density lipoprotein cholesterol levels, and abnormal carbohydrate metabolism, ranging from insulin resistance with and without glucose intolerance to frank diabetes. The use of HAART with and without therapy with protease inhibitors (PIs) is related to carbohydrate abnormalities and changes in body composition. Regimens that include PIs appear to have a higher incidence of insulin resistance (IR) (up to 90%) and diabetes mellitus (up to 40%).

Since the late 1990s, many reports have been published that have described insulin and carbohydrate abnormalities in HIV patients receiving highly active retroviral therapy (HAART).

Prevalence

Existing data suggest that patients receiving therapy with PIs have a greater incidence of insulin resistance (IR) (30%-90%) than patients receiving nonPI-containing regimens (up to 20%).

Potential for morbidity and mortality

The potential consequences of IR in this patient population may be atherosclerosis and other cardiovascular diseases. One important issue is whether body fat changes are independent of the metabolic changes. Data from Mulligan et al. suggest that IR precedes changes in body fat in HIV-positive patients initiating PI therapy.

Nutritional interventions

Patients need to be assessed for risk factors for IR and diabetes mellitus as well as for atherosclerosis (e.g., family history, inactivity, smoking, and body mass index [weight in kilograms divided by height in meters squared as indicator of obesity], hypertension, and dyslipidemia). Diet and exercise, mainstays of therapy for type 2 diabetes mellitus, are also appropriate for HIV-related IR and diabetes. Diet should be composed of 50%60% carbohydrates (mostly complex carbohydrates) and protein intake of 10%20% of all calories; total fat intake should be restricted to 30% of total calories (with saturated fat limited to 10% of total calories and total cholesterol intake <300 mg/d). A word of caution about exercise, particularly in older patients: it may be wise to assess the cardiac status of the patient before starting an exercise program, particularly if the patient has other risk factors for coronary artery disease.

Medical nutrition therapy is integral to total care and management. Achieving nutrition-related goals requires a coordinated team effort that includes the patient.

IR alone (without hyperglycemia) is a major risk factor for atherosclerosis. Hyperglycemia only minimally increases the risk for atherosclerosis above that of IR.. If the patient has diabetes mellitus (defined by fasting glucose values 126 mg/dL or random levels 200 mg/dL), then diet, exercise, and if necessary drug therapy and/or insulin may be required.

Drug therapy in HIV-positive patients with diabetes mellitus should be that recommended for type 2 diabetes mellitus.

Metformin therapy significantly improved IR, and there was a trend toward decreased visceral adiposity as measured by CT scan; however, metformin also decreased peripheral fat. Patients treated with metformin demonstrated significant weight loss, reduced waist circumference, and decreased diastolic blood pressure.

Metformin therapy significantly decreased plasminogen activator inhibitor 1 and tissue type plasminogen activator antigen concentrations, both known to be associated with increased cardiovascular disease risk, suggesting that metformin may improve associated cardiovascular disease risk in this patient population. Importantly, at least over 3 months, metformin did not result in any increase in lactic acidosis, which is a potential side effect of this drug, and, interestingly, the patients randomized to metformin therapy had higher baseline lactate levels than did patients receiving placebo.

Considerations for switching antiretroviral therapies

Decisions about when to switch antiretroviral therapy for patients with IR and/or hyperglycemia should be individualized. For patients receiving PI-containing regimens who develop hyperglycemia that is difficult to control, switching antiretroviral therapy should be considered, especially if it includes a PI. Improvement in insulin sensitivity measured by intravenous insulin-tolerance testing occurred after the substitution of abacavir for a PI.

26. Lactic Acidemia in Infection with Human Immunodeficiency Virus

Lactic acidosis in patients infected with the human immunodeficiency virus was initially identified as a rare complication of therapy with nucleoside analog reverse transcriptase inhibitors (NRTIs). The only patient group that appears to be at greater risk is pregnant women.

Lactic acidemia (defined by venous lactate >2.0 mmol/L) is common to several toxicities associated with nucleoside analog reverse transcriptase inhibitors (NRTIs) and nucleotide analog reverse transcriptase inhibitors that may have a mitochondrial pathogenesis. Virologically active triphosphate forms of NRTIs and nucleotide analog reverse transcriptase inhibitors can inhibit mitochondrial DNA polymerase-, which could in turn lead to impaired synthesis of mitochondrial enzymes that generate adenosine triphosphate by oxidative phosphorylation of glucose and fatty acids.

Prevalence and risk factors

Lactic acidemia with no or mild symptoms was detected in 8%21% of patients receiving at least one NRTI versus 0%1% of patients receiving no antiretroviral therapy. Symptomatic lactic acidemia is less common (1.5%2.5%). Severe lactic acidemia has been described in association with all NRTIs, particularly if treatment duration is >6 months.

Clinical features

The primary clinical features of moderate to severe lactic acidemia are fatigue, weight loss, myalgias, nausea and vomiting, abdominal distension, and pain, dyspnoea, and preterminal cardiac dysrhythmias. The onset is acute or subacute (with symptom duration a median of 4 months in one series). Features of hepatic dysfunction are common and can include soft, tender hepatomegaly, peripheral oedema, ascites, and encephalopathy, but jaundice is rare. Modest elevations in liver enzymes are common, although even in fulminant hepatic failure, these are often not to levels >10-fold above normal, as with other forms of acute hepatic failure. Hepatic steatosis is a common finding on imaging studies and biopsy, with necrosis evident in more fulminant cases. Patients with low-level lactic acidemia (25 mmol/L) may present with a milder constitutional and hepatic illness but are often asymptomatic. Features of NRTI-induced peripheral neuropathy, another mitochondrial NRTI toxicity, may also be present and can include ascending neuromuscular weakness in some cases.

Overall mortality was 80% in patients with HIV-related lactic acidemia >10 mmol/L, whereas no deaths have been reported in those with lactate <10 mmol/L. Prognosis of lactic acidemia depends on the level at the time of diagnosis. In one study, lactate levels (mean, 4.2 mmol/L) returned to normal at a mean of 3 months after NRTI cessation. Clinical features may take longer to resolve.

Treatment

There is no proven intervention for lactic acidemia apart from NRTI cessation. In all patients with confirmed lactate levels >10 mmol/L, as well as those with confirmed lactate levels >5 mmol/L who are symptomatic, all NRTIs should be discontinued if no other cause is evident. All concomitant antiretroviral drugs should be ceased at the same time to avoid development of HIV drug resistance. Non-NRTI or protease inhibitor therapy can be restarted after the lactate level normalizes and the associated illness resolves. Reinstitution of alternative NRTIs in patients with previous lactic acidemia may be possible in some individuals but should be closely monitored, with lactate measured every 4 weeks for at least 3 months.

For symptomatic patients whose levels are <5 mmol/L, lactate levels should be measured regularly. For asymptomatic patients in whom lactate levels are 25 mmol/L, there is no evidence to suggest that any change in antiretroviral therapy is necessary.

27. Osteoporosis and Osteo-necrosis in People with HIV/AIDS

The introduction of highly active antiretroviral therapy (HAART) with the use of protease inhibitors (PIs) has resulted in significant reductions in morbidity and mortality from HIV infection in recent years. Although initial strong enthusiasm for HAART led to its widespread use early in HIV infection, practitioners have now become more cautious in early initiation of HAART in light of reports concerning serious and potentially irreversible toxicities associated with numerous antiretroviral drugs These toxicities include the development of diabetes mellitus, insulin resistance, hyperlipidemia, lipodystrophy, and lactic acidosis

Recently, a high incidence of osteopenia and osteoporosis has been observed in individuals infected with human immunodeficiency virus (HIV). This problem appears to be more frequent in patients receiving potent antiretroviral therapy. Other bone-related complications in HIV-infected individuals, including avascular necrosis of the hip and compression fracture of the lumbar spine, have also been reported. People living with HIV have significant alterations in bone metabolism, regardless of whether they are receiving potent antiretroviral therapy.

Osteoporosis

Worldwide, osteoporosis is a significant cause of morbidity and mortality. It is a skeletal disorder characterized by compromised bone strength predisposing to an increased risk of fracture. Bone strength refers to a combination of bone quantity and quality. Bone quantity is measured by means of bone mineral density (BMD), a commonly used surrogate marker for bone strength.. Osteopenia is defined as a BMD between -1 and -2.5 SDs. Osteoporosis without a history of fracture carries a 45-fold increase in fracture risk compared with individuals with normal BMD. A history of fracture and diagnosis of osteoporosis carries a 20-fold increased risk, and osteopenia alone carries a 2-fold increase in fracture risk .

Gradual bone loss is a common occurrence with aging and is often referred to as primary osteoporosis. Men and women naturally begin to lose bone around the age of 35 years, at a rate of 0.5%1% per year. Women also lose bone at an accelerated rate after menopause. In addition to female sex and age, additional risk factors include white race, low weight, smoking, excessive alcohol use, and history of fracture. A number of secondary causes of osteoporosis are also well known, including corticosteroid use, hypogonadism, hyperthyroidism, prolonged immobility, nutritional deficiencies or malabsorption, chronic illness, and concurrent medications such as anticonvulsants or anticoagulants.

Bone metabolism in HIV-infected individuals

Before the era of HAART, studies indicated that bone mineral metabolism was only minimally affected in HIV-infected individuals. Several studies have indicated the prevalence of osteopenia/ osteoporosis was 28%, compared with the 16% that one would expect in the general population. These studies suggest that HIV infection itself has a significant impact on bone metabolism and may be a contributing factor in the pathogenesis of reduced BMD.

Bone in HIV -infected patients receiving antiretroviral therapy

The use of NRTIs has been associated with mitochondrial toxicity and lactic acidosis. The common risk factors for BMD loss in HIV-infected individuals include history of wasting or poor nutrition, past steroid usage (i.e., for pneumocystis carinii pneumonia or myopathy), hormonal deficiencies, or the potential contribution of HIV-related immune system activation and immune reconstitution

Osteonecrosis

Another emerging bone-related problem in HIV-infected individuals is osteonecrosis, a relatively rare occurrence that is usually the result of lack of an adequate arterial blood supply to the bone. The femoral head is most commonly affected, and patients usually present with pain. However, osteonecrosis in HIV-infected patients has often involved multiple sites.

A few case reports and one small study suggested that osteonecrosis might be related to HAART. Osteonecrosis was more common (55%) in patients with advanced AIDS, but a significant proportion also had suppressed HIV viral loads and relatively high CD4 counts. Medical therapy for osteonecrosis is generally ineffective and surgery is usually needed.

28. Lipid Abnormalities

Dyslipidemia is an important clinical problem in individuals infected with human immunodeficiency virus (HIV) who are receiving antiretroviral therapy. Data suggest that increased cardiovascular disease is occurring in this population. In most situations, the first interventions should be non-pharmacological and should include diet, exercise, and management of other hygienic risk factors. If pharmacologic therapy becomes necessary, the choices of lipid-lowering agents should be limited to agents with the least likelihood of adverse drug interactions.

Prevalence

Abnormalities of lipid metabolism are common in HIV-infected patients and tend to be accentuated in those receiving antiretroviral therapy, particularly with protease inhibitors (PIs).

The introduction of highly active antiretroviral therapy (HAART) with the use of protease inhibitors (PIs) has resulted in significant reductions in morbidity and mortality from HIV infection in recent years. Although initial strong enthusiasm for HAART led to its widespread use early in HIV infection, practitioners have now become more cautious in early initiation of HAART in light of reports concerning serious and potentially irreversible toxicities associated with numerous antiretroviral drugs These toxicities include the development of diabetes mellitus, insulin resistance, hyperlipidemia, lipodystrophy, and lactic acidosis.

Etiology

Abnormalities of lipid metabolism reported before the use of HIV-1 PIs include increases in serum triglycerides and decreases in total and high-density lipoprotein cholesterol (HDL-C) that occurred with disease progression. During therapy with PIs, increases in serum triglycerides may be extreme, particularly with ritonavir therapy

Potential for cardiovascular morbidity and mortality

Many experts speculate that HIV treatment-related dyslipidemia will increase the atherogenic tendency, particularly when combined with other HIV-associated metabolic abnormalities such as insulin resistance, visceral adiposity impaired fibrinolysis, and chronic infection and immune activation.

Evaluation of cardiovascular disease risks(CHD)

Evaluation of serum lipids should be performed after fasting for a minimum of 8 hours, and preferably 12 hours. The standard screening lipid profile should include measurement of total cholesterol, HDL-C, and triglycerides, with calculation of Low Density Lipoprotein Choline (LDL-C) and should be obtained before therapy This should be repeated 36 months after the initiation of HAART, and then yearly. All patients should be screened for other cardiovascular risk factors including family history, smoking, hypertension, menopausal status, physical inactivity, obesity, and diabetes, in addition to potential exacerbating factors such as certain medical illnesses and medications

Thresholds for treatment intervention

For the purposes of initiating therapy for dyslipidemia, these individuals should be treated aggressively.

Management: diet and nondrug therapies

Nondrug interventions should be the first approach for management of abnormal lipid levels. Clinicians should consult with dietary specialists as a first step, when initial attempts at dietary intervention fail to achieve the desired effects, or when intensive dietary modification becomes necessary. Structured exercise plus diet resulted in a 21% decrease in triglyceride levels in HIV-infected patients, and resistance training improved triglyceride levels Smoking cessation and weight reduction for obesity also improve the overall cardiovascular risk profile.

Diet. These diets reduce serum triglycerides. For patients with low HDL-C, reduction of dietary fat is recommended .

Monounsaturated fats (e.g., canola and olive oil) should be substituted for saturated fats. The management of severe hypertriglyceridemia and hyperchylomicronemia requires a verylow-fat diet and avoidance of simple sugars (i.e., use of lowglycemic-index carbohydrates) and alcohol. Fish oils (omega-3 fatty acid supplements) variably decrease triglyceride synthesis and may be tried in patients with severe hypertriglyceridemia.

Weight reduction. In subjects with central (abdominal) obesity, weight reduction through diet modifications and increased physical activity is an important element of therapy for abnormal lipid levels.

Patients with CHD or CHD risk equivalents. The goal for LDL-C is <100 mg/dL in patients with CHD or CHD risk equivalents. In contrast to subjects without CHD, prolonged attempts to lower LDL-C with diet may not be desirable before initiation of drug therapy.

Monitoring the response to therapy. In patients without CHD, after initiation of the therapeutic diet, lipids should be measured and adherence to the diet assessed after 4 to 6 weeks and again after 3 months.

Management: lipid-lowering drugs

If lipid levels remain above the target after intensive dietary interventions have been attempted for at least 12 weeks, drug therapy should be considered. In the absence of other CHD risk factors, especially in patients <35 years of age, a longer period of nondrug therapies may be appropriate. Shorter periods of time may be considered in patients with severe elevations of LDL-C (>220 mg/dL) or with multiple risk factors. Drug therapy should only be added to dietary therapy, never substituted for it.

Lipid-lowering therapies for HIV-infected patients with dyslipidemia are conceptually problematic because of the potential for drug interactions.

Drug therapy for elevated LDL-C or nonHDL-C. When statin therapy is necessary, low initial dosages of either pravastatin (20 mg daily) or atorvastatin (10 mg daily) will be used, along with careful clinical monitoring. Fluvastatin is an alternative statin, but there are no data on fluvastatin interactions with PIs. Therapy with lovastatin and simvastatin should be avoided.

The fibrates (gemfibrozil and fenofibrate) are well-tolerated alternative agents when hypercholesterolemia is accompanied by elevated triglycerides, but fibrates are less effective than statins for reducing LDL-C. Niacin lowers LDL-C and triglyceride levels but produces frequent cutaneous flushing and pruritus.

Drug therapy for elevated triglycerides. Fibrates should be prescribed if drug therapy is necessary for hypertriglyceridemia. Treatment is with gemfibrozil (600 mg bid) or fenofibrate (54160 mg once daily). If treatment with a fibrate results in inadequate lowering of serum triglycerides, or if LDL-C levels remain elevated, a cautious trial of niacin or a statin may be considered, with careful monitoring for symptoms of skeletal muscle toxicity.

Consideration for switching antiretroviral therapies

Where virologically appropriate, substitution of a new antiviral agent with a lesser tendency to induce dyslipidemia for an existing agent with a greater tendency may be considered. In NNRTI-naive patients, substitution of nevirapine for a PI improves serum lipids.

Hepatobilliary Disease

In earlier stage HIV infection (CD4 cell count, >500/mm^3), hepatic complications usually represent liver-specific processes, such as drug-related hepatotoxicity, primary neoplasms, or infection with hepatotrophic viruses. With progression of immunodeficiency to AIDS (CD4 cell count, <200/mm^3), the liver is generally involved as part of a systemic opportunistic infection due to *M. avium* complex, fungi, or cytomegalovirus.

Because the liver is often one of many sites involved with disseminated opportunistic infections in patients with AIDS, liver disease per se is rarely the primary cause of death. Nonetheless, the progressive jaundice, fever, and/or abdominal pain that may accompany hepatobiliary disease can significantly reduce quality of life and therefore merits evaluation in most patients.

- The evaluation of suspected hepatobiliary disease should be tailored to the history, physical examination, pattern of liver tests, and CD4 lymphocyte count.
- Opportunistic infections and neoplasms usually involve the liver secondarily through lymphohematogenous dissemination. Thus, initial evaluation of blood or bone marrow specimens may provide an inferential diagnosis of liver disease.
- Ultrasonography is the test of choice when biliary disease is suspected. Abdominal computed tomographic scan is best reserved for patients with jaundice, marked hepatomegaly, or suspected peritoneal disease.
- Percutaneous liver biopsy should be reserved for patients in whom a treatable cause of parenchymal liver disease is suspected and when blood cultures and other noninvasive tests do not reveal a cause. It is unclear whether percutaneous liver biopsy is associated with a higher rate of complications in these patients.

  Treatment should be initiated according to the underlying cause.

Considerations for selecting antiretroviral therapy

[illegible]

Herpes [illegible]

[illegible]

[illegible] therapy should be [illegible] according to the underlying cause.

12

Tips for Good Nutrition for People with HIV/AIDS

Just because you are HIV positive doesn't mean you can't have a good time; a high "quality of life" surely means you should enjoy yourself. Be relaxed and "take one day at a time". Good nutrition is extremely important if you are HIV positive . Eating well and quality of life are closely related. Quality of life may also be useful to monitor the effectiveness of programmes you use to give you resistance (resilience) against infections.

Every little bit of good may help

Getting enough calories is very important since the HIV virus not only increases your need for energy, but also decreases the proportion of your food that is absorbed from your gut. Moreover, because of the unusual demands on the immune system, your antioxidants, vitamins and minerals are also used up at a faster than normal rate. This means you also need more of them than would a person without HIV. Maintenance of body weight, especially of lean body mass (protein), should be given priority since our immune systems need protein in order to function. While quantity of calories is certainly important, in HIV disease the quality of protein, fat and carbohydrate in your diet is particularly important.

HIV infection is often characterized by nutritional deficiencies and deficiencies of vitamins and minerals as very early symptoms.

Nutrient & Some Possible Deficiency Symptoms

Biotin - anorexia, nausea, dry scaly dermatitis

Chromium - glucose intolerance, abnormal lipid metabolism, neuropathy, encephalopathy

Cobalt - glossitis, anaemia

Copper - neutropenia, leukopenia, failure of erythropoiesis, (high serum cholesterol if caused by high zinc intake), immune suppression

Folic acid - megaloblastic anaemia, diarrhoea, fatigue, confusion, forgetfulness, depression, dementia, apathy, insomnia, irritability, immune suppression

Iodine - increase in blood lipids, thyroid enlargement

Iron - decreased hematocrit, anaemia, immune suppression

Magnesium - muscle weakness, muscle cramps, constipation, oxidative stress, immune suppression, growth retardation

Manganese - impaired central nervous system, defects in lipid and carbohydrate metabolism, immune suppression

Nickel - anaemia

Pantothenate - epigastric distress, anorexia, numbness/ tingling in hands/feet

Potassium - weight loss, growth retardation

Selenium - cardiac myopathy, pancreas degeneration, red blood cell fragility, oxidative stress, immune suppression

Vitamin B_1 - mental confusion, weakness, anorexia

Vitamin B_2 - oedema of pharyngeal and oral mucous membranes

Vitamin B_3 - diarrhoea, mental confusion, glossitis

Vitamin B_6 - dermatitis, glossitis, immune suppression

Vitamin B_{12} - megaloblastic anaemia, peripheral nerve degeneration, mental dysfunction, anorexia, glossitis, elevated mean corpuscular volume (MCV), neutropenia, low folate utilization, skin sensitivity, immune suppression

Vitamin C - appetite loss, fatigue, bleeding gums, capillary rupture, immune suppression

Vitamin E - neuropathy, myopathy, oxidative stress, immune suppression

Vitamin K - defective blood clotting

Zinc - immune suppression, oxidative stress, poor growth, poor wound healing, anorexia, abnormal taste and smell, anaemia, skin inflammation, low plasma zinc levels

Since 1993 , it had been observed that significant slowing of disease progression is associated with vitamin/mineral supplementation.

What does this mean for those living with HIV?

1. In HIV disease, hypertriglyceridemia may occur primarily from carnitine deficiency. Contribution to fatigue and wasting is also highly likely. (Lohninger *et al*, 1987).
2. Oxidation stress is noted to be common with HIV infection. It's logical that this decreases the supply of antioxidants in our bodies. Lipid oxidation products increase with disease progression, and there is a decline in the body's sulphur-containing amino acids, cysteine and methionine. Of the body's amino acids, these are the most susceptible to oxidation and most likely to become deficient in times of nutritional stress (Hommes *et al*, 1991; Millward *et al*, 1990; Revillard *et al*, 1992; Sappey *et al*, 1992; Singer *et al*, 1992; Florence AIDS Conference abstract. TuA66).
3. Oxidation of amino acids is of particular concern since it deteriorates the body's ability to maintain its protein stores.
4. Both cysteine and methionine have been reported to tend to be low in HIV disease. This may be because both cysteine and methionine are readily oxidized, reversibly under lower oxidation stress, but irreversibly under more severe oxidation. The irreversibly oxidized forms are not available for normal body metabolism.
5. Wasting is less of a problem among those who take N-acetyl cysteine (NAC) supplements. The amino acid, cysteine tends to become low in HIV disease, and this is likely at least one of the sources of wasting. Glutathione, in the absence of supplementation with NAC, is a common deficiency with HIV.
6. Serum zinc levels were likely to be severely stressed with HIV disease (Cunningham-Rundles, 1984). Research findings have indicated that decreases in both T4 cells and the T4/T8

ratio are correlated with zinc deficiency (Beach *et al*, 1982; abstract. ThC677, San Francisco AIDS Conference. 1990).

7. Poor wound healing, anorexia, abnormal taste and smell, diarrhoea, skin inflammation, skin stretch marks, nail abnormalities such as white spots or brittleness, anaemia, impaired glucose tolerance, central nervous system malfunction, muscle deterioration, increased oxidative damage of cell membranes, decreased thymic hormone activity, increased apoptosis/cell death, T-helper cell dysfunction, low CD4+ cells, increased CD8+ cells, and reduced natural killer cell activity are some possible results of zinc deficiency. (Badgley, 1986; Chandra, 1984; Cunningham-Rundles *et al*, 1981; Forbes, 1984; Hoffer and Walker, 1978; Hunt and Groff, 1990; Odeh, 1992; Prasad, 1984; Stites and Terr, 1991).
8. Serum zinc deficiencies could be accompanied initially by a simultaneous elevation of serum copper. It is also possible that ***low*** *absorption of zinc across the small intestine mucosal membrane could permit* ***increased*** *absorption of copper* in the stomach. Subsequent supplementation with zinc without copper would be expected to rapidly reverse this.
9. A significant feature of copper deficiency is that it is a possible source of anaemia due to a resulting defective iron metabolism secondary to a defective protein, called ceruloplasmin, which mediates use of iron by the body (Hunt and Groff, 1990).Supplementation with zinc, *especially* at levels of 150 mg per day or higher, without a simultaneous increase in copper intake results in copper deficiencies. These are reversed by appropriate copper supplementation (Black, *et al*, 1988; Prasad *et al*, 1978; Turnlund, 1988).
10. Low zinc levels may be complicated by low metallothionein, the protein that regulates zinc and copper levels in the serum, liver *etc*. This protein is made of about 30% of the amino acid cysteine. This amino acid becomes deficient early in the course of HIV infection.

Eating properly and taking supplements are the first steps:

A "good attitude" is important to keep you healthy. This means having a positive, informed and focused attitude Early, active and positive intervention is essential; an HIV positive person must actively pursue routes that are known to help prolong life and raise the quality of life. Eating properly and taking supplements are excellent first steps.

Many people who are HIV positive take higher than normal amounts of vitamins and some other compounds (minerals such as zinc and selenium, "immune boosters", *etc.*). This may give the body a sort of "store" that provides a sort of "pressure" to work against infections. Antioxidants may be especially important. Those supplements that are water soluble tend not to store in the body so that these should be taken every day; those that are oil soluble store in your fatty tissue and a reservoir is built up - it's not serious if you sometimes miss a day or two.

Eat a good breakfast in the morning, starting with yoghurt; *acidophilus/bifidus* supplements help keep your gut "bugs" plentiful (remember they are your friends). Having an apple or banana provides them with food. Some form of oatmeal cereal is also normally an excellent choice. Be particularly careful if fat content is high; use fats that are not likely to do harm. High levels of soluble fibre (*e.g.*, oatmeal, apples) and reasonably high levels of insoluble fibre are good stuff. Remember that fibre "keeps you regular", helping control both diarrhoea and constipation. Bran types of fibre, however, may make diarrhoea worse. Leafy vegetables, lettuce ,celery, tomatoes, carrots, fresh chopped garlic, green peppers, cucumbers, *etc.* contain antioxidants, vitamins and minerals, and make a good salad that could be eaten *several times a week*.

Foods high in pectins (apples and most fruits, vegetables) are important since these feed the "gut flora". You can make your own salad dressing using vinegar, olive oil and garlic. If it is difficult to maintain weight, remember that salads are not very dense in calories; in this case, it may be necessary to decrease salad intake in favour of extra foods that contain more calories such as eggs, potatoes and supplemental drinks .

Broccoli is an excellent vegetable - lots of good stuff in it. Peas, beans, squash, carrots, cauliflower, etc., etc. - they are all good, preferably cooked only to a "still crisp" stage so that their minerals are not leached out into the cooking water (okay though in soups). Carrots and leafy greens contain vitamin C, are an excellent source of ß-carotene, and contain both soluble and insoluble fibre. Fruits and berries contain good antioxidants. Oatmeal porridge is good - good protein, good fibre, good fat. The carbohydrates are particularly healthy for the walls of the digestive tract (an old remedy for ulcers was to drink gruel made from oatmeal).

Strictly vegetarian diets can cause zinc deficiency, and may be a problem for HIV positive people.

Vegetarian diets are high in phytic acid which binds (chelates) zinc into a biologically unavailable form removing it from the body. The bran fractions of cereals contain very high levels of phytic acid.

Lack of carnitine may also be a problem with vegetarian diets - supplementation with carnitine is likely very important if you are HIV-positive and vegetarian..

It is good to restrict (not necessarily avoid) use of refined sugars (their names end with "ose") since these may encourage you to have yeast and fungal opportunistic infections (e.g., *candidiasis* or thrush). Excessive amounts are not good for your digestion and overall health.

Olive oil is a good oil to use for salads, cooking, *etc.* It is better than many other oils for cholesterol control. It is high in oleic acid which has anti-fungal activity (our elders used warm olive oil treatment for dandruff control).

Main meals - fish and chicken are excellent for protein. Red meats may still be important since they are excellent sources of carnitine and CoEnzyme Q-10. Other proteins from eggs, cheese, yoghurt, chicken/turkey and well-cooked pork provide alternatives to help prevent boredom.

Sometimes it may be necessary to supplement one's food with liquid food supplements. These products contain some or all of the macronutrients, protein, carbohydrate and fat, as well as micronutrients, vitamins and minerals. When they are called "complete", they contain enough of each of the important ingredients considered essential to keep you alive if you eat/drink enough of the product. Criteria of completeness are normally determined without consideration of special nutritional concerns that derive from HIV. Whenever possible, use liquid supplements to supplement regular meals, not to replace regular food. They are low in dietary fibre, if they contain any at all, and don't usually contain important materials such as bioflavonoids which we get in our regular foods. Try to use liquid food supplements at times when they won't rob you of your appetite for regular food. If supplementation supplies a major part of your food, the food supplement needs to be not only "complete", but also should contain these ingredients in high quality forms.

In general, liquid food supplements should be low in simple sugars (those whose names end with the letters 'ose'), and the fat should not contain high proportions of vegetable polyunsaturated oils, such as corn, soy, sunflower or safflower oils. It's best if soy protein is not present, but this is likely important only for some people, for example who have obvious gastrointestinal problems or who know they get bloating, gas, headaches or other negative reaction from soy products.

To help digest your food, it may help to take supplemental digestive enzymes with your meals. Both betaine hydrochloride and glutamic acid hydrochloride may also help digestion by increasing your stomach acidity. Betaine supplies several other useful functions, including giving you a supply of dimethylglycine, often also recommended as a dietary supplement. Some people alternate these, taking betaine HCl once a week and glutamic acid HCl the next. Finally, acidophilus/bifidus supplements with your meal can help digestion and help keep your intestines in good shape.

Always wash fruits and vegetables - dust on them may contain life-threatening bacteria, fungal spores or parasites (if your T-cells are especially low, then special precautions may be necessary.

Having a beer or wine stimulates the appetite for some people - then have a beer or glass of wine (unless there is some medical reason that dictates otherwise)."Excessive" drinking may stress your body - always take plenty of the Vitamin-C and Vitamin B for any amount of alcohol consumption.

Cigarettes result in high exposure of the lungs to cancer-producing compounds, and generally increase oxidation processes in the body - HIV does this also, so why increase this damage?

Drink coffee in moderation. Tea may be a better stimulant; it contains a number of compounds good for the body - perhaps even anti-HIV, such as from gallic, caffeic and chlorogenic acids.

Chew your food until it is liquid to mix it well with your saliva. Make sure even milk is mixed well with saliva. Remember that digestion starts in your mouth-enzymes to break down both carbohydrates and fats are in saliva.Sometimes one needs food in an easy-to-take form. The information here is about things to look for in food supplements you can drink.

A walk in the fresh air may be adequate and is certainly a good idea in any case

- *Eat a diet that is rich in a variety of vegetables (especially the green leafy ones), fresh fruits, whole grains, beans, nuts, and seeds.* These plant foods are rich in essential nutrients and immune-boosting chemicals.
- *Cut out the sweet stuff.* Sugar makes your white blood cells sluggish. Studies show that eating 100 g of sugar (about 3.5 ounces) reduce the effectiveness of a type of white blood cell known as a neutrophil, which engulfs and destroys bacteria, by as much as 40 % within 2 hours after ingestion. Since neutrophils account for about 60 to 70 % of your white blood cells, interfering with them can seriously impair your immune function.
- *Decrease the intake of saturated fats and cholesterol.* A diet high in saturated fat suppresses immunity. Many of my patients initially presenting with high levels of cholesterol and triglycerides also report more frequent colds and flu. When cholesterol and triglyceride levels are normalized, proper immune function is restored.
- *Eat sufficient but not excessive amount of protein.* Adequate protein intake is critical in the making of white blood cells, antibodies, and chemical messengers such as interferon. You also need protein to make antioxidant enzymes such as glutathione, which is found in abundance in white blood cells. Elevated glutathione levels are associated with better immune function. Patients with low immune function can benefit from eating more protein from fish, lean poultry, and lean cuts of meats.
- *Take a high-potency vitamin and mineral supplement.* Doing so will increase your intake of the key nutrients for immune function.

The following are examples of our medically supervised recommendations.

- Include a quality assured , potent multivitamin and mineral supplement daily
- Eat natural, whole foods, the less processed, the better
- Limit simple sugar and refined white carbohydrates
- Use 100% whole grains in moderate amounts divided over meals and snacks
- Use lean, hormone-free meats, poultry and eggs
- Eat cold water fish 3-5 times a week (wild salmon, canned salmon or yellow fin tuna)
- Eat plenty of fresh or frozen vegetables
- Include low-sugar, high-fibre fruits (apples, pears, berries, cherries, citrus)

Use teas or coffees that are organic (processed by water, not chemicals)

Look after yourself

Positive living

- The body needs extra rest. Try to sleep for eight hours every night. Rest whenever you are tired.
- Try not to worry too much. Stress can harm your immune system. Relax more. Relax with people you love, your family, your children and your friends. Do things you enjoy, e.g. listen to music or read a newspaper or a book.
- Be kind to yourself. Try to keep a positive attitude. Feeling good is part of being healthy.
- Take light exercise. Choose a form of exercise that you enjoy.
- Find support and get good advice. Ask for information and assistance from health workers. Many of your medical problems can be treated.
- Ask for help and accept help when it is offered.
- Stop smoking. Smoking damages the lungs and makes it easier for infections to attack your body.
- Alcohol is harmful to your body. You may forget to practise safe sex.
- Avoid unnecessary medicines. They often have unwanted side-effects and can interfere with food and nutrition. If you do take medicines, read the instructions carefully.

Keep active and stay fit

Exercise helps you to gain weight properly.

- Regular exercise strengthens the muscles, makes you feel energetic, helps to relieve stress and increases appetite.
- Cleaning, working in the field and collecting firewood and water may provide enough exercise.
- Find an exercise that you enjoy and can fit into your daily life.
- Walking, running, swimming or dancing are all suitable.

Increase your intake of vitamins and minerals

Your immune system needs vitamins and minerals to function properly. When you are ill with HIV/AIDS you need even more.

- Eat a variety of vegetables and fruit every day, as these are a valuable source of vitamins and minerals.
- Take care not to lose vitamins and minerals when cooking your food. Boil, steam and fry vegetables only for a short time.
- Multivitamin and mineral supplements, usually in the form of pills, can help but they are expensive and leave less money for food.
- Too many vitamins and minerals can harm you. If you take supplements, follow the instructions on the label.
- *During infection*
- It is very important to try to eat, even though you may not feel like eating, to avoid weight loss.
- Treat infection as early as possible. If you are ill for more than a couple of days see a health worker.

Eat staple foods with every meal

These foods are relatively cheap and supply not only energy and protein but also small amounts of vitamins and minerals. Staples include cereals (such as rice, maize, millet, sorghum, wheat and barley), starchy roots (such as potatoes, sweet potatoes, cassava and yams) and starchy fruit (such as plantains).

Eat legumes if possible every day

These foods include beans, peas, lentils, groundnuts (including peanut butter) and soybeans. When eaten with staple foods the quality of protein is increased.

Eat animal and milk products regularly

Foods from animals and fish should be eaten as often as you can afford them. They supply good-quality proteins, vitamins, minerals and extra energy. All forms of meat, poultry (birds), fish, eggs and dairy products such as milk, sour milk, buttermilk, yoghurt and cheese should be included. If insects, such as caterpillars or grasshoppers, are part of your eating patterns, they also provide good nutrients.

Eat vegetables and fruit every day

These foods are important for a person to grow well and fight infection. A recommended list is provided below.

Yellow, orange, red or dark green	*Other vegetables and fruit vegetables and fruit*
Green leafy vegetables (spinach, pumpkin, cassava leaves), green peppers, squash, carrots, yellow peaches, apricots, papaya and mangoes	Tomatoes, cabbage, oranges, mandarins, grapefruit, lemons, guavas mangoes, passionfruit, pineapples, mulberries and baobab fruit
• Good sources of vitamin A	• Good sources of vitamin C; help to fight infection

Use fats and oils as well as sugar and sugary foods

Fats, oils and sugar are good sources of energy and are important for maintaining weight or regaining weight lost. They add flavour to food, thereby stimulating the appetite.

Fats and oils include butter, lard, margarine, cooking oil (vegetable, coconut and palm oil), cream, mayonnaise and coconut cream. They are also found in avocados, oilseeds (sunflower, groundnut and sesame), fatty meat and fish, curds and cheese.

Sugars and sugary foods include honey, jam, table sugar, cakes and biscuits.

Drink plenty of clean and safe water

Drink about eight cups of water per day and even more if you are suffering from diarrhoea, vomiting or fever. You can also drink fruit juice, soups and other beverages. Collect your water from a protected source and store it in a clean container. If the water is not from a protected source it should be boiled for ten minutes and cooled down afterwards before drinking. Avoid drinking tea or coffee with a meal, as they reduce the iron the body gets from your food.

Nutritional Protocol for Enhancing Immune Function

- Nutrient-rich, whole foods
- Include the right dietary fats
- Eliminate bad dietary fats
- Vitamin/mineral/antioxidant supplementation

Nutritional Protocol for Treating Diarrhoea and Other Gastrointestinal Side Effects

- Take out offending foods
- Eliminate wheat and gluten-containing foods
- Consider options for replacing cow milk dairy
- Switch to hormone-free or organic dairy products
- Consider fortified soy, rice or almond nut milk
- Add soluble fibre
- Food sources: ground flax meal, 100% whole grains, legumes, peas and lentils, low-sugar fruits and vegetables
- Include Supplements
- Drink plenty of hydrating fluids including water and decaffeinated tea
- Limit, or avoid, caffeine, sodas and alcohol
- Add probiotics (a blend of acidophilus and bifidobacteria)
- For severe diarrhoea associated with weight loss, use L-glutamine up to 30 g (2 Tbsp. worth) a day in divided doses

Nutritional Protocol for Treating High Cholesterol and Triglyceride Levels

- Limit sugar and refined, white carbohydrates
- Include the right dietary fats (avoid processing or high heat): flax/borage oil blend — add to foods or liquids without heating it; cold water fish; olives; avocado; cold-pressed oils (olive, sesame, canola, walnut, sunflower and safflower); raw nuts and seeds; flax meal/oil; raw nut butter (peanut, almond or cashew)

- Eliminate bad dietary fats: saturated animal fats and hydrogenated (trans) fat (typically found in processed, long shelf-life convenience foods like popcorn, crackers, snack cakes, many salad dressings and margarines, etc.)
- Improve dietary fiber intake
- Add quality assured supplements including fish oil, policosanol or non-flush niacin
- Improve physical activity

Nutritional Protocol for Improving Glucose Tolerance and Managing Diabetes

- Limit sugar and refined, white carbohydrates
- Include the right dietary fats
- Ensure adequate protein and "good fats"
- Divide meal intake into small portions, eating every 3-4 hours
- Limit starches at meal based on blood sugar levels before and 2 hours after a meal
- Include chromium and vanadium supplement with each meal

There are several good products you can use to make your own liquid food supplement, including:

- Bananas - a medium-sized banana gives about 100 calories, a moderate amount of protein, good dietary fibre (even for diarrhoea), low fat, and is a source of magnesium and potassium; bananas rarely cause allergies.
- Apples - a medium-sized apple gives about 80 calories, excellent carbohydrate that includes dietary fibre, low protein and fat; good source of potassium; apples rarely cause allergic reactions.
- Hard boil an egg or two and use the yolk part in your blender drink.. You can eat the white separately, as it may not be easy to blend it into your drink.
- Cold-pressed flax oil - high in calories; available in nutritional supplement stores. Use this sparingly, for example a teaspoonful or two per blender drink.
- The medium-chain triglyceride product from coconut oil may be good for the immune system, and is easy to digest; available in nutritional supplement stores.

- By adding flax meal, you can thicken the supplement so that you can eat it like a pudding; about one heaping teaspoonful per cup or glass of drink should provide you with a nutritious pudding.

You can try your own combinations considering the needs of the body .

What are the experts saying ?

"Multivitamin supplements ... may be helpful" for "debilitated ARC or AIDS patients who suffer from malabsorption" (Dwyer *et al*, ***1988***, Tufts University) .

"Supplementation of vitamins and trace minerals in amounts one or two times the recommended daily allowance (RDA) may offset possible deficits..." (RJ Raiten, Life Sciences Research Office of the Federation of American Societies for Experimental Biology, ***1990***).

"vitamin E supplementation should always be done in the presence of an adequate selenium] level. An adequate level of Selenium is indispensable for potentiating vitamin E" (Tengerdy, ***1990***, Colorado State University).

"supplements of vitamins and minerals, especially vitamins A (as ß-carotene), E, C, riboflavin, B_6, and B_{12}, and the minerals zinc and selenium, should be part of any oral regimen" (Gorbach *et al*, ***1993***, Tufts University)

"..daily use of a multivitamin supplement was associated with a 40% reduction in the risk of a low CD4 T-lymphocyte count ...those whose supplement consumption was within the highest tertile of intake were about half as likely to develop AIDS compared to those in the middle or lowest tertiles". .. "intake of vitamin E and iron from supplements alone was also significantly associated with a reduced risk of AIDS". ... there was "no statistically significant association between AIDS and intake from food alone of micronutrients or the macronutrients fat and protein" (Abrams et al, **1993**, University of California, Berkeley)

"the highest levels of intake (from food and supplements) of vitamins C and B_1 and niacin were associated with a significantly decreased progression rate to AIDS", and "the progression rate to AIDS was also decreased in subjects in the highest quartile of intake for vitamins B_1, B_2, B_6, and C" (Tang *et al*, ***1993***, Johns Hopkins University)

"the apparent protective effects observed from the B-group vitamins were *primarily due to the intake of vitamins from supplements rather than food*" ...."quartiles of food intake showed no association with survival" (Tang/Graham, ***1995***, Johns Hopkins University)

"we have recommended multivitamin supplementation for *all* HIV-infected patients" (Coodley *et al*, ***1993***, ***1994***, ***1996***, Oregon Health Sciences University). "we agree that a single multivitamin a day may not be sufficient.." (Coodley *et al*, ***1994***)

"Supplementation of vitamins and trace minerals in amounts one or two times the RDA may offset possible deficits..." (RJ Raiten, Life Sciences Research Office of the Federation of American Societies for Experimental Biology, ***1990***)

"vitamin E supplementation should always be done in the presence of an adequate Se [selenium] level. .. an adequate level of Se is indispensable for potentiating vitamin E" (Tengerdy, ***1990***, Colorado State University).

"supplements of vitamins and minerals, especially vitamins A (as ß-carotene), E, C, riboflavin, B_6, and B_{12}, and the minerals zinc and selenium, should be part of *any oral regimen*" (Gorbach *et al*, ***1993***, Tufts University)

"..daily use of a multivitamin supplement was associated with a 40% reduction in the risk of a low CD4 T-lymphocyte count ...those whose supplement consumption was within the highest tertile of intake were about half as likely to develop AIDS compared to those in the middle or lowest tertiles". .. "intake of vitamin E and iron from supplements alone was also significantly associated with a reduced risk of AIDS". ... there was "no statistically significant association between AIDS and intake from food alone of micronutrients or the macronutrients fat and protein" (Abrams et al, **1993**, University of California, Berkeley)

"the highest levels of intake (from food and supplements) of vitamins C and B_1 and niacin were associated with a significantly decreased progression rate to AIDS", and "the progression rate to AIDS was also decreased in subjects in the highest quartile of intake for vitamins B_1, B_2, B_6, and C" (Tang *et al*, ***1993***, Johns Hopkins University) "the apparent protective effects observed from the B-group vitamins were *primarily due to the intake of vitamins from supplements rather than food*" ...."quartiles of food intake showed no association with survival" (Tang/Graham, ***1995***, Johns Hopkins University)

"we have recommended multivitamin supplementation for *all* HIV-infected patients" (Coodley *et al*, ***1993***, ***1994***, ***1996***, Oregon Health Sciences University). "we agree that a single multivitamin a day may not be sufficient.." (Coodley *et al*, ***1994***)

"across the spectrum of this disease many patients have micronutrient deficiencies but it was also shown that *enhanced supplementation of these micronutrients was associated with longevity*", (P Cimoch, ***1994***, Center for Special Immunology, California)

13

Nutrition for the HIV-Positive Woman

Proper nutrition plays an important role in overall health care. For the HIV-infected woman, adequate nutrition is critical, and efforts must be made to optimize nutritional status. Without good health, we are putting family, job/financial security, and ourselves on the line. Kids want and need healthy moms, and co-workers need healthy colleagues. Proper nutrition is one way to help obtain and keep good health. It is a crucial part of the overall healthcare of the HIV-infected person, and should be taken seriously.

Since women in today's society are pulled in so many different directions by taking on many roles, playing homemaker, mother, caregiver, wife, and career women all in the same day, often we neglect ourselves. Part of that neglect may be in our diet habits. Reasons such as too busy, too tired, and forgetting to eat are some of the more common phrases used to explain why proper diet is often lost during the day.

Eventually something serious occurs, most obviously presented by unexplained weight loss. This is a visible indication of what has already been a progression of body changes from HIV disease itself.

HIV-infected women are all at risk for poor nutrition status. Women who play "superwoman" and do not take care of their health may be at increased risk for compromised nutritional status. Unfortunately, unless there has been some significant weight loss, we may not know what's going on inside the body. It is not until this time that a woman thinks about her diet and food intake.

The building blocks of good nutrition include an appreciation of the basic food groups and principals of a well-balanced diet. When making a nutrition and exercise plan, it's probably best to start with small improvements over what you already do.

- Do you eat three healthy meals a day? If not, try to incorporate that third (or even second) meal into your day.
- Do you exercise? If not routinely, then commit to walking around the locality or stretching in your home each day. Once you've made these small changes, then try another set of healthful new activities. The key to success is not to create unrealistic goals and expectations, but rather real and do-able goals that you find enjoyable and fit within your lifestyle. And like any basic programme, periodically check and adapt your strategy to your changing needs.

Nutritional Concerns of Women With HIV

Women often tend to the nutritional needs of their families and neglect their own nutritional health. For women with HIV, this lapse can lead to increased instances of AIDS-related conditions, a general lack of energy and depression; serious consequences which may result in hospitalization.

By addressing their basic nutritional needs, HIV-positive women can maintain a healthier, stronger immune system; mount a better defense against infections; increase effectiveness of medicines and medical procedures (also minimizing their side effects); prevent the breakdown of soft body tissues and maintain the energy needed to lead an active, full life.

Here are a few conditions affecting HIV-positive women which can be controlled and enhanced through proper nutrition:

Why focus on women, nutrition, and HIV ?

HIV is said to have the face of a woman. The vulnerability of women and girls to HIV is increased by biological, economical, social, and cultural factors. In addition, in some countries the legal and political status of women makes them more vulnerable to HIV/AIDS. HIV spreads rapidly, particularly among young women. The stigma associated with HIV can cause isolation and depression, particularly if governments, religious leaders, and community leaders do not discuss the disease (UNAIDS 2001). Silence also contributes to the general impact of HIV/AIDS on food security and nutrition, because infected people may be discriminated against in the workplace or be unable to work because of illness, personal isolation, and difficulty coping with their status. In addition, the burden on women who must care for HIV infected children or other family members is especially great and increases the family's vulnerability to food insecurity and malnutrition.

Good maternal nutrition is important for the health and reproductive performance of women, as well as the survival and development of their children . However, these reproductive years are periods of nutritional stress for many women. Pregnancy-related health and nutrition problems have an effect on the quality of their lives and the lives of their newborn infants well beyond delivery. Malnourished women have high reproductive risks and subsequently poorer pregnancy outcomes than women who are well nourished. Well-nourished women have healthier babies and a lower risk of maternal morbidity and mortality. The physiological changes that occur during pregnancy require extra nutrients and energy to meet the demand of an expanding blood supply, the growth of maternal tissue, the developing foetus, loss of maternal tissue at birth, and preparation for lactation. Malnutrition weakens the immune system and therefore increases vulnerability to infections and may hasten the progression of HIV to AIDS. HIV compromises the nutritional status of infected people and increases their susceptibility to other infections (Piwoz and Preble 2000. For women who are HIV infected, the effects of malnutrition and HIV increase poor clinical outcomes and poor birth outcomes. The nutritional status of an HIV-infected woman or adolescent girl prior to, during, and after pregnancy may influence her own health as well as risk transmitting HIV to her infant.

Heavy Menstrual Periods

Some HIV-positive women experience heavier bleeding during their periods. This may be due to low platelets. For women taking

AZT, there is a greater risk of iron-deficient anaemia. Eating lean meats, liver, egg yolk, legumes, green leafy vegetables, whole grains, molasses, fortified cereals and other iron-rich foods may be helpful.

Low Iron Levels

To increase absorption of iron from non-animal sources, combine foods with those high in vitamin C such as citrus fruits, tomatoes, cabbage, strawberries, green leafy vegetables, broccoli, green and red peppers, potatoes and supplements.

Lighter or Missed Menstrual Periods

This condition often appears in women who are extremely underweight or overweight. When a woman is underweight and under stress, while not getting enough calories and nutrients, the body functions conservatively and slows or stops menstruation (called amenorrhea). To help alleviate this, concentrate on eating "three square meals" a day, including each of the food groups, with additional healthy snacks and weight-gain supplements (drinks or bars are fine). Increase fluid intake and take time for both physical movement and rest each day.

Premenstrual Syndrome (PMS)

This condition can be improved through proper diet. Eat starchy and protein rich foods every three hours to avoid food jags and sharp drops in blood sugar. Choose from each of the basic food groups, including liver, meat, eggs and vegetables for B-vitamin values. Add a bit of vegetable oil (sunflower, safflower or corn) to ensure intake of fatty acids. It may be beneficial to eliminate, or cut back on, caffeine (including chocolate) to reduce breast-swelling and pain. Also, avoid high sodium foods (added salt, chips, processed foods) which can cause bloating. It may be a relief to know it is common to eat 300-500 more calories premenstrually, but choose this food wisely and resume your normal caloric intake after your period.

Menopause

As with all menopausal women, HIV-positive women at this stage lose bone calcium and need to increase calcium in their diet with calcium (such as Tums). As women get older, they tend to eat more and exercise less. Including a good protein source at each meal and snack, and participating in a physical activity each day, such as stretching and walking, as advised.

Good maternal nutrition during both pregnancy and lactation is vital for the survival and well-being of the developing infant. Well-nourished mothers have healthier babies and a lower risk of maternal mortality and morbidity. In contrast, malnourished women have higher reproductive risks and subsequently poorer pregnancy outcomes than their well-nourished counterparts.

Malnutrition and HIV work in tandem, with malnutrition weakening the immune system and increasing vulnerability to infection and HIV compromising nutritional status and increasing vulnerability to infection. Consequently, the nutritional status of an HIV-infected woman or adolescent girl before, during, and after pregnancy may influence her own health as well as the risk of transmitting HIV to her infant. Improving nutritional status and food security for all, including HIV-infected pregnant and lactating women or adolescent girls, so that they remain productive is a challenge for policymakers.

Malnutrition and HIV

Malnutrition HIV Infection Weakens the immune system, increases vulnerability and susceptibility to infection and increased nutrient requirements. Malnutrition during pregnancy increases maternal morbidity and mortality and affects birth outcomes. For the HIV-infected pregnant woman, HIV infection causes nutrient losses that increase nutritional requirements and the risk. of malnutrition, which increases the risk of mother-to-child transmission (MTCT) of HIV.

Vitamin A deficiency, even in mild and moderate forms, is independently associated with HIV viral load in blood, genital secretions, and breast milk, increasing the risk of MTCT. Vitamin A deficiency is common among women.

Anaemia already affects half of all pregnant women in the developing countries and is common in HIV infected women. Anaemia is a risk factor for pre-term delivery and low birth weight, and both of these conditions increase the risk of MTCT.

The pregnant or lactating adolescent

A young maternal age (11-18 years) increases nutrient needs above the ordinary demands of pregnancy. This is a result of the combined needs for adolescent growth and foetal growth and development. For the HIV-infected pregnant or lactating adolescent, nutrient requirements increase as a result of HIV infection. Thus the requirement for energy, protein, and other nutrients increases overall to ensure continued growth of the adolescent mother, growth and development of the foetus, and fulfillment of then increased demands on the body by HIV infection. The HIV-infected pregnant or lactating adolescent is at high risk of malnutrition and should be closely monitored. Improving nutrition prior to pregnancy should be the main goal to minimize the impact of HIV on nutrition.

Nutritional requirements of HIV–infected pregnant or lactating woman

During pregnancy and lactation the requirements for energy, protein, and various micronutrients increase to meet the demands for adequate gestational weight gain, growth and development of the fetus, and milk production. HIV infection causes excess nutrient loss and malabsorption, further increasing the nutritional requirements of HIV-infected pregnant or lactating women. The requirements may be higher if the HIV-infected pregnant woman is suffering from secondary infections. These requirements are in addition to those needed to support a normal and healthy pregnancy and lactation. As a result, the HIV-infected pregnant or lactating woman is at greater nutritional risk than the non-HIV-infected woman.

The HIV infected pregnant and lactating women have the following nutritional risks :-

- Increased need for energy, protein, and other nutrients secondary to the demands of pregnancy or lactation
- Increased need for energy, protein, and other nutrients secondary to HIV infection
- Increased risk of opportunistic infections and malnutrition
- Increased risk of weight loss and delivery of a lowbirth weight baby as a result of HIV infection

- Increased risk of inadequate dietary intake and hence malnutrition as a result of depression, isolation, or stigmatization
- Increased risk of MTCT with poor nutritional status
- Increased risk of transmitting the virus to the baby through breastfeeding
- Increased need for energy, protein, and other nutrients secondary to the demands of pregnancy or lactation.

Recommended nutritional requirements for the HIV infected pregnant or lactating woman

Similar to HIV, common secondary infections such as fever and diarrhoea increase energy and nutrient requirements. Fever, a common symptom in HIV-infected people, increases energy requirements by about 10 percent for every degree rise above normal body temperature. The energy and nutrient requirements imposed by a co-infection such as fever may need to be taken into account when assessing the nutritional requirements of someone infected with HIV, just as they would be for someone who is not HIV infected. HIV infection increases the energy requirements of a pregnant or lactating HIV infected woman, and fever increases them further.

Micronutrient supplementation for pregnant and lactating women and adolescent girls

Pregnant women and infants are the most vulnerable to iron deficiency. Anaemia is common during HIV infection (Levine et al 2001), and in the HIV-infected mother Anaemia increases the risk of mortality. The causes of anaemia in HIV infection are complex. In developing countries anaemia in pregnant or lactating women may be a result of poor dietary intake, poor absorption of iron or other vitamins such as folate and vitamin B12, and co-infections such as malaria and hookworm. For the HIV infected pregnant woman, prolonged use of some antiretroviral drugs (ARVs), such as AZT (Zidovudine), can cause anaemia that presents as megaloblastic anaemia like that seen with folate or vitamin B12 deficiency. Anaemia during pregnancy is a risk factor for infant and probably maternal morbidity and mortality. Iron deficiency anaemia of up to 80 percent is found in developing countries. Because anaemia is so prevalent, iron and folic acid supplementation is recommended during pregnancy and lactation for 6 months in pregnancy. If started late, this supplementation should extend into the post-natal period for 6 months where the prevalence of anaemia is < 40 percent. Where the prevalence is > 40 percent, supplementation is recommended for 6 months in pregnancy and 3 months post-partum for a total of 9 months (WHO/BASICS/UNICEF 1999). Iron and folic acid supplements should be provided to HIV-infected pregnant women as per existing national standards for antenatal care for all pregnant women. In many developing countries iron supplementation during pregnancy and lactation is recommended. Excessive amounts of iron may contribute to HIV disease progression (Clark and Semba 2001; Gorduek et al 2001; Semba et al 2001).

The use of high levels of supplements is not recommended because it can lead to nutrient toxicity that can be harmful to the body. Nutrients that may become toxic if taken in large amounts include iron, zinc, selenium, and vitamins A, B, C and D. For the HIV-infected pregnant or lactating woman, a high intake of these nutrients could do more harm.

In many developing countries, many pregnant adolescent girls are already undernourished. Getting more than the recommended 2,000 kcal/day to meet the demands of adolescent pregnancy may be difficult, especially where food security is a significant concern.

Pregnancy and HIV have a negative synergetic effect on the immune function.

- Both impose physiological stress on the body.
- Both affect immune response in women, which increases their vulnerability to viral, bacterial, and fungal infections.
- Both increase metabolism, which increases the requirements for energy, protein, and micronutrients.

The risk of malnutrition increases in teenage pregnancies because of the combined needs of the growing adolescent and the growing fetus, especially if the pregnancy occurs less than 2 years after the start of menses. Nutrition requirements should consider energy needs for normal growth of the adolescent and weight gain needed for the pregnancy. Pregnant adolescents need an extra 300 kcal/day in the second and third trimesters

Nutritional care and support for the HIV-infected pregnant or lactating woman or adolescent girl

It is well established that the nutritional well-being of a healthy mother is critical for an uncomplicated pregnancy and positive outcome. Nutritional status has even greater implications for the HIV-infected woman or adolescent, who is at higher risk of delivering premature or low-birth weight infants and being malnourished than the uninfected woman. Poor nutritional status of the HIV-infected mother during pregnancy may also increase the risk of vertical transmission during pregnancy. For all women, improving nutritional status before and during pregnancy and during lactation can help ensure adequate gestational weight gain and decrease the risk of premature delivery and low birth weight. For the HIV-infected woman in particular, improving nutrition can help strengthen the immune system, prevent weight loss during lactation, prevent maternal malnutrition, and delay disease progression, allowing the woman to remain productive and prolong her quality of life. Nutritional care and support plays an important role in the overall care of the pregnant or lactating woman or adolescent girl living with HIV/AIDS.

Purpose of nutritional care

HIV-infected pregnant or lactating women or adolescents should be able to maintain good nutritional status throughout pregnancy to carry their pregnancies to term. HIV infection increases not only the pregnant woman's nutrition requirements but also her susceptibility to infection, which in turn puts her at high risk for malnutrition and pre-term delivery. This vicious cycle can be controlled to some extent through good nutritional care and support. This should be done as early in the pregnancy as possible to minimize the impact of HIV on the woman's nutritional status and delay disease progression. The woman can then remain productive and able to take care of her infant, herself, and her family. Psychological support for the HIV-infected pregnant or lactating woman or adolescent girl is integral to this care.

During pregnancy nutritional care is needed to meet the demands of expanded blood volume, growth of maternal tissues, a developing foetus, and loss of maternal tissues at birth, as well as to prepare for lactation. During lactation nutritional care is needed to meet specific nutrient needs to optimize maternal post-natal nutritional status, the quality and quantity of breastmilk production, and infant growth and development. Nutritional care during pregnancy and lactation is needed for all pregnant and lactating women or adolescents, regardless of their HIV status.

Practical considerations

1. Antenatal contacts with mothers can be used for voluntary counseling and testing (VCT) to determine as early in the pregnancy as possible whether the mother is HIV infected. Antenatal contacts can also be used for nutritional assessments to determine whether eating patterns provide adequate nutrient intake and to allow for early nutrition interventions, monitor weight gain during pregnancy, and support successful infant feeding post-partum.
2. Actions have been identified for the health sector can carry out to improve the nutrition of pregnant and lactating women, including those who are HIV infected. These Essential Health Sector Actions aim to ensure the following outcomes (Huffman et al 2001):
    - Adequate food intake during pregnancy and lactation
    - Adequate micronutrient intake during pregnancy and lactation
    - Reduction in malaria infection in pregnant women in endemic areas
    - Reduction of hookworm infection in pregnant women in endemic areas
    - Birth spacing of 3 years or longer

The Essential Health Sector actions can be achieved through contacts with women during antenatal care, delivery and post-partum care, child health visits, and family planning services. Each contact point can be used to provide nutritional care and support to improve the nutrition of the pregnant and lactating women and adolescent girls.

Management of secondary infections is important to minimize their impact on the mother's nutritional status. This management includes promoting the treatment of opportunistic infections and management of common HIV symptoms that are diet related, such as nausea, vomiting, diarrhoea, fever, anorexia (loss of appetite), taste changes, sores in the mouth or throat (thrush), constipation, heartburn, and bloating. Some of these common HIV symptoms (i.e., nausea, vomiting, constipation, heartburn, and bloating) are also common in pregnancy. Anorexia, nausea, vomiting, oral thrush, constipation, heartburn, and bloating can have a serious impact on the HIV-infected pregnant woman's nutritional status because they reduce food intake. Diarrhoea and vomiting increase nutrient losses, and fever increases nutrient requirements. Management of these symptoms should be prompt to minimize their impact on the nutritional status and health of the mother. Nutritional care should be part of a comprehensive programme that provides health care as well as emotional, psychological, and spiritual support for the HIV-infected mother and her family.

Goals of nutritional care and support for the HIV-infected pregnant or lactating woman or adolescent girl

The following goals should be achieved regarding the nutritional care and support for HIV infected pregnant women

- Improve nutritional status. Maintain weight, prevent weight loss, and preserve lean body mass.
- Ensure adequate weight gain during pregnancy. A pregnant woman should gain at least 1 kg per month during the second and third trimesters.
- Ensure adequate nutrient intake by improving eating habits and building stores of essential nutrients (both macronutrients and micronutrients). These nutrients include carbohydrates, protein, important antioxidant nutrients, and other vitamins and minerals necessary for the functioning of the immune system.
- Prevent food-borne illnesses by promoting hygiene and food and water safety.
- Enhance the quality of life by promptly treating infections and managing the symptoms that affect food intake to minimize the impact of secondary infections on nutritional status.

- Provide palliative care as necessary during advanced stages of the disease.

Components of nutritional care and support for the HIV-infected pregnant or lactating woman or adolescent girl

The HIV-infected pregnant or lactating woman or adolescent girl needs regular nutritional assessments and early nutrition interventions. Programmes that provide nutritional care and support for HIV-infected pregnant and lactating women should include the following components:

Nutrition screening and assessment

The nutritional assessment is important to gather information on the nutritional status and adequacy of the diet and to identify risk factors for developing nutritional complications. The earlier in the pregnancy this assessment can be done the better. The information gathered should be interpreted to identify problems that put the woman at high nutrition risk or contribute to the malnutrition. The nutritional assessment should help counsel the mother on her diet to ensure adequate gestational weight gain, improve eating habits, and identify and address food insecurity issues. The goal of the nutritional assessment and interventions are to improve nutritional status, enhance quality of life, and prolong survival of the mother .

Nutritional assessments include the following:

Nutrition history

- Dietary intake and adequacy
- Eating habits
- Food intolerance and aversions to related symptoms
- Dietary problems (e.g., poor appetite, difficulty chewing and swallowing, gastrointestinal problems, and pain in the mouth and gums)
- Hygiene and food preparation and handling practices
- Psychosocial factors contributing to inadequacy of intake, such as social isolation, depression, stigma, and inability to prepare food

- Fatigue
- Physical activity
- Knowledge of food and nutrition issues
- Use of vitamin and mineral supplements and alternative practices

B. Physical assessment

- Anthropometric measurements
- **Pregnant woman**: Height, pre-pregnancy weight, weight gain during pregnancy (at least 1 kg per month in the second and third trimesters)
- **Lactating woman**: height, current weight, pre-pregnancy weight, weight during pregnancy and 6 weeks post-partum;
- **body mass index (BMI) of less than 18.5 indicates nutrition risk**
- Measurement of mid-upper-arm circumference (MUAC) for evidence of loss of muscle mass; **less than 23 cm indicates nutrition risk**
- Screening for oral or pharyngeal inflammation or pain
- Screening for pallor (inner eyelids and palms)

C. Medical history

- Gastrointestinal problems (e.g., diarrhoea, abdominal pain, nausea, vomiting)
- Pattern of bowel movements (constipation or diarrhea)
- Presence of opportunistic infection
- Concurrent medical problems (e.g., diabetes, hypertension, malaria)

D. Medication profile

- Drug use (ARVs, alternative therapies, and other medications)
- Side effects of medications with nutritional implications
- Nutrition-medication interactions
- Traditional herbs or medicine interactions

E. Biochemical data (laboratory data where available and feasible)

- Serum albumin
- CD4 and viral load counts

- Evaluation of anaemia: Iron (Hb), vitamin B12, and folate status

F. Psychosocial profile

- Living environment and functional status
- Income, housing, amenities for cooking, access to food, attitude towards nutrition and food preparation, age, family or support system, and educational level

G. Profile of lactating woman

- Family and other support for breastfeeding
- Breastfeeding pattern: Exclusive breastfeeding, mixed feeding (breastmilk and formula), breastfeeding during pregnancy

Practical considerations for nutrition interventions :

1. Encourage women to eat a varied diet with extra food and get additional rest, particularly in the third trimester of pregnancy. The HIV-infected pregnant or lactating adolescent may require even more food than the HIV-infected pregnant or lactating woman. However, all interventions should be based on the individual nutritional assessment.
2. Conduct nutritional assessments for women with weight gain below the recommended range. This may indicate a possible medical problem (e.g., an opportunistic infection), inappropriate energy intake, or food insecurity. Identify and implement appropriate interventions.
3. Monitor weight gain during pregnancy. Pregnancy weight gain of less than 1.5 kg per month in the second and early third trimesters, or less than 10.5 kg during the entire pregnancy, is of serious concern, and the mother should be referred for further care. **Note:** This applies to all pregnant women. The gestational weight of HIV-infected pregnant women or adolescents should be monitored more regularly because of the impact of the infection on the body. In this way any faltering can be addressed early and good nutritional status maintained.
4. Be aware of community services and programs (e.g., food distribution programs, women's groups for psychosocial support) that may benefit nutritionally vulnerable women. Establish links and refer women who need these services.

5. Assess the HIV-infected pregnant woman for other risk factors that can affect nutritional status and pregnancy outcome. These factors include adolescence, previously existing malnutrition, underweight status at the start of pregnancy, anaemia, gestational diabetes, and opportunistic infection.
6. Discuss with the mother dietary management and appropriate interventions of diarrhoea, nausea, vomiting, malabsorption, loss of appetite, oral thrush, and opportunistic infections. These conditions may prevent weight gain in the HIVinfected pregnant woman or adolescent and have a profound impact on nutritional status and disease progression in an HIV-infected pregnant woman.
7. Be aware of cultural foods, traditional therapies, and practices that are harmful during pregnancy and lactation and counsel the mother about them.
8. Counsel the mother on foods to avoid, especially foods that expose her to bacterial or enteric infection, which can hasten disease progression. These foods include raw eggs or foods with little nutritional value or that do not improve nutritional status. For example, coffee and alcohol decrease appetite, interfere with metabolism, and in the case of alcohol, may interact with some medications to decrease their efficacy.
9. Note the medications, including ARVs, that the HIV-infected pregnant or lactating woman is taking and be aware of the food and drug interactions that can have a negative impact on the woman's nutritional status by reducing food intake. Provide appropriate interventions as required.
10. Improving micronutrient status is an important step to decrease maternal malnutrition, although the additional amounts required by the HIV-infected pregnant or lactating woman have not been determined. Provide multivitamins and other vitamin or mineral supplements as per the country guidelines or WHO/UNICEF guidelines for all pregnant women. Stress the use of iodized salt to prevent iodine deficiency.
11. If multivitamins are recommended to improve the adequacy of the diet or the mothers' nutritional status, carefully analyze their composition. High doses of many nutrients (more than

10 times the usual recommended dietary allowance) may harm the immune system rather than benefit the mother. For example, vitamin C in excess of 1,000 mg may cause or exacerbate diarrhoea. In summary, it is important to improve the diet and eating habits of HIV-infected pregnant or lactating women and adolescent girls. If the diet is not varied, a multiple nutrient supplement, where available, may be needed. Managing barriers to weight gain is important. Ensure that the woman eats sufficient food daily and that the types of food used to prepare meals and snacks provide her with enough critical nutrients to meet her daily needs for pregnancy and lactation. Provide information and counseling on managing feeding and appetite problems during pregnancy and, if necessary, during lactation.

Nutrition education and counseling

Nutrition education and counseling should be an integral part of nutritional care and support of the HIV-infected pregnant or lactating woman or adolescent. Nutrition education and counseling are important to help the mother understand the need to maintain an adequate diet and how to manage common gastrointestinal problems related to HIV and pregnancy that may have a negative impact on nutritional intake. Counseling on the dietary management of common symptoms that affect intake is essential to ensure continued adequate energy and nutrients to maintain lean body mass, ensure optimal gestational weight gain during pregnancy, and delay disease progression. In addition, counseling and education should address vitamin and mineral supplementation (particularly iron and folate supplementation) during pregnancy, malaria and hookworm treatment as required, and adequate diet to support lactation and prevent weight loss.

Nutrition counseling in the context of HIV/AIDS

Many people think counseling is giving information and advice. But counseling an HIV-infected pregnant woman or adolescent girl may involve more than imparting information and advice on diet, nutrition, and healthy eating. The counselor may also help the mother address her feelings about and reactions to being HIV infected. A counselor who understands how clients react to HIV infection can provide nutrition counseling to help them examine their options and make the best choices. In this way the clients are more likely to comply with the nutrition information and advice. An effective counselor must:

- Build a trusting relationship with the client
- Maintain professionalism and confidentiality at all times
- Treat the client with respect and acceptance (avoid being judgmental)
- Respect the client even if the counselor does not agree with the client's attitudes, beliefs, and life choices

Nutrition counseling and education to prevent malnutrition during pregnancy and lactation and improve reproductive health and birth outcomes can benefit all pregnant and lactating women, regardless of their HIV status.

Food safety and hygiene

Improper food handling can cause infection in anyone, but for people infected with HIV, food-borne illnesses can cause even more damage because their weakened immune systems increase their susceptibility to other infections . Therefore, the main goal of nutritional care and support for HIV-infected pregnant or lactating women or adolescents is to avoid food-borne illnesses by educating and counseling on hygiene. This can help prevent infections that cause diarrhea, a common cause of HIV disease progression. Hygiene includes water and sanitation and proper food handling and safety. During the counseling and education session, based on the analysis of the nutritional assessment, the counselor should stress safe food handling practices to avoid food-borne illnesses.

Management of diet-related HIV problems :

Common diet-related HIV problems include anorexia, nausea, vomiting, diarrhea, constipation, bloating, mouth or throat sores, fever, malabsorption, fatigue, and taste alterations. These can all be barriers to gaining weight during an HIV complicated pregnancy.

Dietary modifications to manage the conditions that affect food intake can minimize the impact on the woman's nutritional status, maximize nutritional intake, ensure adequate gestational weight gain, maintain weight and muscle mass during lactation, and improve quality of life for the infected woman. Appropriate locally available and affordable dietary interventions should be explored and used as much as possible. Use of medications together with dietary interventions to manage common dietary problems should be an integral part of nutritional care and support for HIV-infected pregnant or lactating women or adolescent girls. Safe traditional therapies that help relieve symptoms should also be considered and encouraged. a guide on the dietary management of some common HIV symptoms.

Physical activity

Maintaining physical activity has been shown to improve body composition and quality of life in people living with HIV/AIDS. Exercise can also help stimulate the appetite and increase energy. The pregnant or lactating woman should be encouraged to maintain physical activity as much as possible. Exercise as simple as a daily walk should be encouraged. However, as pregnancy advances the pregnant woman or adolescent girl should be encouraged to get more rest and, if possible, avoid strenuous physical activity or work.

Safer sex and reproductive health practices

Education and counseling on HIV prevention is important. Safer sex practices such as condom use should be promoted and VCTC services provided. These are especially important for the HIV-infected pregnant or lactating woman or adolescent girl because acute infections, including sexually transmitted infections (STIs), may increase maternal viral replication, causing a higher maternal viral load. There is strong evidence that a high viral load increases the risk of vertical transmission of HIV during pregnancy and lactation and further weakens the immune system, making women even more susceptible to opportunistic infections. Condom use may help HIV-positive women avoid infecting their uninfected partners or prevent repeated exposure to infection from HIV-infected partners. Repeated exposure to HIV can increase maternal viral load and increase the risk of MTCT.

Psychosocial support

Psychosocial support is an important part of nutritional care and support for the HIV infected pregnant or lactating woman or adolescent. Malnutrition with wasting has an impact on self-esteem, which can lead to depression, isolation, lack of appetite, and an aversion to food. For the HIV-infected pregnant or lactating woman or adolescent, this can increase the risk of malnutrition. It is important to explore feelings such as guilt, fear, and denial when providing psychosocial support. The woman should receive emotional, spiritual, and social support in a supportive environment. Encourage access to peer support where available. Counsel and support the woman on coping with possible stigmatization and discrimination, especially if she has not disclosed her HIV status to her partner,family, and friends.

Antenatal and post-natal care

Good antenatal and post-natal care are integral components of nutritional care and support for women infected with HIV. The antenatal clinic is a good place to start early nutrition interventions to minimize the impact of HIV on a woman's nutritional status. Monitoring weight and diet at all antenatal contacts can help ensure adequate weight gain and food intake during pregnancy

Early nutrition interventions for HIV-infected pregnant women may help improve their overall pregnancy outcomes. Where available, ARVs should be provided to reduce mother-to-child transmission of HIV. Antimalarial prophylaxis and deworming medications should be provided as per national protocols to reduce the risk of anaemia and low birth weight. Inclusion of the traditional birth attendants can help reduce the risk of MTCT.

Infant feeding options and risks

All pregnant women and adolescents should be counseled on infant feeding options and risks. HIV-infected women and adolescents should be informed about ways to reduce risk of HIV transmission to the infant and counseled on related infant feeding options and risks. HIV-infected mothers who choose to breastfeed should be counseled on how to make breastfeeding safer, and mothers who decide not to breastfeed should know the options and risks of replacement feeding. For breastfeeding women who are at risk of malnutrition, programmes should consider providing nutritional support to prevent nutritional depletion, weight loss, and disease progression, as well as to enhance the success of exclusive breastfeeding(the efficacy of this is now being studied).

Medications and ARV therapy

Medications used to treat HIV-opportunistic infections may result in negative drug nutrient interactions or cause side effects. As access to ARVs increases, more women will be treated with ARVs to delay disease progression and reduce the risk of transmission of the virus to their infants. Many ARVs and medications prescribed to treat opportunistic infections have side effects that may affect dietary intake. These side effects include nausea, vomiting, diarrhoea, constipation, anorexia, and changes in taste. The side effects of medications should be managed to ensure continued food intake and adherence to the medications

Associated with HIV in Adults for details on managing common problems in HIV infection). In addition, some food and drug-nutrient interactions have to be taken into consideration, and proper counseling should be provided on the use of these medications by the pregnant or lactating HIV-infected woman or adolescent. For example, supplements containing iron and zinc should not be taken with the antibiotic Ciprofloxacin.

Young women 15 to 24 years old are two-and a-half times more likely to be infected than

young men of the same age. HIV-infected pregnant and lactating women have increased

nutritional requirements compared to their healthy HIV-negative counterparts due to a combination of the virus replication process and disease symptoms that limit dietary intake and reduce nutrient absorption. Medications used to treat HIV and associated infections can also create side effects that cause an individual to reduce food intake, while opportunistic infections associated with HIV contribute to additional nutrient losses. Good nutrition is important for all pregnant women and contributes to maternal health and optimal birth outcomes. Inadequate food intake, poor dietary quality, and untreated infections before and during pregnancy increase the risk of maternal mortality and morbidity and are risk factors for negative birth outcomes such as infants with low birth weight (LBW) or intrauterine growth restriction (IUGR). Because the nutritional requirements of women are greater during pregnancy, they need to consume adequate quantities of nutritionally dense foods to meet their own nutritional requirements and the requirements of the growing fetus and prepare for lactation. This section presents a brief review of the nutritional requirements of all pregnant women in the context of HIV/AIDS and provides dietary recommendations to ensure women's health and improve birth outcomes. A healthy and normally active pregnant woman requires approximately 285 additional kcal each day. She also needs to eat increased amounts of protein and take a daily supplement containing 60 mg of iron and 400 mg of folate, according to national protocols. A diverse, micronutrient-rich diet should be consumed, including fortified foods if available. A daily multi micronutrient supplement containing upto 1. recommended dietary allowance (RDA) 2 of all essential nutrients may be recommended when an adequate and balanced diet is not available. A pregnant woman should gain approximately 12.5 kg during the pregnancy.

Ensuring Good Nutrition for all Pregnant Women and Adolescent Girls

Benefits for the mothers:

- Decreases the risk of complications during pregnancy and delivery;
- Prevents or controls anaemia in the mother; lowers the risk of mortality/morbidity during delivery and in the early postpartum period; and
- Ensures energy storage for lactation.

Benefits for the infant:

- Prevents intrauterine growth restriction (IUGR), micronutrient deficiencies, and LBW and contributes to healthy growth and development.

Benefits for the household

- Well-nourished, healthy mothers are more available for child care and contribute more fully to the functioning of the family; and
- Improved work productivity is associated with improved nutritional status.

Benefits for the community and the nation

- Increases productivity; and
- Decreases maternal and infant morbidity and mortality

Energy Requirements. Healthy pregnant women need an extra 285 kcal per day if the pre-pregnancy activity level is maintained. The additional 285 kcal per day translates approximately into one additional serving of the staple food each day. The extra daily energy requirement is reduced to 200 kcal per day if the activity level is reduced.

Protein Requirements. A pregnant woman requires more protein for the development of foetal and maternal tissue, including the placenta, and an increased red blood cell mass.

Non-pregnant women need 0.8 g protein/kg per day, while pregnant women require 1.1 g/kg per day, or approximately 71 g each day3. In addition to the consumption of staple foods, pregnant women should eat foods that provide protein, such as pulses (e.g., chickpeas, lentils, cowpeas, beans), oil seeds (e.g., pumpkin, sunflower, melon), and foods of animal origin (e.g., meat, eggs, milk). Foods of animal origin provide protein, zinc, selenium, and iron that is more bio-available than the same nutrients derived from plant sources. Pregnant women need to eat a variety of foods to meet their macronutrient and micronutrient requirements.

Micronutrient Requirements. Many micronutrient requirements increase with pregnancy. Pregnant women have higher iron requirements because of the mother's increased red blood cell mass and the iron needed by the developing fetus. They are therefore at higher risk of developing iron deficiency anaemia than non-pregnant women. In order to meet both foetal and maternal iron requirements, an adequate dietary intake of iron plus supplementation with iron/folate is necessary for pregnant women.

Anaemia and Iron. Anaemia in pregnant women is associated with pre-term delivery, LBW, and increased perinatal mortality. The risk of maternal mortality is increased in pregnant women with decreasing haemoglobin levels. In resource limited settings, anaemia affects half or more of all pregnant women. WHO recommends that pregnant women consume a supplement containing 60 mg of iron and400 micrograms of folic acid on a daily basis for six months during pregnancy where the prevalence of anaemia is less than 40 percent and for an additional three months postpartum where anaemia prevalence is equal to or greater than 40 percent to prevent anaemia.

Take an Integrated Approach to Anaemia Prevention and Control Services for Pregnant Women

- Provide iron or iron/folate supplements to pregnant women according to international or national protocols.
- Promote animal sources of iron, iron-fortified foods, and enhanced bioavailability of iron in the diet.
- Deliver malaria prevention and treatment services to pregnant women, especially in first and second pregnancies.
- Provide helminth control—once in the second trimester with hookworm prevalence 20 to 30 percent; repeat once in third trimester with prevalence greater than 50 percent—in areas with endemic helminth infections:

  " Albendazole—400 mg single dose;

  " Mebendazole—500 mg single dose or 100 mg twice daily for three days;

  " Levamisole—2.5 mg/kg single dose; best if dose repeated on next two consecutive days; and

  " Pryantel—10 mg/kg single dose, best if dose repeated on next two consecutive days.
- Treat other infectious diseases.
- Provide birth spacing information and access to modern family planning methods.

Vitamin A. Pregnant women are particularly vulnerable to vitamin A deficiency, making them more susceptible to infection and, in one study in Nepal, increasing the risk of maternal death.

In addition, low maternal stores of vitamin A compromise breastmilk quality and negatively affect the vitamin A stores of their infants. Improving vitamin A status may also contribute to a reduction of anaemia.

Iodine. In areas where iodine deficiency is a problem, women are more likely to miscarry or give birth to stillborn children. Both the mental and physical growth and development of children may be impaired and children born to iodine deficient women may suffer

irreversible mental retardation. Universal consumption of iodized salt by all household members should be encouraged. Additional micronutrients of particular importance to pregnant women are zinc, folate, calcium, and vitamin D. Eating a varied diet including locally available fruits and vegetables will help pregnant women meet their micronutrient requirements and add fibre to their diet. Micronutrient-fortified staple foods such as wheat also help to increase the dietary sources of micronutrients for women.

Pregnancy's Discomforts Pregnancy may be accompanied by changes in eating habits. Some pregnant women have cravings for or aversions to specific foods. Additionally, many women suffer from nausea, vomiting, and constipation at different points in pregnancy. Though normal, the body's reaction to pregnancy can be of special concern in HIV-infected women since the virus places an added stress on their bodies. **Cravings and Aversions.** Craving and eating only specific foods and avoiding others because of the flavour, odour, or colour may lead to nutrient deficiencies. Some pregnant women eat unusual items such as clay, chalk, and cola nut leaves that can be harmful for the mother and the infant. Health workers can help women identify nutrients that may be missing from their diets and suggest healthful alternatives to the unusual substances being consumed to correct the deficiency.

Nausea. Some women suffer from nausea and vomiting during the first trimester of the pregnancy, which may lead to reduced food intake and limited gestational weight gain. Health workers can counsel women on how to manage nausea and vomiting during pregnancy so that they are able to maintain or increase food intake and meet their nutritional requirements.

Constipation. Constipation may result from a reduction in activity level, a change in eating habits or as a side effect of iron/ folate supplements. Health workers should encourage women to drink plenty of fluids, eat a variety of locally available fruits and vegetables every day, and maintain physical activity as much as possible.

Tips for Pregnant Women, Suffering from Frequent Nausea and Vomiting

- Eat small and frequent meals. Nausea is worse if nothing is in the stomach.
- Eat dry food such as dry bread, roasted or boiled groundnut, plantain, yam, potato, or any other available tuber before getting out of bed.
- Drink fluids between meals rather than with meals.
- Avoid drinking beverages containing alcohol and caffeine.
- Avoid lying down for at least twenty minutes after eating.
- Rest between meals.

Special Considerations for Adolescent Pregnancy

A pregnancy during adolescence often increases the risk for malnutrition, complications during pregnancy and delivery, and poor birth outcomes, including death of the mother and child. This section will address nutritional considerations for pregnancy during adolescence. The nutritional requirements of pregnant adolescent girls are greater than the requirements of pregnant adult women because an adolescent is usually still growing. Her daily intake must satisfy both the requirements of the developing girl and those of the developing fetus. Completion of linear growth may take up to seven years after menarche, and pelvic bone growth continues even after full height is achieved. This places pregnant adolescents at increased risk for prolonged and/or obstructed labor leading to increased maternal and infant mortality as well as the potential for crippling injuries such as vaginal fistulae. Adolescent mothers are also more likely to have LBW babies because of the competition for nutrients between mother and fetus, as well as poorer placental function. This perpetuates the intergenerational cycle of malnutrition.

By addressing the special requirements of adolescents—before they become pregnant as well as during pregnancy—there is a potential opportunity to break the cycle.

Pregnant adolescent girls are at a very high risk for mortality. For adolescent girls less than 18 years, the risk of dying in childbirth is 2 to 5 times greater than for women between the ages of 18 and 25.

HIV-infected pregnant women and adolescent girls, like other PLWHAs, have increased energy requirements due to infection with HIV. Attention to nutrition for HIV-infected pregnant women and adolescent girls is doubly important in order to maintain weight, prevent weight loss, and continue adequate weight gain during pregnancy. Improved nutritional status will help to maintain a strong immune system, decrease susceptibility to infections, and slow the progression to AIDS. It is important that health workers are able to provide guidance to HIV-infected pregnant women and adolescent girls on the range of locally available nutrient dense foods that they can eat to meet their daily increased energy and overall nutrient requirements. This means being familiar with the energy and micronutrient content of local foods. Heath workers may need to work with agencies in the community to find ways to meet the nutritional requirements of HIV-affected women and their families to improve or maintain their health and nutritional status. Options include the direct provision of food rations, either on-site or take-home, distributed through maternal and child health programs, food-for-workand food-for-training programs. Income generation activities may be funded through limited cash resources from food-assistance programs to improve household food security and the means to acquire food.

Energy Requirements. Energy requirements of HIV-infected pregnant adolescents and adult women vary according to the stage of the disease.

Nutritional Care and Support for HIV-infected Pregnant Women and Adolescents

HIV-infected asymptomatic pregnant adolescents and adults (WHO stage 1) should increase energy intake over the level recommended for healthy non HIV-infected pregnant adolescents and adult women by an amount equaling 10 percent of the intake level recommended for non-pregnant adolescents or women of the same age and activity level plus the additional energy (i.e., approximately 285 kcal per day) needed to support pregnancy. HIV-infected symptomatic pregnant adolescents and adults (WHO stage 2 and above) should increase energy intake over the level recommended for healthy non HIV-infected pregnant adolescents and adult women by an amount equaling 20 to 30 percent of the intake level recommended for non-pregnant adolescents or women of the same age and activity level plus the additional energy needed to support pregnancy. The amount of increased energy is the same for HIV-infected persons taking ARVs. The level of additional energy intake for the HIV infected pregnant woman depends on the presence and severity of symptoms.

Protein Requirements. At this time, there is not enough evidence to suggest that HIV infected pregnant women require more protein than the level recommended for healthy non-HIV-infected pregnant woman. Meeting the protein requirements of HIV-infected pregnant women will help prevent muscle wasting and support the additional protein demands of pregnancy including the growth of the placenta and increased red blood cell mass.

Micronutrient Requirements. Micronutrients play important roles in the healthy functioning of the immune system and therefore are particularly important for PLWHAs. At the same time, in populations with high AIDS prevalence, micronutrient deficiencies are often common World.

Health Organization advise HIV-infected pregnant adolescents and adult women to consume varied diets to ensure that they meet the RDAs for micronutrients. The results of vitamin A supplementation trials for HIV-infected women are mixed. The current WHO guidelines advise that vitamin A intake by HIV-infected pregnant and lactating women not exceed the existing RDAs. No additional vitamin A should be provided. In areas of endemic vitamin A deficiency, WHO continues to recommend administration of a single high dose (i.e., 200,000 IU) vitamin A supplement within the first six to eight weeks4 of delivery to the new mother. Although a varied, nutritionally adequate diet is the best source for micronutrients, there will be women for whom a multiple micronutrient supplement is recommended. Some studies have shown improvements from specific multivitamin and mineral supplements to HIV-infected women for a range of outcomes, including increased maternal weight gain during pregnancy, increased haemoglobin concentration, HIV progression to AIDS and improved CD4 cell counts. For children, improved birth weight, reduced postnatal transmission of HIV, and decreased mortality have been shown, particularly among nutritionally vulnerable women with advanced HIV disease. The optimal composition of multiple micronutrient supplements for HIV infected women has yet to be determined and is currently being studied.

Some HIV-infected pregnant women may take ARV medications to prevent MTCT and reduce their viral loads. There are different types of ARV regimens that may be administered.

Nutritional Care and Support for Pregnant and Lactating Women and Adolescent Girls

By six weeks after delivery if a woman is not breastfeeding to avoid any risk of harm to a new foetus; by eight weeks after delivery if she is breastfeeding.

Single-course regimens such as nevirapine may have minimal food and drug interactions.

Food and drug interactions may occur more often with medium- and long-course regimens and the side effects of these interactions can negatively impact the nutritional status of HIV infected pregnant women. Appropriate dietary management can help to maintain food intake and the efficacy of the medication. HIV-infected pregnant women may also take other medications in combination with ARVs to treat opportunistic infections. These medications may interact with food and the side effects may cause decreased food intake, thus affecting nutritional status and the efficacyof the medication or medications. For example, pregnant and/or HIV-infected women are more susceptible to the side effects of the TB drug, isoniazid. HIV-infected pregnant women who are also being treated for TB may be advised to take vitamin B6 (i.e., pyridoxine) supplements to prevent or treat drug-induced peripheral neuropathies (e.g., numbness or burning in the feet). The recommended preventive dose is 10 mg B6/day; 100 mg B6/day is prescribed for treatment.

Additional Recommended Care Practices Food Safety and Handling. Proper food handling and safety practices for HIV-infected pregnant women are the same for all PLWHAs. HIV infected women and adolescent girls are more susceptible to harmful bacteria and viruses in contaminated food and water as a result of their infection with HIV. Food poisoning can cause weight loss and further lower their resistance to future infections. Hygienic food handling should be accompanied by sanitary disposal of faeces, good personal hygiene, including hand washing and covering of wounds, and the use of clean water for drinking and food preparation.

The Essential Nutrition Actions

The following essential nutrition actions may be considered to improve the nutrition of women and children:

1. Promotion of optimal breastfeeding during the first 6 months
2. Promotion of appropriate complementary feeding beginning at 6 months with continued breastfeeding to 2 years and beyond
3. Promotion of appropriate feeding of the child during and after illness
4. Prevention of vitamin A deficiency (breastfeeding, consumption of fortified and vitamin A-rich foods, maternal and child supplementation 6-59 months)
5. Prevention of anaemia (maternal and child iron supplementation, deworming, malaria control, and consumption of fortified and iron-rich foods)
6. Promotion of iodized salt consumption by all families

7. Promotion of improved women's nutrition (increased food intake during pregnancy and lactation, iron and folic acid supplementation, treatment and prevention of malaria, deworming during pregnancy, post-partum vitamin A supplementation).

Ensuring good nutrition during pregnancy and lactation

Vitamin A deficiency has been associated with a significant increase of HIV in breast milk and increased mortality of HIV-infected adults (Nduati et al 1995). Vitamin A supplementation, however, has not resulted in reduced MTCT (Coutsoudis et al - 1999). Iron deficiency is associated with low birth weight and prematurity. Both are risk factors of infant HIV infection. One study (Fawzi et al 1998) found that multivitamin supplements resulted in a 44 percent reduction in low birth weight, 39 percent reduction in prematurity, and improved maternal haemoglobin and CD4 counts after delivery.

Breastfeeding techniques

It is especially important for PMTCT programming that staff members are trained in lactation management skills. The risk of cracked nipples may be reduced by improving positioning and attachment (i.e., latching onto the areola rather than nipple). The use of abrasive creams and soaps, which may result in cracked nipples, should be discouraged by counselors and health workers. The pain of cracked nipples may cause the mother to avoid emptying her breasts, resulting in engorgement and eventually leading to mastitis. Gentle expression techniques may be required to assist the mother with emptying her breasts.

Voluntary and confidential counseling and testing

Voluntary counseling and testing (VCT) has been shown to be a cost-effective approach to reducing HIV-related risk behaviours. Stigma is an important issue to consider for this intervention. Sensitivity counseling, community education, and involvement of partners in the VCT process may help alleviate the stresses caused by the stigma of HIV .

- Men should be properly counseled about MTCT

- Health workers must be properly trained in MTCT.
- Counseling programs should be offered to support HIV-infected women and men. Peer counselors, service providers, and social workers must be properly trained.
- Prevention messages should be included with VCT, especially in the context of MTCT, because newly infected women are twice as likely to transmit the virus to their infants.

Psychosocial Support. HIV-infected pregnant women and adolescent girls need special care and attention. In addition to dealing with a life-threatening disease, they must also deal with the usual discomforts that can accompany pregnancy. They may also have to confront discrimination and stigmatization by their family and community. Psychosocial support from caregivers and health workers is important. Mental health interventions may be needed to address depression. Program staff should work with communities to raise awareness about the need to support HIV-infected pregnant women to improve pregnancy outcomes and the survival of the mother.

Safer Sex Practices. Unprotected sex may expose HIV-infected pregnant adolescents and adult women to sexually transmitted diseases and/or re-exposure (i.e., surinfection) to HIV, resulting in an increased viral load. This, in turn, results in an increased risk of MTCT and can speed up the disease's progression o AIDS by further weakening the immune system. Unprotected sex can also expose women's partners to infection. Health workers should advise HIV-infected mothers on safer sex practices, such as abstinence, involvement with one committed partner who has tested negative for HIV and remains faithful and use of condoms during every sexual contact.

Other Issues to Consider The Low Social Status of Women. Poor health and nutritional status of girls and women, especially in limited resource settings, may be due in part to gender inequality and the low status of women in certain societies. Women may need the approval of husbands or mothers-in-law to obtain nutrition and health services. Differential access to education and income generation opportunities for adolescent girls and women may be a barrier to their ability to improve dietary intake and/or treat and control infections. Community-level programme staff should carry out a situation analysis of women's health and nutrition and identify and address problems that affect their nutritional status, especially during pregnancy and lactation.

Food Insecurity in the Context of HIV/ AIDS. In many resource limited settings that have been hit hard by the HIV/AIDS epidemic, access to sufficient food may be limited, especially for families affected directly by HIV/AIDS. Strengthen linkages and refer women to programmes that provide nutritional care and support and support food security and coping strategies of HIV/AIDS-affected households and individuals.

Inequity in Intra-household Food Distribution. In many cultures, women frequently serve themselves last at meals. Husbands and male children are often the first to get food and mothers and girls eat what remains. For HIV-infected pregnant women and adolescent girls, problematic intra-household food distribution patterns may compound already existing inadequate nutritional intake due to increased energy needs of HIV infection and pregnancy.

Food Taboos. Pregnant women may observe culturally dictated dietary guidelines that prohibit certain foods. These food taboos may restrict nutrient dense foods, such as eggs or a specific type of meat. Avoiding such foods deprives pregnant women of an important source of protein and micronutrients and can contribute to malnutrition. Although culturally sensitive, programmes should work with communities to address taboos that may deprive women of foods they need to ensure good nutritional status and birth outcomes.

Cultural Beliefs: Fear of Having a "Big Baby." In some cultures, women restrict food intake during the final months of the pregnancy. This limits weight gain to reduce the size of the baby and, thus, decrease the risk of obstructed labor. In addition to LBW, inadequate diets can contribute to a weakened immune status of the mother with resulting increased risk of morbidity and possibly mortality of both mother and baby.

High Physical Activity Workloads. Women in resource limited settings routinely have heavy workloads that do not diminish with pregnancy. To compensate for the high amounts of energy expended on household and agricultural work, in addition to the energy used by the virus and by the growing baby, HIV-infected pregnant women must increase their energy intake. Alternatively, their workloads can be reduced and periods of rest can be added to reduce their energy expenditure. However, continued physical activity at usual/moderate levels remains important for HIV-infected women to preserve lean body mass.

The Perception of the Pregnancy. Pregnancy may be viewed in some settings as a condition that does not require special attention. The need for increased energy intake and/or decreased energy expenditure may go unrecognized, as could the need for improved dietary quality or the importance of accessing antenatal care services. Raising the awareness of household and community members about the nutritional requirements of pregnancy and lactation and the importance of health care during these periods may help women gain access to the food and health/nutrition services that they need to remain healthy and improve birth outcomes.

Stigma and Discrimination. Family members or other community members may stigmatize HIV-infected pregnant women and adolescent girls. Stigmatization may result in neglect by or estrangement from the family, which can cause the health of these women to decline rapidly. Communities and family members may be particularly intolerant of pregnancy or HIV in adolescent girls leading to the need for programmes to target HIV-infected pregnant adolescents for specialized services that may include supplementary food.

Energy Requirements. Lactating women need extra energy to support the production of breast milk. The extra energy required for lactating women is about 500 kcal per day for the first six months, assuming that their nutritional requirements were met during pregnancy. This translates approximately into eating an extra meal each day. A woman who has been able to consume the recommended quantities of energy and nutrients during pregnancy will have stored adequate amounts of fat, which is used for lactation. The same recommendation, an extra 500 kcal per day, applies to the second six months of breastfeeding when children have begun to consume complementary foods in addition to breast milk. If energy requirements were not met during pregnancy, which is often the case with women who were undernourished prior to pregnancy, a lactating woman may need up to an additional 700 kcal per day to produce the necessary quantity of milk without affecting her own nutritional status. The energy requirements for lactating adolescent girls are greater than for adult women of the same size and activity level because of their continuing growth.

Protein Requirements. Protein requirements are the same for lactation and pregnancy: approximately 71 g per day or 1.1 g/kg of maternal weight per day, according the U.S.National Academies of Science in 2002.

Micronutrient Requirements. Micronutrient requirements are also increased during lactation because of the transfer of micronutrients to breast milk. Lactating women should eat a variety of fruits and vegetables, and foods from animal origin daily to meet their micronutrient requirements. In areas of endemic vitamin A deficiency, lactating women should be provided with a high dose vitamin A supplement within the first eight weeks postpartum to increase the vitamin A content of their breast milk. Current WHO recommendations are to provide 200,000 IU vitamin A in a single dose.

Energy Requirements. The energy requirements of HIV-infected lactating mothers vary according to the stage of the disease. HIV-infected asymptomatic (WHO stage 1) lactating adolescents and adults should increase energy intake over the level recommended for healthy non-HIV-infected lactating adolescents and adult women by an amount equaling 10 percent of the intake level recommended for non-lactating dolescents or women of the same age and activity level plus the additional 500 kcal to support lactation.

HIV-infected symptomatic (WHO stage 2 and above) lactating adolescents and adults should increase energy intake over the level recommended for healthy non HIV-infected lactating adolescents and adult women by an amount equaling 20 to 30 percent of the intake level recommended for non-lactating adolescents or women of the same age and activity level plus the additional 500 kcal to support lactation. The necessary energy intake increase is the same whether or not the HIV-infected person takes ARVs. The level of additional energy intake for the HIV-infected pregnant woman depends on the presence and severity of symptoms.

Protein Requirements. HIV-infected lactating women and adolescents need the same level of daily protein intake as healthy HIV-negative lactating women, which is estimated to be 1.1 g/kg body weight per day or approximately 71 g of protein per day, according the U.S. National Academies of Science in 2002.

Micronutrient Requirements. HIV-infected lactating women and adolescents need the same amounts of micronutrients as healthy HIV-negative lactating women. HIV-infected lactating women should be encouraged to eat a variety of foods, including animal products, fruits, and vegetables, to help ensure adequate micronutrient intake.

Possible Problems and Nutritional Support required for Women with HIV infection

Cracked Nipples

Cracked nipples, mastitis, and breast abscesses increase the risk of HIV transmission through breast milk. Health workers should demonstrate proper latching-on techniques to prevent the development of cracked nipples and counsel on how to prevent and manage other types of breast problems such as mastitis.

Unintentional Weight Loss :

Unintentional weight loss is called wasting. Society's glamorizing of thin women might lead doctors — and some women with HIV — not to be alarmed by unplanned weight loss. Although some women initially may be somewhat excited about some weight loss, it is not something to be taken lightly. Weight loss may indicate an infection or other problem, and can become life threatening. Any weight loss that is unplanned and can't be explained should be cause for alarm. Your weight should be monitored with the same watchful eye as your lab results. Malnutrition and weight loss are common problems with HIV disease. Malnutrition can result from loss of appetite and food intake due to depression, fatigue, illness or side effects from therapy. Without monitoring, it can persist undetected for a long time.

Weight loss is an obvious sign of malnutrition. It can begin and become severe anywhere in the course of HIV infection, though it's an increasing threat when CD4+ cell counts fall below 100. Wasting is an extreme type of weight loss and is an unexplained loss of 10% or more of a person's normal weight.

In the context of HIV disease, it can be considered AIDS-related wasting. The cause of wasting can be complex and varied. Researchers believe that aside from the changes in food intake, absorption, and metabolism all playing a role in wasting, hormonal changes may also contribute to the difference in body wasting in women. Wasting in a woman appears different than in a man. Women tend to lose fat tissue, whereas men appear to lose lean tissue quicker. It is important not only to monitor weight and to measure what the body is made of, or your body composition (body fat, body cell mass), but we must preserve body cell mass, and preserve a certain amount of fat to live and function.

What can we do to help prevent wasting? Apart from visiting your doctor regularly, nutritionally you can do a number of things. First, you can eat a variety of foods. Make sure you are getting enough vitamins and minerals, calories, and protein daily.

If you need to gain weight, or to keep from losing weight, eat the higher number of servings for extra calories.

Bone Health

When we're young, our bones get stronger as we grow. At some point, perhaps around age 30, we stop building bone. Our bones get weaker as we get older, and women in general experience bone loss at a much higher rate than men.

Even without HIV, you're at higher risk of losing bone quickly if you are: female, over age 50, are in or have been through menopause, slender or have a family history of osteoporosis. Bone loss also happens faster if you smoke, drink alcohol or a lot of caffeine, use corticosteroids like prednisone, or don't exercise. Our bodies need both calcium and vitamin D to build bone. People with HIV seem to experience bone loss more often than people without HIV. Being a female and having HIV are both risk factors for bone loss. Recently, two bone conditions have been seen in people living with HIV.

Osteoporosis (sometimes called brittle bones) is a loss of the mineral in bones, which makes them more porous and likely to fracture. Osteonecrosis refers to the death of bone, due to a lack of blood supply to the bone. You can have osteoporosis without any symptoms, but there are tests to diagnose it. This is very important if you're at high risk (many positive women are) or if you've been experiencing bone pain. A special X-ray, called a DEXA scan, is used to measure bone mineral density. It's also important to ask your doctor to check your hormone levels, since estrogen deficiency can increase your risk of bone loss.

There are several things you can do to slow down bone loss: stop smoking, reduce or stop drinking alcohol and caffeine, and increase your intake of vitamin D and calcium (by using calcium supplements and/or eating foods like leafy green vegetables and dairy products). Regular exercise that requires you to bear weight, such as walking or lifting weights, also helps strengthen your bones.

Drugs called biphosphonates — Fosamax (alendronate) and Actonel (risedronate) — are often used to prevent and treat bone density loss in postmenopausal women. These drugs haven't been studied in pre-menopausal women with bone loss, but some healthcare providers offer them to positive women who have low bone density. Evista (raloxifene) is a selective estrogen receptor modulator (SERM) that may offer bone and heart benefit for women with low estrogen, without the increased risk of breast or endometrial cancer.

Because women are more susceptible to osteoporosis, it is essential we get enough calcium. Calcium is a mineral responsible for bone health. Lack of adequate calcium can lead to loss of bone mass and tissue. Calcium is found in dairy foods, and can also be found in calcium-enriched juices and cereals, sardine (with bones), salmon (with bones), collard greens, broccoli, and turnip greens. Women need 1000 mg daily of calcium, 1200 mg for pregnant women and the elderly (51+years). This is equal to 3 cups of milk or calcium-fortified orange juice.

Gynaecological Care in HIV: Finding Good Care

One of the most important things you can do for yourselves is to find a gynecologist you feel comfortable with. If you don't trust or understand your doctor, how can you get answers? Many women being treated for their HIV don't receive adequate gynaecological care. This is a serious problem. Be sure your gynecologist has experience treating women with HIV. One way to do this is to talk to other positive women and get a reference to a gynaecologist from someone you know. If you don't know other women with HIV, you can always call the HIV positive network or the state AIDS Control Society or the state or district hospitals.

Genital Tract Infections

Your vagina, cervix, ovaries, uterus and fallopian tubes are all part of your genital tract. Most genital tract infections begin in the vagina, where they're usually treated relatively easily. Many — but not all — of these infections are sexually transmitted, including chlamydia, gonorrhea, trichomonas (trich), human papilloma virus (HPV), herpes, and syphilis.

If left untreated, simple vaginal infections can progress up the vagina to your cervix, where they may cause inflammation (cervicitis), cellular abnormalities (dysplasia), or both. Since these conditions are already more common in positive women, it's important to seek prompt diagnosis and treatment for *any* symptoms you experience. Untreated infections can also progress further up your genital tract, infecting your uterus, ovaries, or fallopian tubes. Here, they can cause pain, inflammation, and reproductive complications.

PID (pelvic inflammatory disease) is a general term that refers to inflammation somewhere in your upper genital tract. Most cases begin with easy to treat infections like chlamydia or bacterial vaginosis. Though no more common in positive women, PID can seriously threaten your health when it does occur. The best way to prevent PID is to have regular gynaecological examinations every six months — sooner if you experience a symptom such as: ongoing stomach and/or lower back pain; irregular periods; abnormal bleeding; cervical tenderness (during sex or on exam); painful urination; abnormal vaginal discharge; or fever.

Even when you don't have symptoms, make sure to have regular and thorough gynaecological check-ups.

- If you're having sex, at least one of your examinations a year should include a pelvic examination and a cervical swab (different from a Pap smear) for chlamydia, gonorrhea, and other common infections, and a blood test to check for syphilis.
- A simple vaginal sample can identify yeast and bacterial levels in the vagina and can also measure your vaginal pH.

- Pap smears only look for cervical abnormalities. If you're having problems in other parts of your genital tract, you may need a combination of blood test, cultures, pelvic exam, sonogram, colposcopy, or biopsy to diagnose the problem.
- If you have Human Papilloma Virus (HPV), ever had genital warts, or have had anal sex, it's important to have:
- A Pap smear every six months — sooner if results show abnormalities.
- A rectal (butt) exam to check for warts in the anus.
- An anal Pap smear to check for anal abnormalities.
- If you've never had hepatitis A or hepatitis B, and you haven't been vaccinated against them, ask your doctor to test you to see if you should receive this simple series of shots — they can prevent you from getting these two viruses.

Herpes

Many positive women have problems with genital herpes, an infection caused by a virus (called herpes simplex virus) that lives inside nerve cells. Since herpes is transmitted through skin to skin contact, condoms may not always protect you from infection during sex. You can get herpes sores on your labia, buttock, or the area between your vagina and anus. If you develop any pain, ulcers or sores, be sure to see your gynaecologist . Your doctor may take a small fluid sample from the area of your sore to try to grow herpes virus in a culture.

Once you have it, herpes is usually present for life. Sores can be treated using antiviral drugs, but the body rarely gets rid of the virus itself. Like other gynaecological conditions, herpes symptoms can reflect the status of your immune system. If your immune system's weakened, herpes virus can be reactivated, and you may develop painful sores. Herpes outbreaks can occur more frequently in positive women and are sometimes more difficult to treat. Herpes sores that persist for over one month are linked to severe immune weakness and are an AIDS-defining illness.

There are several different antiviral treatments for herpes, including Zovirax (acyclovir), Valtrex (valacyclovir), and Famvir (famciclovir). These drugs come in pill, gel, and cream form, in a variety of doses. Treatment can help with sores, manage the pain, and, hopefully, delay additional flare-ups. For severe and painful sores, your doctor can prescribe a lidocaine ointment or a numbing gel such as Neosporin Plus. Many women find that applying a facial clay directly to the sores can also help ease the pain.

Yeast Infections (Vaginal Candidiasis)

Your immune system, hormones, and "friendly" bacteria in your vagina all play an important role in keeping your vagina lubricated and healthy. Changes in your immune status, hormonal balance, or the amount of bacteria in your body can result in a range of vaginal symptoms, including yeast infections.

Yeast infections are overgrowths of a fungus called candida, normally found in small amounts throughout your body. When there's too much candida, your vagina can become inflamed or painful. You may see a thick, white, itchy discharge around your vagina, labia, or anal area.

Antibiotics, steroids, birth control pills, and foods high in sugars or starches (breads, pastas, and alcohol) all promote the growth of yeast. So can douching, which reduces levels of "helpful" bacteria in your vagina and is not recommended for women with HIV. In HIV positive women, recurrent yeast infections are often the result of immune suppression. You are more likely to develop these infections, or see them return after treatment, if you have a decreasing CD4 count.

Many women self-diagnose and treat yeast infections with over-the-counter anti-fungal creams . Creams come in different strengths and are used for 3 to 10 days depending on the formulation. Positive women often need longer courses of treatment with anti-fungal drugs, or prescription-strength creams. Your doctor can recommend the right strength for you (3% or 5%, for example).

Some yeast infections just don't respond to topical creams. This is more likely if your CD4s are low, if you use over-the-counter drugs frequently to treat yeast infections, or you don't finish the full course of treatment. For difficult-to-treat infections, your doctor can prescribe oral antifungal drugs such as Nizoral (ketoconazole), Diflucan (fluconazole), or Sporanox (itraconazole). Keep in mind that drugs taken by mouth reach far more parts of your body than a cream or suppository, can interact with HIV medications, and sometimes cause side effects.

Since yeast infections can resemble bacterial infections sometimes seen in positive women, it's a good idea to see your gynaecologist if you notice any unusual discharge or odour — especially if you've already tried over-the-counter drugs and you're still having symptoms. Your gynecologist may collect a sample of your discharge to make sure it's just yeast that's causing the inflammation. A similar vaginal sample can show whether you have healthy levels of acid in your vagina (called vaginal pH). If your pH levels are too high or too low, your doctor may suggest simple remedies to help restore a healthier vaginal pH level.

Since HIV can lead to a number of vaginal conditions, consider dietary and other changes that will support your overall vaginal health. Dietary changes include less sugars and starches, more soy products, and a multivitamin supplement. If you take antibiotics or birth control pills, you may also want to consider acidophilus supplements to restore supportive bacterial levels in your vagina. Try to wear loose, cotton underwear and clothes that won't trap moisture in your vagina. You may also want to steer clear of chemicals (found in scented soaps, detergents, douches) that throw off the vaginal pH. Douching can change bacterial and fungal levels in your vagina and should be avoided unless your doctor specifically recommends it.

HPV and Cervical Dysplasia

HPV (human papilloma virus) is the most common sexually transmitted infection. Most women have at least one type of HPV during their lifetime, but only a few of you know you have it. There are over 100 strains, and it's possible to have more than one strain at the same time. Some HPV strains cause warts to develop on your skin and genital area. Others infect cells inside our cervix, vagina, or anal canal, where you can't see them, but they can cause lesions to develop. Lesions are areas of abnormal tissue. If untreated, lesions can lead to invasive cervical, anal and genital abnormalities (called dysplasia) and cancer in some women.

In addition to higher rates of HPV infection, HIV-positive women with HPV are more likely to have:

- Chronic HPV infection
- Infection with the HPV strains more likely to cause cancer

- HPV in both the cervix *and* anus
- Several strains of HPV at once
- Reactivated HPV infections that were previously under control

Any of these factors alone can make you more likely to develop cervical and anal abnormalities. Immune suppression from HIV also plays a role. It seems that with lower CD4 counts and higher viral loads, you are increasing the risk for developing HPV-related lesions — including high-grade lesions — in the cervix and anus.

Smoking and untreated sexually transmitted infections, especially chlamydia, can make your cervix more vulnerable to damage from HPV and other infections. So can low levels of certain nutrients including beta-carotene, folic acid, and vitamins A and C. It's not clear yet if supplementation helps, but if you have HPV, it's at least a good idea to maintain normal levels of these nutrients, either through food sources or a multivitamin.

Screening Methods

Pap smears are the first step in screening for abnormal cell changes in the cervix and in the anus. Pap smears collect cells — called squamous cells — from the transition zone of your cervix or anus, the area most likely to be infected by HPV. Pap smears can detect inflammation and, in most cases, predict cervical or anal abnormalities.

In HIV-negative women, annual Paps are frequent enough to detect any changes that may have occurred since the last exam. This isn't the case in HIV. As a positive woman, it's important to evaluate your individual risk for cervical and anal dysplasia and consider more frequent screening. How frequently depends on a lot of individual factors, including your previous Pap result and whether you've been treated for warts or abnormalities. If your CD4 count is below 300 or has been dropping, have Pap smears at least once every six months. In HIV, any Pap smear result showing abnormal cells needs to be further evaluated by colposcopy.

Colposcopy is an examination of your cervix using a low-powered microscope to look at the tissue more closely. This procedure allows your doctor to see your cervix (or anus) and identify any areas of abnormal tissue. Lesions, warts, and inflammation are usually visible during colposcopy. But it's still hard to tell the difference between low and high-grade lesions. This is why a biopsy is often taken if any lesions are seen during colposcopy.

Biopsy is a procedure that takes a small tissue sample from an area of your cervix. Biopsy is the most reliable way to tell the difference between mild lesions and those that are more likely to progress to cancer. Be prepared — biopsy can be uncomfortable, even painful, and some women have mild bleeding afterwards. Ask your provider about your pain management options *before* the procedure begins.

Many positive women have more than one biopsy, either during diagnosis or as part of follow-up care. Understandably, this can make it hard to go back. But it's important to stay involved in your care and give input to treatment decisions that affect you.. If you're feeling resentful, angry, or scared, tell your gynecologist. Remember, your gynaecologist wants to keep you healthy. The more she or he knows about what's going on with you, the better they'll be able to work with you.

Anal HPV and Anal Dysplasia

Anal Human Papilloma Virus(HPV) is common in women with HIV, especially women who've had genital warts, anal sex, or cervical dysplasia. One large study (called the Women's Interagency HIV Study) found anal HPV in 70% of positive women studied. When these women had anal Pap smears, abnormal cells were found in 42% of the women with CD4 counts less than 200, and 25% of the women with CD4 counts between 200 and 500. Although anal sex is the most direct way to get anal HPV, you can have anal HPV even if you've never had anal sex.

If you have HPV, ever had cervical dysplasia, or you've had anal sex, ask your doctor for a anal examination and an anal Pap smear to check for anal HPV. Anal Paps are like cervical Paps — they collect cells to screen for lesions in the anus. If ASCUS, ASC-H, or any other abnormalities are found, your doctor can use an anoscope (similar to a colposcope) to look inside your anal canal and identify any lesions, warts, or abnormal tissue that might need treatment.

Routine cervical screening, followed by treatment of high-grade dysplasia, has dramatically cut the rate of cervical cancer in women. Despite possibly high rates of anal dysplasia in HIV, no comparable screening guidelines exist for anal abnormalities. An anal screening and treatment programme, similar to cervical screening, could help prevent anal cancer in both women and men with HIV. As positive women, it's important that we keep being evaluated regularly for cervical HPV, and for anal HPV.

Treatment Options for Dysplasia

For those of you with Human Papilloma Virus(HPV) , there's no simple pill or treatment to prevent you from getting warts or developing cervical and anal abnormalities. So it's important to screen carefully and regularly for changes in the cervix and anus and deal with any high-grade abnormalities, so that they don't progress to cancer.

Treatments for HPV can remove genital warts, destroy HPV lesions, and get rid of abnormal tissue. Genital warts can be treated with topical solutions or by laser, freezing or burning. Most treatments for dysplasia focus on destroying the abnormal tissue so that it doesn't progress to cancer. Treatment options include:

- LEEP: removes abnormal tissue with a wire loop
- Cone biopsy: removes a cone-shaped piece of tissue from the cervix by surgery or laser. This is done under anesthesia. It's frequently used to treat high-grade dysplasia in positive women.
- Electrocautery (burning)
- Topical solutions
- There are additional challenges to treating cervical and anal abnormalities in positive women:
- Many women respond poorly to standard therapies used to treat HSIL.
- Some of us need multiple treatments using different methods.
- Treatment of HSIL can only try to manage HPV — it won't prevent a recurrence.
- There is low success treating LSIL.
- Anal/cervical dysplasia and cancer are more common in positive women.

Both cervical and anal dysplasia can return after treatment. Recurrences may be more likely if you have a higher viral load, but it's not clear that antiretroviral therapy slows the progression of cervical disease. Even when the immune system is partially restored by anti-HIV treatment, anal and cervical dysplasia may progress to cancer. So be careful, regular monitoring is the best way for you to ensure that any problems are detected and treated as soon as possible.

Menstrual Period Problems

Many positive women experience an abnormal or changing menstrual cycle. Although it's easy to want to forget about them, you need to pay attention to your menstrual periods — especially any changes in the amount of bleeding or pain. The following lists some of the most common menstrual changes and things to consider if you experience them:

Special Considerations for Women Using Birth Control Pills

Birth control pills are often used in HIV to regulate abnormal menstrual cycles or for women entering menopause. The pill comes in many different formulations; some contain progesterone, others contain both estrogen and progesterone. Every woman responds differently to the pill, and you may need to try several types or doses before you find the best fit.

Combined pills contain high amounts of ethinyl-estradiol, a synthetic version of the strongest estrogen in your body. While necessary to prevent pregnancy, high doses lead to side effects in many women and are not safe if you're over 50. If you use the pill to regulate periods rather than to prevent pregnancy, you can consider much lower-dosed tablets.

Many of the currently prescribed anti-HIV drugs interact with ethinyl-estradiol, the main ingredient in most birth control pills. If you're taking Norvir, Kaletra, Viracept, Viramune or, possibly, Agenerase, the pill may be less effective. Crixivan, Sustiva and, possibly, Rescriptor can increase ethinyl-estradiol to levels that are higher than you need. Remember, many women take these drugs in combinations, where the effect on the pill is even less clear.

Since too much blood loss can lead to anaemia, it's important to identify all possible sources of heavy bleeding and try to correct

Menstrual Symptom	*Possible Causes*	*What to Do About It?*
Lighter bleeding Missed periods No periods at all	• Chronic infection like HIV • Malnutrition • Regular heroin, methadone, or amphetamine use • AIDS-related wasting • Steroid use • Menopause • Cysts and other problems in the ovaries	• If you miss two or more periods in a row, have a pelvic exam and blood tests to identify possible infections in your reproductive tract. • Check hormone levels. • Get a pregnancy test.
Heavy bleeding	• Low platelets • Fibroid tumorus • A complication of PID • Other genital tract infection • Drugs used to treat HIV such as Norvir (ritonavir), Retrovir (AZT), Hivid (ddC), or others	• Check your platelet counts through blood work. • Review list of drugs and contraceptives you're taking with your doctor. • Monitor closely for anemia. • Your provider may want to do a sonogram. • Check progesterone levels.
Bleeding between periods or after sex	• Chlamydia in the cervix • High-grade cervical dysplasia • Problems with the pill • Tearing from sex • Atrophy (thinning or weakening of vaginal tissue)	• Get a pelvic exam. • Your doctor may need to look at your vagina/cervix to see where the bleeding's coming from. Have a sonogram or colposcopy. • Check hormone levels.

the problem. Heavy bleeding — along with bleeding between periods — may signal an infection in your cervix, vagina, or ovaries. If you have any of the above symptoms, be sure to discuss them with both your GYN *and* HIV medical providers.

If you're using the pill with any of these drugs, ask your doctor about whether you need to alter the dose of your pill in order to maintain effectiveness or to reduce side effects from the pill. If a dose adjustment isn't possible and you're using the pill to prevent pregnancy, you'll need to use condoms or another form of contraception.

As you can see, there's the potential for drug interactions in almost every HIV treatment decision. That's why it's so important to tell your doctor about any medications, Buprenorphine, Methadone, street drugs, herbs or hormones you're taking along with your HIV regimen. Any time you are prescribed a new medication, be sure to ask your doctor and pharmacist about possible interactions.

Treatment Issues for Women

Muscle Mass

There is more benefit to having muscle than just looking good. Muscle provides important fuel for the day-to-day operations of the body, including fighting infections.

If you lose more than 5% of your weight without trying and you can't explain it, you should get help to figure out what's happening. Many of us are praised and told we look great when we lose weight, but much HIV-related weight loss is often a loss of muscle. Reduced muscle mass can be a sign of wasting, which is linked to faster disease progression. Weight loss may also be happening along with other changes in your body shape and metabolism that need to be watched.

There is a simple test — called BIA (bioelectrical impedance analysis) — to see if you have healthy levels of overall muscle, fat and water in your body. To measure the fat or muscle in any one part of your body, you would need a CT scan or DEXA scan. If these tests are not available, it's also possible to measure body dimensions with calipers, a tool that gently pinches flesh at different points on your body. You may want to measure your body composition periodically, since body shape changes aren't always immediately visible. Gaining and maintaining muscle mass is critical to surviving HIV, because muscle helps keep hormones regulated and helps your body fight infection. It's also necessary to get enough calories from healthy foods and to drink plenty of water. A combination of resistance exercise (like lifting weights) and aerobic exercise (like climbing stairs or swimming) is important, since resistance work builds muscle and aerobic work burns fat.

There are unanswered questions about using testosterone in women, but human growth hormone (Serostim) or the anabolic steroid oxandrolone (Oxandrin), combined with exercise, may be options for women who need extra help to build muscle. Both of these treatments are extremely expensive, and Oxandrin can be particularly difficult to get. If you're considering either of these drugs, you may want to talk to other women about their experience using them.

Lipodystrophy

Lipodystrophy is the name given to a cluster of body changes that sometimes occur in people living with HIV, especially people taking antiretroviral drugs. Antiretroviral drugs certainly play a major role, but HIV itself may also contribute. You may experience an increase in fat in some areas (breasts, belly and neck) and a loss of fat in other areas (face, arms, legs, or butt). Sometimes, your overall body weight can stay the same, but your body shape can change significantly. Both men and women can experience all of these symptoms, but we're more likely than men to have fat accumulation — particularly in the abdomen and breasts.

In addition to changes in body shape, some people experience changes inside the body, too. Fats in the blood, like cholesterol and triglycerides, can increase. Sometimes, the body becomes less able to process glucose and may become diabetic. Women who are overweight, don't exercise, smoke, and/or are over 40 are already at higher risk for diabetes and heart disease, even without lipodystrophy. So it's very important — especially if you're taking combination therapy — to monitor your lipid and glucose levels through regular blood work.

Cholesterol and triglyceride measurements are most accurate if you don't eat at least 10-12 hours before having your blood drawn. This usually means a morning blood draw.

It's still not entirely clear what to do about lipodystrophy. Some people with increased cholesterol, triglycerides, or glucose levels stop taking their antiretrovirals or switch them, but this isn't possible for everyone. Plus, there's not a lot of evidence yet that switching regimens necessarily helps. There are medications that help control diabetes, and cholesterol/triglyceride levels.

One thing you *can* do for yourself is maintain a good diet and exercise regularly — at least three times a week. Exercise doesn't have to involve joining a gym; there are many ways to get your body moving without using a gym. Dietary changes that support your heart health include eating less animal fats like butter, cheese, and red meat, and adding more fish oil (especially salmon and sardines), nuts, whole grain cereals and breads. You may also want to reduce or try to quit smoking, and avoid progesterone-dominant birth control pills. Some women experience one or more of the symptoms of lipodystrophy, while others experience all of them. In addition to checking lipid levels, try to pay attention to your overall body shape (how your clothes fit is generally a good guide) and tell your health care provider about any changes you notice, however small they may seem.

In addition to learning as much as possible about HIV, treatment options, it's important to take care of yourself emotionally. For many women, HIV is just one of many daily struggles. Poverty, addiction, and violence are common. While we're often talking about physical health in HIV, we rarely talk about the grief, loss, fear, and isolation so many positive women feel at one point or another. Without support, these feelings can seem overwhelming. Regardless of where you're at, we encourage you to reach out and find support wherever you can.

14

Nutrition and HIV/AIDS Among Young Children

The first case of AIDS in children was reported in 1982.. Since then, 3.2 million children have been infected by the end of December, 2002 as reported by UNAIDS. In 2002 alone , out of 5 million people newly acquiring HIV infection in 2002 alone, 800,000 were children.

Out of 27.9 million deaths since the beginning of the epidemic upto December, 2002 , 5.5 million were children below 15 years of age. In 2002 alone, out of 3.1 million people died of AIDS , 610,000 were children. Approximately 13.4 million children have lost one or both parents to AIDS .

Children are the victims and orphans of AIDS. Children are the victims of exploitation and abuse . Children are the victims of war and violence . Children are living in the street . Children are denied good quality education and health care . Children are the victims of political, economic , cultural, religious and environmental discrimination

The voices of the children are never heard . How can we achieve a world fit for children ? Kofi Annan , Secretary General of the United Nations once said " We must put the best interest of children at the heart of all political and business decision making and at the centre of our day to day behaviour and activities"

What kind of women are likely to have children with HIV infections ?

Only HIV infected women give birth to children with HIV infection. The women is infected first before they give birth to HIV infected children.

The following categories of women are at increased risk of HIV infection :-

- Injecting drug users through sharing of needles and syringes
- Commercial sex workers - due to unprotected sex , sex without condom and multi partner sex
- Women whose sexual partner or husband are injecting drug users or HIV infected .

Does breast milk contains HIV DNA ?

In a Haiti study, HIV DNA is detected in 70% of the 47 colostrums samples and 50% of the breast milk samples . HIV DNA was also detected in 47% of 147 breast milk samples collected 15 days after delivery and in 20% of the 96 samples collected six months after delivery.

What are the factors which affect mother to child HIV transmission :-

The following conditions may facilitate mother to child HIV transmission :-

- Recent infection with HIV
- Severity of HIV infection
- Infection with STDs
- Obstetrical procedures
- Duration of breast feeding
- Exclusive breast feeding or mixed feeding
- Conditions of the breast
- Condition of the baby's mouth

What are the risk factors which increase the risk of HIV transmission from mother to child ?

Many research have indicated that the following maternal conditions constitute increased risk of HIV transmission to the newborns :-

- High maternal viral load
- Low CD4 count - Maternal immune deficiency
- Vial characteristics
- Advanced HIV disease of the mother
- Severe immune deficiency of the mother
- HIV infection acquired during pregnancy or breast feeding period
- Vaginal delivery of the child
- Prolonged rupture of the membrane
- Infant immaturity
- Breast feeding of the child
- Invasive procedures at the time of delivery
- Episiotomy
- STDs
- Chorloamnionitis
- Vitamin- A deficiency
- Anaemia
- Injecting drug use
- Lesions of the skin or mucus membrane
- Oral thrush
- Mixed feeding in the first 6 months (i.e., combining breastfeeding with breastmilk substitutes)
- Breastfeeding duration (i.e., long term breastfeeding increases the risk of HIV transmission)
- Improper latching and positioning during breastfeeding
- Breast conditions (i.e., fissured and bloody nipples, mastitis, and breast abscess)
- Sores in infant's mouth
- Maternal malnutrition
- New HIV infection

(WHO). HIV and Infant Feeding: A guide for healthcare managers and supervisors, 2003).

What is the schedule of Vitamin A Supplementation among children ?

For children from six to 12 months , 100,000 IU of vitamin – A should be given every four to six months and for children between 12 to 59 months 200,000 IU of vitamin should be given for every six months

How to diagnose HIV infection in a child ?

Diagnosis of the child for HIV infection is done after 18 months of age. The diagnosis is done by ELISA test and other supplemental tests like Western Blot or Rapid or Simple. It is easy and simple. Anti HIV antibodies can be detected in a child's blood for a median of 13.3 months (range is 10.4 months to 16.6 months). Before 18 months of age , we have to depend on PCR test for HIV antigen (p24) or HIV culture or we have to see whether the child meets the criteria for AIDS case definition

In children, the progressive loss of CD4 lymphocytes is the hall mark of the course of HIV disease.

How to diagnose a child with AIDS ?

A diagnosis of AIDS can be made in children in presence of at least two major and two minor signs from the flowing list :-

Major Signs :-

- Weight loss or abnormally slow growth
- Chronic diarrhoea for more than one month
- Prolonged fever for more than one month

Minor Signs :-

- Generalized lymph nodes enlargement
- Fungal infections of the mouth and or throat
- Recurrent common infections (e/g ear , throat)
- Resistant cough
- Generalized rash

Confirmed HIV infection of the mother is a minor criterion.

What may be the complications in a child with HIV/AIDS ?

The complications may be any of the following :-

- **Respiratory Diseases :** Viral pneumonia , parainfluenza, measles and herpes virus or bacterial pneumonia due to infections with streptococcus pneumonia , H. influenzae, K. Pneumonia and pseudomonas aeroginosa are very common.
- **Growth failure :**This is a common finding among children with HIV infection. This may be due to low birth weight or

HIV associated anorexia and hypermetabolism. There may be oropharyngeal ulcerations, severe neuralgic dysfunction, which may lead to poor food intake and poor nutrition or malnutrition.

If the child is not gaining weight, what to do ?

If the child is not regularly gaining weight or not growing well, you have to consider the following points :-

- Is the child eating often enough ? A child needs to eat three to five times a day .
- Is the child receiving enough food ? If the child finishes his or her food and wants more , the child needs to be offered more .
- Do the child's meals have too little growth or energy foods. Foods that help the child to grow are meat, fish, egg, nuts, grains and pulses .
- Is the child refusing to eat ? New food should be offered if the child does not like the taste of food.
- Is the child sick ? A sick child needs encouragement to eat small, frequent meals.
- Is the child getting enough food with vitamin-A to prevent illness ? Breast milk is rich in vitamin -A. Other foods with vitamin -A are liver, eggs, dairy products , red palm oil, orange, vegetables.
- Is the child being given breast milk substitutes from the age of 6 months to 24 months .
- Are food and water kept clean ?
- Are faeces being put in a latrine or toilet or buried ?
- Is the young child left alone much of the time or in the care of an older child.

Treatment should be given accordingly .

Has antiretroviral therapy any role in the treatment of children with AIDS ?

Yes. Antiretroviral therapy is recommended for the following categories of children :-

- all infants and children with symptomatic HIV infection
- all children whose CD4 count falls below the following values

- less than 1500 cells /cmm for infants
- less than 1000 cells /cmm for infants of 18-24 months
- less than 750 cells /cmm for children 2-6 years
- less than 500 cell /cmm for children above 6 years
- CD4 count less than 20% in infants less than one year
- CD4 count less than 25% children between 1-2 years
- CD4 count less than 20% in all children above 2 years.

Highly Active Antiretroviral Therapy (HAART) should be initiated early to slow down viral replication and disease progression. The theory of antiretroviral treatment is same as those of adults . The antiretroviral treatments available in paediatric formulations include AZT, ddI, d4T, STC, ritonavir, neifinavir . Anti-retroviral therapy(ART) is given free to all children below 15 years in India under the National AIDS Control Programme under the Government of India Policy announced in 2004 .

Antiretroviral Therapy(ART) may have side effects .

Children need antiretroviral therapy to reduce viral load and delay disease progression. However, ARVs may have side effects (nausea, vomiting, diarrhoea, constipation, and changes in taste) that may affect the dietary intake of the infected children. The side effects may be caused by the interaction between food or nutrients and the drugs . Side effects should be managed to ensure continued food intake and adherence to medication regimens.

Can we immunize or vaccinate a child with HIV/AIDS ?

Immunization protects the child from specific diseases. It can protect the child from tuberculosis, diphtheria , whooping cough , tetanus, poliomyelitis and measles . If the child is not immunized , he or she is more likely to become malnourished , sick and die. Vaccines may be given only once or several times . To receive all the necessary immunizations, the child should be immunized on five occasions in his or her first year of life as per national immunization schedule. The child should be immunized in the first year of life . The child is mostly vulnerable to diseases at this time. The child should complete the immunization course even if there is a long delay between doses . Routine immunization can be given to a sick child. Children with mild illness such as fever, cough and cold, diarrhoea, malnutrition should be immunized

What is the role of breast milk?

Breast milk is the best food for babies for the first four to six months of life. Breast milk meets all the food and fluid needs of an infant for the first six months of life. It protects the baby from diseases and malnutrition Colostrum, the first milk that comes out of the mother's breast after delivery should be given to the baby. It helps protect the baby against infection and prepares the baby's stomach to digest milk. There is no need to give anything else such as sugared water to the baby while waiting for the breast milk to come in. Breast feeding should continue even if the baby is sick, unless there is a medical restriction. In addition to breast milk, complementary (weaning) foods should be given to the baby starting from four to six months of age. If possible breast milk should be given up to two years of age.

What are the strategies for Prevention of transmission through breast milk ?

The following strategies must be considered for prevention of HIV transmission through breast milk.

No breast feeding

breast feeding followed by early cessation of breast feeding

heat treatment of expressed milk

wet nursing by a tested HIV negative woman.

Several studies have indicated that HIV is inactivated when milk is left to stand at room temperature for half an hour.

Expression of breast milk and heat treatment may be another possible option. Wet nursing by a member of the family or community is also practiced. It may be advisable that the wet nurses agree to and understand the implications of voluntary counselling and HIV testing.

When is Infant feeding counselling needed?

Infant feeding counselling is needed:-

Before a woman is pregnant.

During her pregnancy

Soon after her baby is born

When her baby is older or

When a woman fosters a baby whose mother is very sick or has died.

A woman may believe that she is HIV positive despite a negative test. She needs reassurance that she is unlikely HIV positive. She needs counselling to discuss her worries and generally should be encouraged to breastfeed.

All woman who are HIV positive need infant feeding counselling, to discuss breast feeding options and to decide what is best for them in their situation.

What are the infant feeding options to be discussed with the HV positive pregnant women ?

HIV-positive mothers should be made aware of the risks and benefits of different infant feeding options, including the risk of transmission of HIV through breastfeeding. Mothers who can provide replacement feeding that is acceptable, feasible, affordable, sustainable, and safe are advised to do so. When these criteria cannot be met through family or community resources, particularly in resource-limited settings, women are advised to exclusively breastfeed. Essential nutrients, breastmilk contains antibodies and enzymes that protect against infections and strengthens the infant's immune system. However, HIV may also be transmitted to an infant during breastfeeding. On average, approximately one out of seven infants born to an HIV-infected mother will become infected through breastfeeding up to 24 months. WHO, the United Nations Children's Fund (UNICEF) and other United Nations agencies currently recommend that HIV-positive mothers avoid breastfeeding if replacement feeding from birth is acceptable, feasible, affordable, sustainable, and safe (AFASS). If these conditions are not met, then it is recommended that HIV-positive mothers practice exclusive breastfeeding for the first months of life. If circumstances change and the AFASS criteria can be met, shortening the period of exclusive breastfeeding and transitioning as quickly as possible to another breast milk option or replacement feeding will reduce the risk of exposure to HIV.

How to decide the infant feeding options for Infants and Children born to HIV positive mothers ?

For infants of HIV-positive mothers, WHO (2003) advises that: When replacement feeding is acceptable, feasible, affordable, sustainable and safe(AFASS), avoidance of all breastfeeding by HIV-positive mothers is recommended. Otherwise, exclusive breastfeeding is recommended during the first months of life. To minimize HIV transmission risk, breastfeeding should be discontinued as soon as feasible, taking into account local conditions, the individual woman's situation and the issues of replacement feeding including infections other than HIV and malnutrition. When HIV-positive mothers choose not to breastfeed from birth or stop breastfeeding later, they should be provided with specific guidance for at least the first two years of the child's life to ensure adequate replacement feeding.

(AFASS) Acceptable, Feasible, Affordable, Sustainable, and Safe These terms should be adapted in the light of local conditions and formative research. The following may serve as a starting point::-

Acceptable: The mother perceives no barrier to replacement feeding. Barriers may have cultural or social reasons, or be due to fear of stigma or discrimination. According to this concept the mother is under no social or cultural pressure not to use replacement feeding; and she is supported by family and community in opting for replacement feeding, or she will be able to cope with pressure from family and friends to breastfeed, and she can deal with possible stigma attached to being seen with replacement food.

Feasible: The mother or family has adequate time, knowledge, skills, and other resources to prepare the replacement food and feed the infant up to 12 times in 24 hours. According to this concept, the mother can understand and follow the instructions for preparing infant formula and, with support from the family, can prepare enough replacement feeds correctly every day and at night, despite disruptions to preparation of family food or other work.

Affordable: The mother and family, with community or health-system support if necessary, can pay the cost of purchasing/ producing, preparing, and using replacement feeding, including all ingredients, fuel, clean water, soap, and equipment, without compromising the health and nutrition of the family. This concept also includes access to medical care if necessary for diarrhoea and the cost of such care.

Sustainable: Availability of a continuous and uninterrupted supply and a dependable system of distribution for all ingredients and products needed for safe replacement feeding for as long as the infant needs it, up to one year of age or longer. According to this concept there is little risk that formula will ever be unavailable or inaccessible, and anotherperson is available to feed the child in the mother's absence and can prepare and give replacement foods.

Safe: Replacement foods are correctly and hygienically prepared and stored and fed in nutritionally adequate quantities, with clean hands, and using clean utensils, preferably by cup. This concept means that the mother or caregiver:

- Has access to a reliable supply of safe water (e.g., from a piped or protected-well source);
- Prepares replacement feeds that are nutritionally sound and free of pathogens;
- Is able to wash hands and utensils thoroughly with soap and regularly boil the utensils to sterilize them;
- Can boil water for preparing each of the baby's feeds; and
- Can store unprepared feeds in clean, covered containers and protect them from rodents, insects, and other animals.

(WHO, What are the Options? Using formative research to adapt global recommendations on HIV and infant feeding to the local context, 2004.)

The Infant feeding options to be discussed with women who are HIV positive are :-

- exclusive and continued breast feeding
- stopping early with a change to another form of feeding
- expression of breast milk and heat treatment of her breast milk
- breast feeding from a HIV negative wet nurse
- replacement feeding either with a home prepared formula or with commercial formula .

Replacement feeding is the process of feeding a child who is not receiving any breast milk , with a diet that provides all the nutrients the child needs until the child is fully fed on family foods.

Adequate complementary foods from about six months of age will be required in all cases.

- Provide HIV-positive mothers with information on different infant feeding options to enable them to make an informed choice for their infants.
- Inform HIV-positive mothers of the advantages and the risks associated with the infant feeding option they have chosen.
- Provide HIV-positive mothers with the support required to implement their choice.
- Where possible, involve the mother's partner or other members of the family in the counseling and decision-making process.

When to Counsel on Infant Feeding Options

- After an HIV-positive test, but prior to delivery, to assist the mother to select the best option for her infant
- Within 10 days of delivery to assess the ability of the mother to successfully implement her infant feeding choice
- At routine postpartum visits, well-child checks, and sick-child service delivery points
- When mothers plan to change her current feeding practice (WHO, HIV and Infant Feeding: A guide for healthcare managers and supervisors, 2003)

If the mother decides to breastfeed, she should:

- Breastfeed exclusively for not longer than six months and prevent and manage breast problems and sores in the infant's mouth to prevent HIV transmission from mother to child during breastfeeding; and
- Transition to replacement feeding when it is AFASS. This means feeding infants who are not receiving breast milk with a nutritious diet that meets their nutrient requirements until they are old enough to consume a diet of family foods. From birth to six months, replacement feeding is a suitable breast milk substitute. After six months, this means giving a breast

milk substitute plus appropriate complementary foods to support optimal growth and development. Exclusive breastfeeding practices for children of HIV-positive others are the same as for children born to HIV-negative mothers or mothers of unknown IV status. Infants are fed only breast milk for up to six months. No other foods, teas, water, juices, milks, or infant formula should be given to the infant.

What are the advantages of breast feeding ?

The advantages of breast feeding are :-

- if the baby is put on breast milk immediately after delivery, the sucking helps the uterus to contract and reduces bleeding.
- breast feeding lowers maternal risk of developing breast and ovarian cancer.
- Breast milk does not require preparations
- breast milk provides ideal nutrition for her infant
- breast feeding protects the child against many infections
- breast feeding delays the return of her fertility , helping to space the next child
- breast feeding provides the closeness and contact between her and her baby which helps psychological development .
- breast milk comes in attractive containers .

Compliance with Exclusive Breastfeeding.

Exclusive breastfeeding for six months is rarely practiced even when programmes actively promote and support it. In the context of HIV, the practice of mixed feeding may be especially harmful because of the increased risk of transmission. The exact mechanisms fostering this increased risk are not known but several have been suggested: the gut may become inflamed as a reaction to new food allergens, or germs from the food and water may damage the gut, increasing susceptibility to infection by HIV carried in breast milk. Exclusive breastfeeding helps to maintain a healthy gut epithelium that acts as a protective barrier against infectious agents. Through awareness raising activities, counseling, and community mobilization, programmes need to create a supportive environment in which mothers can successfully practice exclusive breastfeeding.

Feeding Expressed, Heat-treated Breast milk.

An alternative to exclusive breastfeeding s collecting expressed breast milk and heat treating it. This is accomplished by bringing it to a boil and cooling the milk immediately by standing the clean container in cold water. Untreated expressed breast milk may be stored for up to eight hours at room temperature in a cool place and 72 hours in a refrigerator. Once the milk is heat treated, it must be used within an hour. The mother or caregiver feeds the heat-treated breast milk to the infant with a cup in order to avoid the risk of contamination from bottles. This method of feeding infants of HIV-infected mothers requires resources for heating and storing the milk, time to prepare the feeds, and a supportive environment to successfully feed children in this manner.

Breastfeeding by an HIV-negative Wet Nurse.

This infant feeding option requires that the mother and family of the child consider wet nursing only if the wet nurse is offered HIV testing and counseling, takes the test voluntarily, and is found to be HIV negative. She must then practice optimal exclusive breastfeeding and safer sex practices to ensure that she is not infected with HIV while breastfeeding the infant. She will need to be available to feed the infant frequently and on demand throughout the day and night and she must receive services to prevent and treat any problems such as cracked or bleeding nipples, mastitis, or abscesses that may occur.

Keeping Breasts Healthy.

Mastitis, nipple lesions, and breast abscesses may increase the risk of HIV transmission through breast milk. Health workers should counsel HIV-positive mothers on how to prevent, manage, and seek treatment for breast problems to reduce the risk of HIV transmission to the infant.,

What are the risks of not breast feeding ?

The risk of not breast feeding may be the following :-

- The child is likely to get sick very often
- preparing and giving replacement feeding takes more time , less convenient than breast feeding .

- to feed the baby in another way is expensive . She has to buy breast milk substitutes, fuel and water .
- A woman who does not breast feed her baby may be criticized by her family or others in the community and told that she is not a good mother
- No breast feeding may lead to stress in family relationships –particularly between husband and wife
- Not breast feeding may identify a woman as HIV positive . She may be blamed , avoided or punished by the members in her family or community . This is a social sigma .
- A woman who does not breast feed her baby may feel less close to her infant . She may feel sad and disappointed if she is not able to breast feed her baby. Breast feeding is a pleasurable experience . Most women grow up expecting to breast feed and they look forward to it.

Sores in an infant's mouth may increase the risk of HIV transmission from breastmilk. Health workers should show HIV-positive lactating mothers how to check for sores and, if found, advise them to promptly seek medical care. Where possible, refer mothers to a breastfeeding counselor or a breastfeeding support group.

Infants at Birth through Six Months Born to HIV-positive Women:

Replacement Feeding with Appropriate Breast milk Substitutes

HIV-positive mothers who do not breastfeed are advised to exclusively feed their infants with appropriate breast milk substitutes (i.e., replacement feeding). These can be either commercial infant formula, the most nutritionally complete substitute for breastmilk, or home-modified animal milk.

Early Cessation of Breastfeeding.

The risk of HIV transmission during breastfeeding continues for as long as breastfeeding is practiced. Because this risk is cumulative, early breastfeeding cessation is recommended for HIV positive mothers. A transition from exclusive breastfeeding to exclusive replacement feeding will decrease the risk of HIV transmission. The best time to stop exclusive breastfeeding varies from one situation to another and is dependent on such factors as the mother's health status, the physical environment, economic status of the household, and risk factors for disease and death due to alternative feeding practices. Health workers and mothers should discuss and decide the most appropriate time for transition to replacement feeding based on case-specific circumstances. Health workers should then provide the necessary guidance to make the transition to exclusive replacement feeding as safe as possible.

Transitioning from Breastfeeding to Replacement Feeding.

Mothers usually transition gradually from exclusive breastfeeding to breastfeeding plus complementary foods after an infant is six months old. However, in cases where a mother is HIV-positive, it is recommended that the transition from breastfeeding to replacement feeding occur as quickly as possible. While some mixed feeding is usually necessary during the transition, it should be strictly avoided once the baby has switched to replacement feeding. Healthcare workers can provide guidance and support to mothers when they have decided to make the transition to replacement feeding: • Begin by expressing breast milk to familiarize the baby with cup feeding by offering the expressed breast milk by cup between regular breastfeeds;

- When the infant has accepted cup feeding, ,eliminate one breastfeed at a time and replace with expressed breast milk fed by a cup;
- Express and discard breast milk if breasts become engorged during the transition process. Apply cold compresses to reduce swelling;
- Once all feeds are accepted by cup, feed only breast milk substitutes;
- Health care workers can advise mothers on comforting infants with alternative methods to breastfeeding such as massaging, swaddling, carrying, rocking, singing, sleeping with, and talking to the baby; and
- Counsel women on adequate protection against pregnancy in the absence of the contraceptive protection of breastfeeding.

When using breast milk substitutes, mothers need to be assisted in the prevention of breast engorgement, plugged milk ducts, or mastitis as lactation is suppressed in the early days following delivery. The infant should not be allowed to suckle; breasts should be well supported but not tightly bound, and mothers can express small amounts of breast milk to relieve discomfort.

Commercial Infant Formula

Commercial infant formula is usually available as powder and needs to be reconstituted with clean water according to the instructions on the tin before being fed to the infant. Over-concentration can cause health problems such as diarrhoea, and over-dilution can lead to malnutrition due to insufficient nutrient intake. Safe feeding of commercial infant formula includes:

- Utensils for measuring/preparing the formula;
- Clean water to prepare the formula and clean all utensils;
- Fuel in adequate amounts to boil water for reconstituting the formula and cleaning utensils;

Commercial infant formula Home-modified animal milk

- Wash hands with soap and water.
- Clean all utensils, containers, and cups with soap and water.
- Read or have someone read instructions on the formula tin.
- Boil water vigorously for a few seconds and let it cool. Boil as much water as needed for the whole day and store in a clean covered container.
- Measure the amount of milk powder needed for one feed and mix it with the correct amount of boiled water.
- Prepare fresh commercial formula before each feed if refrigeration is not available.
- Feed the infant by cup about 150 ml of correctly prepared formula per kg per day, divided into six to eight feeds. The infant will have to learn to drink from a cup.
- Wash hands with soap and water.
- Clean all utensils, containers, and cups with soap and water.
- Boil water vigorously for a few seconds and let it cool. Boil as much water as needed for the whole day and store in a clean, covered container.

- Measure the amount of water and milk needed .
- Measure the exact amount of sugar and mix it with the liquid.
- Prepare formula before each feed if refrigeration is not available.
- Feed the infant by cup the appropriate amount based on the infant's weight. The infant will have to learn to drink from a cup.
- Give the infant multivitamins specially formulated for the non-breastfed child. The multivitamin can be in the form of liquid syrup (i.e., 5 ml per day) or powder. The multivitamin can be mixed with the formula or given separately.

Both commercial and home-prepared formulas require time and knowledge to prepare safe replacement feeds, and equipment and fuel to clean utensils and the preparation environment.

Home-modified Animal Milks

When commercial infant formula is not readily available, too expensive, or otherwise not acceptable, home-prepared modified animal milk can be used as a replacement feeding option. Families need to have access to at least one half liter or the equivalent of animal milk or milk product per day. Home-modified animal milk is used exclusively, and the infant does not receive breast milk. Modified animal milks can be made from fresh animal milk, evaporated milk, dried full cream milk powder, or ultra high-temperature (UHT) milk. All of these milks need to be modified to become suitable for the infant by diluting with water and adding sugar.

Resources for hand washing and food preparation hygiene include :-

- Ability to read or follow directions for correct reconstitution of infant formula;
- Caregiver time to prepare at least eight feedings per day if refrigeration is not available; and
- Correct use of cup for feeding prepared infant formula. Mothers need to have access to consistent and affordable supplies of commercial formula for at least six months. WHO estimates that 20 kg of commercial infant formula are required per infant during the first six months of life for replacement feeding.

Programmes should assess the types and costs of replacement feeding options that are available in the area as well as the reliability of supply. Many households in resource limited settings may not be able to afford replacement foods. In such cases, programmes should work to identify mechanisms to help households access the required foods.

Infants and Young Children from Six through 23 Months Born to HIV positive Mothers:

Complementary and Replacement Feeding Foods

Appropriate complementary feeding for children of HIV-positive mothers ages six though 23 months consists of feeding breast milk or breast milk substitutes (e.g., milk, milk products) with complementary or additional semi-solid and solid food/liquids. All infants require foods in addition to milk by six months in order to meet their nutritional requirements for energy, protein, and micronutrients. By about six months of age, infants are able to digest undiluted animal milk as well as semi-solid foods, making replacement feeding less difficult and less expensive for mothers than during their child's first six months. HIV-positive mothers have the following options for feeding their children from six months of age:

- Continued breastfeeding until transition to other options are safe and feasible (e.g., cessation of breastfeeding and transition to breast milk substitutes), plus appropriate complementary foods;
- Expressing and heat-treating breast milk plus appropriate complementary foods;
- Wet nursing by an HIV-negative woman plus appropriate complementary foods;
- Breast milk substitutes (e.g., commercial infant formula, fresh animal milk, powdered full-cream or evaporated milk, UHT milk) plus appropriate semi-solid and solid foods; and
- Appropriate semi-solid and solid foods plus clean drinking water in circumstances

where milk is not available. As discussed earlier in this chapter, complementary foods include a variety of locally available foods and liquids that are fed on a daily basis to children from six months as a complement to breast milk. Complementary

Micronutrients for Home-modified Animal Milk

The minerals and vitamins needed in a micronutrient supplement to fortify 100 kcal of home-modified animal milk (i.e., 100 mL of milk + 10 g sugar = 50 mL water) are listed below.

Minerals:

Manganese 7.5 ìg
Iron 1.5 mg
Copper 100 ìg
Zinc 205 ìg
Iodine 5.6 ìg

Vitamins:

Vitamin A 300 IU
Vitamin D 50 IU
Vitamin E 1 IU
Vitamin C 10 mg
Vitamin B1 50 ìg
Vitamin B2 80 ìg
Niacin 300 ìg
Vitamin B6 40 ìg
Folic acid 5 ìg
Pantothenic acid 400 ìg
Vitamin B12 0.2 ìg
Vitamin K 5 ìg
Biotin 2 ìg

(WHO, HIV and Infant Feeding: A guide for healthcare managers and supervisors, 2003)

.Foods can be mixtures of a staple such as cereals (e.g., rice, wheat, maize, millet) or starch foods (e.g., plantain, banana, cassava, potato) with beans, groundnut paste, meat, chicken, fish, eggs, fats and oils, fruits, and vegetables. Children should receive four to five meals of nutritious foods each day from six months of age, with additional nutrient-rich snacks one to two times a day as desired. Meals may be a combination of milk-only feeds, other foods, or a mix of milk and food. It is optimal to include milk in the diets of children through at least the first year of life.

Mother and Child Relationship.

Psychosocial stimulation through skin-to skin contact may be lacking when a child is fed by replacement feeding. Programmes and health workers should discuss with caregivers the importance of psychosocial contact and encourage them to hold, talk, and play with infants to help ensure adequate psychosocial stimulation. Health workers should also discuss with mothers how to avoid breast engorgement following the end of breastfeeding.

Stigma Associated with Replacement Feeding.

In many communities, mothers who do not breastfeed or stop breastfeeding early may be suspected of being HIV-positive and, subsequently, may be discriminated against because of the stigma often associated with HIV. Programme managers should assess the socio-cultural acceptability of replacement feeding and work with the community and partners to support mothers who choose replacement feeding. Because of the stigma associated with replacement feeding, mothers who choose replacement feeding may feel compelled to breastfeed in public. This type of mixed feeding may increase the risk of HIV transmission or other infections to the child. Programme managers and health workers should work with community support groups to raise awareness about the risks of mixed feeding. Health workers should also provide support and guidance to mothers on how to deal with situations where she may be asked why she stopped breastfeeding her infant.

Replacement Feeding and Child Spacing.

Women who do not breastfeed are at a higher risk of becoming pregnant. For an HIV positive mother, an early pregnancy can put the new baby at risk of malnutrition and increase the energy and other nutrient requirements of the mother. Mothers who decide not to breastfeed should be provided with family planning services to ensure adequate child spacing and all women in the context of HIV need information and support to practice safer sex to avoid sexually transmitted infections including HIV.

Nutritional Care Recommendations for Infants and Children

HIV infection is often difficult to diagnose in very young children. Infants born to HIV infected mothers have HIV antibodies made by the mother's immune system that cross the placenta to the baby's bloodstream before birth and may persist for up to 18 months. Because these maternal antibodies reflect the mother's but not the infant's infection status, an HIV antibody test is not reliable for children under 15 to 18 months. More definitive tests can determine whether a younger infant is actually infected with HIV but these tests are still expensive and are not typically available in ,resource-limited settings.

Unacceptable Options for Replacement Feeding.

The following fluids are not acceptable options for use in replacement feeding of infants because of their inadequate energy and micronutrient content: sweetened condensed milk, skimmed milk, coffee creamers, soy milk, fruit juices, sugar water, or diluted porridges.

What are the goals of nutritional care and support of children born to HIV-infected women ?

The goals of nutritional care and support of children born to HIV-infected women are as follows :-

- Improving nutritional status—maintaining weight, preventing weight loss, and preserving lean body mass
- Building stores of essential nutrients (macronutrients and micronutrients) necessary to boost immunity for resistance to infections and speedy recovery in case of infections
- Preventing food-borne illnesses by promoting hygiene and food and water safety
- Enhancing the quality of life by promptly treating infections and managing the symptoms that affect food intake to minimize the impact of secondary infections on nutritional status

What are the components of nutritional care and support for HIV-infected children and children born to HIV-infected women ?

The risk of malnutrition among children born to HIV-infected women or childreninfected with HIV requires regular nutritional assessments and early nutrition interventions. Programmes that prøvide nutritional care and support for affectedchildren should include the following components:

- Prevention of mother-to-child transmission of HIV (including maintaining appropriate weight gain in pregnancy and avoiding behaviours that increase risk of low birth weight and length)
- Periodic nutritional assessment of infants and young children
- Nutrition support and behaviour change communication to improve nutrition for the mother and the child
- Proper food hygiene and handling (plus periodic deworming)
- Diversification of the child's food (or the use of micronutrient supplements and fortified foods) to increase energy density and micronutrient availability
- Prompt treatment of infections and opportunistic infections that affect food intake and nutrition
- Use of ARVs where available or affordable

What are the good obstetric care and maternal nutrition ?

The good obstetric care and prevention of mother-to-child transmission of HIV are vital to prevent transmission of HIV to children and maintain good nutrition. Actions include supporting women to maintain appropriate weight gain in pregnancy, take multivitamin supplementation, and avoid behaviours that increase the risk of low birth weight and length.

What is the role of periodic nutritional assessment (growth monitoring) ?

The goal of nutritional assessment and intervention is to improve nutrition status, prevent further complications, and enhance the child's quality of life and survival.

The nutritional assessment is important to gather information on the current nutrition status and adequacy of the diet and to identify risk factors for developing nutritional complications. The earlier and more consistently this can be done the better. The information gathered should be interpreted to identify problems that put the children at increased nutrition risk and to design the best intervention with caregivers.

The periodic nutritional assessment should capture the following information:

- Changes in nutritional status (weight for height and height for age)
- Changes in eating behaviours associated, for example, with food availability issues, feeding pattern changes, and appetite changes
- Morbidity that may result in nutritional changes Components of the nutritional assessment The nutritional assessment should cover the child's physical assessment and biochemical (laboratory) data, nutrition history, medical history, and medication profile.

1. **Physical assessment**
   - Anthropometric measurements- Growth monitoring measures normally include weight and age but should also include height. Weight changes are assessed monthly basis (a child should grow parallel to the growth curves).
   - Measurements to assess changes in muscle mass
   - Screening for pallor (inner eyelids and palms) to assess anaemia
2. **Biochemical data (where available and feasible)**
   - Serum albumin and Prealbumin
   - CD4 and viral load counts
   - Evaluation of anaemia: iron (Hb), B12, and folate status
   - Transferrin/Total Fe and % saturation
   - B12/Folate
   - CBC with Differential
   - Electrolytes
   - Liver and Renal functions
3. **Nutrition history**
   - Dietary intake, frequency and adequacy of food consumed (including breastmilk)
   - for infants who are breastfed), exclusiveness of breastfeeding among infants
   - who are breastfed, exclusiveness of replacement feeding among infants who are not breastfed, adequacy of breastmilk substitutes for infants who receive

- replacement feeding, foods given, and hygiene practices
- Dietary problems such as poor appetite, difficulty chewing and swallowing, gastrointestinal problems, oral thrush, and sores
- Food intolerance and aversions, especially related to dietary symptoms
- Hygiene and practices in preparing and handling baby foods
- Use of vitamin and mineral supplements (e.g., vitamin A, iron supplementation), deworming, and alternative practices
- Medical history
- Recent gastrointestinal problems (e.g., diarrhoea, abdominal pain, nausea, and vomiting)
- Pattern of bowel movements (e.g., incidence of constipation)
- Opportunistic infections
- Concurrent medical problems (e.g., malaria, worm infestation, oral thrush and sores)

4. Medication profile

Drug use (e.g., ARVs, alternative therapies, and other medications)

- Side effects of medications and their nutrition implications
- Nutritional support, education, and counseling of caregivers
- Caregivers need not only nutrition education but also a sense of empowerment and confidence to apply the knowledge in their contexts. Nutritional support and counseling of caregivers should:
- Address issues relevant and of concern to most caregivers and their children
- Allocate time for individual evaluation and counseling
- Provide practical suggestions
- Use a list of local, affordable, and accessible foods to show mothers how much extra food they need to eat or to feed their children
- Provide advice on how to manage symptoms such as loss of appetite, diarrhoea, vomiting, and weight loss

- Address harmful traditional feeding practices and practices that do no harm that should be encouraged
- Be respectful and confidential at all times

Proper food hygiene and handling practices is important .

The aim of proper food hygiene and handling is to avoid food- or water-borne infections such as diarrhoea, dysentery, cholera, and typhoid that can further weaken the immune system and thus foster HIV disease progression.

Food diversification for the child with HIV is important.

Children's food can be diversified by increasing energy density and providing micronutrient supplementation or fortification. This meets the energy requirements of children infected with HIV or born to HIV-infected mothers and optimizes their nutrient intake. Asymptomatic HIV-infected adults require 10 percent more energy than non-infected adults of the same age, sex, and activity level, and symptomatic HIV-infected adults require 20 percent-30 percent more energy. Children with HIV/AIDS also have increased energy needs, but there is no current recommendation specific to children. Most of the energy for a young child may come from breast milk if then mother chooses to breastfeed. The breastfeeding mother needs adequate food intake and nutrition to benefit both herself and her child . Optimizing intake For a child infected with HIV to consume enough calories, proteins, and nutrients, intake needs to be optimized by:

- Increasing the frequency of feeding (probably to 5-8 small servings per day)
- Providing higher energy- and nutrient-dense foods (germinated or fermented foods, fortified foods)
- Modifying the diet to enable the child to increase consumption (e.g., by pureeing or slightly spicing the food)

Prompt treatment of infections and opportunistic infections is important .

Prompt treatment of diseases such as malaria, diarrhoea, acute respiratory infections, sore mouth, and ulcers minimizes the impact of the infection on the child's nutritional status. The possible effect of infections on food intake and absorption is also important.

The following common opportunistic infections may affect food intake among children infected with HIV:-

- Sore throat and problems in the gastrointestinal tract
- Thrush
- Fever

Children need medications to treat opportunistic infections and other diseases. The medicines themselves may affect food intake through side effects, discomfort, changes in taste.

What nutrition actions the service providers can take in care and support of children with HIV ?

HIV-infected children are more likely experience growth failure and face an increased risk of death. These risks require early intervention and continual follow up.

Nutritional Care Recommendations for Infants and Children For All Children

- Ensure that the infant has received all vaccinations by one year of age, according
- to national protocols.
- If the prevalence of anemia in children six to 24 months in the community is less than 40 percent, give 2 mg iron/kg body weight +50 ìg folic acid each day from six through 11 months of age. If anemia prevalence is equal to or higher than 40 percent, give 2 mg iron/kg body weight +50 ìg folic acid daily from six through 23 months of age.
- In vitamin A-deficiency risk areas, encourage the intake of vitamin A-rich foods.
- Encourage the intake of iron- and vitamin C-rich foods.
- During diarrhoea, continue breastfeeding and give children extra fluids and oral rehydration salts (ORS) properly mixed with clean boiled water.
- Seek appropriate healthcare for fever, diarrhoea, chronic cough, malaria, hookworm, and other parasitic infections.
- Regularly and accurately monitor growth (weight and height) to recognize
- growth failure, malnutrition, and its possible causes.

- Counsel caregivers to identify any opportunistic infection (e.g., oral thrush or
- sores, fever, gastrointestinal problems) or other infection (e.g., malaria, acute
- respiratory infections, diarrhoea) and seek early support from a health worker.
- Counsel caregivers to identify support services and programmes in their
- communities (e.g., home-based care, food distribution, psychosocial support)
- that may improve their or their children's nutrition.
- Review the child's diet at every clinic visit to ensure appropriate feeding.
- Counsel caregivers on cultural feeding habits, traditional therapies, and other
- practices that may be harmful to young children.
- Promote good food hygiene and food handling practices to make food safe and
- prevent food-born infections.
- Refer caregivers to programmes that may have available medications, including ARVs for young children.

For infants 0-5 months

- If the mother is breastfeeding, promote ONLY exclusive and frequent breastfeeding (> 8 times/day).
- If the mother is not breastfeeding, ensure infants receive ONLY replacement feeding and that proper hygiene is maintained. Provide the child with multivitamins or counsel on giving foods fortified with micronutrients .

For children 6-35 months

- If the infant is HIV negative or of unknown status, educate and support the mother on early weaning at or before 6 months of age.
- Promote adequate and proper feeding to 24 months or beyond. Review the child's diet at every well- and sick-baby clinic visit to ensure appropriate feeding (crucial if the mother is formula feeding).

- Promote good hygiene and proper food safety and handling.
- Counsel the caregiver to increase the amount and variety of foods given to the child, emphasizing the use of locally available, energy-dense foods (e.g., germinated or fermented flours to make porridge), fortified foods (e.g., fortification sachets), and increased use of fruits and vegetables.

For severely malnourished children

Severely malnourished HIV-infected children rarely respond to conventional rehabilitation or take much longer to rehabilitate.

- Refer children with severe malnutrition to an appropriate nutritional rehabilitation institution.
- Treat severe malnutrition according to new WHO guidelines, following the following steps:
- Categorize the extent of malnutrition by both anthropometric (e.g., body weight, skinfold measures, height) and clinical and biochemical methods. Also try to determine current intake patterns to assess adequacy and determine optimal intervention.
- Treat any infections, especially those that affect food intake and absorption.
    - Prevent and control hypoglycemia (also a common complication of ARVs).
    - Use oral rehydration therapy to replace lost fluids.
    - Regulate body temperature to prevent hypothermia.
    - Use antibiotics as necessary to treat any infections.
- Give adequate nutritional therapy.
    - Provide locally available and culturally acceptable high-energy and nutrient-dense diets.
    - Promote breastfeeding where appropriate during rehabilitation.
    - Provide vitamin A supplements according to national protocols (e.g., 200,000 IU on admission, a second dose the next day, and a follow-up dose 14 days later).
    - Use gastrotomy tube supplementation for HIV-infected children if other oral methods fail.
- Provide nutrition counseling to the caretakers.
- Provide follow up after discharge while monitoring weight and other infections

The Centers for Disease Control and Prevention (CDC) and World Health Organization (WHO) recognize malnutrition or growth faltering as an important sign of AIDS infection in children (CDC 1987). Malnutrition is a problem not only for children infected with HIV but also for HIV-negative children born to infected mothers. Numerous factors known to clinically indicate HIV infection in children have been used to define the essential actions for care of HIV-affected children, though many other factors are still unknown.

Malnutrition:

Malnutrition is a common complication of HIV infection and AIDS. Malnutrition places added stress on an already weakened immune system and may complicate the treatment of the disease by affecting the intestinal tracts ability to absorb drugs, not to mention its inability to absorb proteins, carbohydrates and fats.

Malnutrition in children is particularly devastating because children are still growing and developing, placing even higher energy demands on their bodies and immune systems. All children, regardless of the stage of their infection, should be seen by a registered dietitian (RD) for a thorough assessment and evaluation. It has been estimated that over 90% of children with HIV infection/ AIDS will experience delayed growth. The reason for this is multifactorial including poor socioeconomic situations, poor nutritional intake, malabsorbtion and the disease itself.

What are causes of Malnutrition in children with HIV ?

- Changes in Metabolism
  - alterations in the function of the gastrointestinal tract and the ability to use food in an efficient way
  - increased use of body fat stores
  - recurrent fevers and infections causing a rise in metabolic rates
  - depletion of vitamin and mineral stores
- Changes in Oral Intake
  - decreased intake due to medication schedules that require the child to be without food (NPO) for a period of time before and after the medications are given, as well as potential problems with nausea, vomiting and mouth sores

- altered intake due to oral infection with *Candida* (thrush.) Bear in mind that *Candida* can invade the oesophagus (throat), as well as the small intestine without being present in the mouth
- lack of adequate food supply in the home
- caregivers that may be infected as well and not able to care for the child properly
- inability to tolerate fats and lactose (milk sugars)
- diarrhoea, the cause of which may or may not be known

- Functional Impairment
  - chewing and swallowing may be greatly affected in children with HIV involvement of the nervous system. An evaluation by a speech pathologist can be very beneficial.

What are the risks of malnutrition among children born to HIV-infected women and HIV-infected children

Low birth weight and stunting are common among children born to HIV-infected others. HIV-infected women are likely to give birth to low birth weight children

Four factors seem to be associated with reduced birth weight among children born to HIV-infected women:

- Shorter gestational age among HIV-infected women
- Severity of maternal HIV disease, a factor of viral load
- Intrauterine growth retardation and micronutrient deficiency, most likely occurring late in the pregnancy. Infection with HIV increases demand for energy and nutrients. If food intake is not adequate to compensate for the increased needs, a negative energy and micronutrient balance may result.
- Prenatal drug or alcohol use during pregnancy (Arpadi 2000).

Progressive post-natal stunting is common among HIV-infected children

Although uninfected infants born to HIV-infected women start with lower birth weights, they show rapid weight gain and "catch-up" growth immediately after birth. Mainly this is facilitated by fat mass deposition. By the third month most uninfected children born of HIV-infected women have caught up in height and weight with children born to HIV-negative women (Agostoni et al 1998). Poor growth, however, is common among children infected with HIV. As many as 50 percent of children with HIV fail to thrive (Arpadi 2000). In fact, since 1994 the CDC has used failure to thrive as an AIDS definition condition in children. By the third month, linear growth (height) is proportionately decreased among HIV-infected children. The difference in linear height is significant and evident by the second year of life. By that time, HIV-infected children have a growth velocity of less than the fifth percentile, an indication of severe growth failure. Along with stunting, symptomatic HIV-infected children commonly show HIV-related wasting, mainly marasmus.

What are the causes of growth failure among HIV infected children ?

What explains the slow linear growth among HIV-infected children? The etiology is not well understood and may involve many factors. Some documented factors are listed below:

- The rate of HIV replication has a reciprocal relation to the rate of growth.
    - o HIV-infected children with poor growth also have higher viral loads than infected children with normal growth curves (Pollack et al 1997).
    - o Suppression of viral load with antiretroviral drugs (ARVs) appears to have a favourable effect on growth, especially weight gain (Arpadi 2000a).
- Underlying disease activity seems to be a major factor in children's growth (Bailey et al 1999). Gastrointestinal dysfunction (including persistent diarrhoea) and malabsorption are key factors in the nutrition of children in resourceconstrained areas.
- Inadequate energy and micronutrient intake (simple starvation) affect growth. For most HIV-infected children, daily intake may not be sufficient to meet increased metabolic demands. In addition, during this period of rapid growth there is normally increased demand on available nutrient pools. HIV-infected children or children born to HIV-infected parents

may not be able to consume adequate foods to meet all their needs, for various reasons:

- o High social risk of being born to poor households and having mothers with HIV/AIDS who are unable to access enough food for themselves and their babies or to provide quality care
- o Gastrointestinal dysfunction, including infections and malabsorption
- o Infections and use of medicine affecting child food intake
- o Micronutrient deficiency associated with growth failure
- o Additional nutrient and energy needs for growth and development, even in the absence of abnormal eating habits

- Children infected with HIV also show preferential decreases of fat-free mass (lean body mass) compared to uninfected children . This is also seen among children (especially boys) depicting normal rates of growth. This may be associated with:
  - o High viral load, also associated with decreased proportion of free fat mass
  - o Host immune response to the replication of the virus, which may increase the basal metabolic demands (and thus increased energy expenditures) in HIV-infected children. Unlike in adults, hypermetabolism is rarely reported in HIV-infected children. However, the lack of hypermetabolism may partly result from a lower amount of FFM, which is preferentially decreased in children infected with HIV, especially those with growth failure.
- Maternal vitamin A deficiency influences infant linear growth during the first year of life. Increased mortality is associated with vitamin A deficiency during human immunodeficiency virus infection (Semba, Miotti, Chiphangwi, et al 1997).
- The following additional factors may be associated with the etiology of growth failure and altered body composition:
  - o Metabolic and endocrine alterations or disorders associated with stress
  - o Growth hormone deficiency
  - o Hypothyroidism

What are the consequences of growth failure among HIV-infected children ?

Poor growth is associated with poor survival. HIV-infected Ugandan infants with weight-for-age below –1.5 Z-scores have five times the risk of dying before the age of 25 months compared with non-infected children (Berhane et al 1997). growth failure among HIV-infected children is associated with retarded cognitive development and functional deficits such as delayed sexual development among boys. Micronutrient deficiencies will result in functional consequences similar to those reported in uninfected children.

What Interventions are required for Nutritional Problems among children with HIV?

- Poor Oral Intake:

As mentioned earlier, there are many reasons why intake can be affected. It is critical to establish those reasons, then develop strategies to help the patient.

A frequently used and tolerated intervention is to encourage small, frequent feedings instead of a traditional three meal pattern. Parents and caregivers may feel that unless the child is eating three meals they are not getting adequate nutrition. It is important to remember that if smaller meals and snacks are planned appropriately. sufficient calories and protein can be provided.

Infants may require having their formulas concentrated to 24, 26 or even 30 calories per ounce. It will be imperative to teach parents how much free water the child needs to have as well. Formulas can also be boosted with medical nutritional such as carbohydrate sources , protein sources , or fat sources . If parents are going to use vegetable oil for boosting calories, it is important to keep shaking the bottle gently during the feeding. (Vegetable oil will rise to the top of the formula. If the infant receives the oil in this concentrated form, it may cause diarrhoea.)

It is common practice at the Clinical Center to recommend vitamin and mineral supplements for all children, regardless of the stage of infection. One that provides 100% of the recommended daily allowance for the age range of the child is appropriate. For older children and adolescents, an adult vitamin is appropriate.

- Oral Lesions:

Good oral hygiene is crucial regardless of the reason for the oral lesions. Your doctor may be able to prescribe some type of topical medication to use that will numb the mouth so meals will be better tolerated. Usually children will require modified textures of soft, moist, easily chewed and swallowed foods such as casseroles, ground meats, egg dishes, and/or pasta products, extra gravies added to meals, vegetables, potatoes or rice.

Foods and fluids should be served as close to room temperature as possible to reduce heat intolerance. Fluids may be better tolerated through a straw. Non-acidic beverages are better tolerated. Supplements will be very beneficial in this instance as they can provide good sources of all nutrients in small volumes.

What to do if there is Diarrhoea/Malabsorption ?

As always, it is crucial to determine the underlying cause of the diarrhoea and if possible, have it medically treated.

If the symptoms come from infectious causes, supplemental feedings via tube feedings and or Total Parenteral Nutrition may be indicated on a short term basis. There are specific formulas available on the market that may be better tolerated. Most tube feedings are lactose-free, but some also have modified forms of fat. Others are elemental and easily digested . The dietitian, Case manager and physician should all have suggestions as to what type of formula is appropriate, and the best means of delivering the formula to the patient.

For acute periods of diarrhoea it may be necessary to limit the amount of lactose and fat in the diet:

1. Offer lactaid milk and yogurt products.
2. Soy milk may be offered.
3. Offer small frequent meals.
4. Try to include soluble forms of fibre in the diet (i.e. oatmeal; rice; bananas; applesauce.)
5. Replace fluid losses with electrolyte solutions such as Peidialyte® or Ricelyte®.

Potassium and sodium are two electrolytes, in particular, that may need added replacement. For sodium: try foods such as broths, bouillon, and crackers. For potassium: foods such as bananas, apricots, potatoes, and meats (prepared plainly).

You may consult with your dietitian. The case manager can provide a referral to a dietitian. A dietitian can help personalize a plan just for your child to make sure they are getting all the nutrition they need.

Safe Drinking Water is important :

In India, there has been an increased occurrence of a water-born illness known as Cryptosporidiosis. The organism *Cryptosporidium* is found in wells, lakes, rivers, and in some water supplies. People with depressed immune systems, especially those with CD4 counts less than 200, are at increased risk of infection from this organism. The symptoms of Crytopsporidiosis include large amounts of watery diarrohea. For children this is a potentially life threatening situation if they become too dehydrated.

Bottled mineral waters are okay, but not all manufacturers have safeguards in place to be sure that *Cryptosporidium* is not present. To be on the safe side boil water for 30 minutes then place in containers to be used when needed. If children are going to be swimming in lakes, pools etc., it is important that they do not swallow any water.

15

Protect the Quality and Safety of Your Food

People living with HIV/AIDS are more vulnerable to infection because their immune systems have already been weakened. Properly handling food and water is especially important to avoid infections caused by bacteria and viruses in contaminated food and water. Food can be contaminated with harmful bacteria and viruses (called germs), which produce poisonous toxins. A person eating this food may be infected by the germs and made sick from the toxins. Because HIV affects the immune system and the body's resistance to disease, people with HIV/AIDS are more vulnerable to germs and should be careful to avoid eating contaminated food. If they get food poisoning, they will lose weight and become even weaker, which will lower the body's resistance to future infection.

Most food poisoning can be prevented by following some basic rules of hygiene. Food hygiene measures have two aims:

1. to prevent contamination in food preparation areas;
2. to prevent germs from multiplying in food and reaching dangerous levels.

The food safety and hygiene practices suggested below will achieve both these aims and ensure maximum protection from the risk of harmful germs.

Food and water safety precautions

The following precautions for preventing or minimizing food- or waterborne diseases are important (*Nutrition and Your Health: Dietary Guidelines, USA)*

- Do not eat raw or undercooked meat, poultry, fish, or shellfish (clams, oysters, scallops, and mussels). Whole poultry should be cooked to 180°F, poultry breast and well-done meats to 170°F, and medium-rare beefsteaks, roasts, veal, and lamb to 140°F.
- Reheat sauces, soups, marinades, and gravies to a boil. Reheat leftovers thoroughly to at least 165°F. Use a food thermometer to determine temperature. If a microwave oven is used, cover the container and turn or stir the food to make sure it is heated evenly throughout.
- Do not eat raw or partially cooked eggs, or foods containing raw eggs, raw (unpasteurized) milk, or cheeses made with raw milk. Cook eggs until whites and yolks are firm.
- The risk of contamination is high from undercooked hamburger and from raw fish (including sushi), clams, and oysters. Cook fish and shellfish until it is opaque; fish should flake easily with a fork. When eating out, order foods that have been thoroughly cooked and make sure they are served piping hot.
- When cooking, keep hot foods hot (140°F or above) and cold foods cold (40°F or below.) Harmful bacteria can grow rapidly in the danger zone between these temperatures. Whether raw or cooked, never leave meat, poultry, eggs, fish, or shellfish out at room temperature for >2 h (1 h in weather 90°F or above). Chill leftovers as soon as possible. Use refrigerated leftovers within 3-4 days.
- Freeze fresh meat, poultry, fish, and shellfish that cannot be used in a few days. Thaw frozen meat, poultry, fish, and shellfish in the refrigerator, microwave, or cold water changed every 30 min. Cook foods immediately after thawing.
- Avoid cross-contamination of foods. Uncooked meats should not come in contact with other foods. Hands, cutting boards, counters, knives, and other cooking utensils should be washed thoroughly after contact with uncooked foods.

- Listeriosis is a serious disease that occurs frequently among HIV-infected persons who are severely immunosuppressed. Some soft cheeses and some ready-to-eat foods (e.g., hot dogs and cold cuts from delicatessen counters) have been known to cause listeriosis. Reheating these foods until they are steaming before eating them can prevent listeriosis.
- HIV-infected persons should not drink water directly from lakes or rivers because of the risk for cryptosporidiosis and giardiasis. They should avoid swimming in water that may be contaminated with human or animal waste, and they should avoid swallowing water during swimming.
- Boiling water for 1 minute will eliminate the risk of acquiring cryptosporidiosis infection. The use of submicron, personal-use water filters or the drinking of bottled water might also reduce the risk for acquiring cryptosporidiosis. Current data are inadequate to support a recommendation that all HIV-infected persons boil or otherwise avoid drinking tap water in nonoutbreak settings. Persons choosing to use a personal-use filter or bottled water should be aware of the complexities involved in selecting the appropriate products, the lack of enforceable standards for destruction or removal of oocysts, the cost of the products, and the difficulty of using these products consistently.
- Nationally distributed brands of bottled or canned carbonated soft drinks are safe to drink. Commercially packaged noncarbonated soft drinks and fruit juices that do not require refrigeration until after they are opened are also safe. Nationally distributed brands of frozen fruit juice concentrate are safe if they are reconstituted with water from a safe source. Only juices labeled as pasteurized should be considered free of *Cryptosporidium* risk. Other pasteurized beverages and beers are considered safe to drink.

Food safety

People living with HIV/AIDS need to be especially careful about germs and the food that they eat, because their severely weakened immune systems might not be able to cope as effectively as a normal, healthy immune system and opportune diseases can set in.

Germs in food and water

Eating food or drinking water that is contaminated (i.e. it contains harmful germs) can cause various infections.

"Food poisoning" is a general term for infections contracted through food. Typical symptoms of food poisoning include stomach cramps, diarrhoea, nausea and vomiting. Bacteria are the most common cause of food poisoning, followed by viruses and parasites. There are several hundred food-borne diseases, many of which cause other symptoms besides food poisoning. Poisonous chemicals that get into food can also make you ill.

People with HIV/AIDS are particularly vulnerable to infections from germs in food and water, and need to take extra care. You can't always tell if food or water is contaminated by how it looks, tastes or smells, but you can greatly reduce the risks by following the simple steps outlined below.

Personal hygiene

- Wash your hands regularly and thoroughly with soap and water, particularly after going to the toilet
  - after touching animals
  - after sneezing or blowing your nose
  - before and after food preparation
  - after touching raw meat, fish or poultry
- Try to avoid coming into contact with animal faeces. If you do, wash your hands very well - with anti-bacterial soap if possible.
- Cover wounds on your hands to prevent contamination when working with food. Make sure bandages or plasters are clean. Rubber gloves are useful for keeping both wounds and food clean.

Drinking water

- Boil drinking water first if you are unsure about whether it is safe to drink. Tap water is usually safe, but water from other sources, such as rivers and wells, is not. If boiling isn't possible, treat the water with bleach, as follows: Mix 1 teaspoon (5 ml) of bleach with 25 litres of water (a large basin-full). Leave it to stand at least two hours before drinking.

- Store safe water in a clean, covered container, preferably in the fridge.
- Make sure cold drinks and ice cubes have been made with safe water.
- Remember not to swallow unsafe water while bathing or swimming.

Food shopping

- Buy foods in amounts that can be eaten before they go off.
- Don't buy or use dented, bulging or leaking cans.
- Pre-packaged, sealed cold meats and cheeses are safer.
- Don't buy cracked eggs: the cracks allow germs to enter.
- Don't buy foods after their "sell by" date. Throw out foods at home that have reached their expiry date, and don't even taste food if you suspect it has gone off.
- Avoid foods that have been home-bottled.

Choosing, preparing and storing food

- If you're not sure where food comes from or how it's been prepared, don't eat it.
- Keep food away from animals.
- Cover food to keep insects off it.

Fruits and vegetables

  - Peel fresh fruits and vegetables or wash them with clean water.
  - Throw out moldy or rotten fruits or vegetables.

Milk and milk products

  - Use pasteurised milk. (Milk is heated to high temperatures to destroy germs.) Home-produced milk should be boiled before use.
  - Throw out moldy cheese. Avoid cheeses that contain live molds, like blue cheese, Brie and Camembert.
- Don't eat wild mushrooms, unless you are absolutely sure they are safe.

Meat

  - Never eat raw meat, poultry or fish.

- Cook meat thoroughly. (It shouldn't be pink inside.) Ask to have your meat well done when eating at restaurants or friends' houses.

- Avoid seafood that does not come from a known, safe source.

Eggs

- Never eat raw eggs. Cook eggs until the white and yolk are firm.
- Don't use cracked eggs.
- Wash eggs before breaking them.

Frozen food

- Food should be kept either hot or cold. Keep cold foods cold:
- Keep frozen foods frozen until you're ready to eat them.
- Pick up frozen foods last, and hurry home with them or pack them with ice in a cooler bag.
- Don't keep foods in your freezer longer than a month.
- Once food has defrosted, it should be used as soon as possible, and not refrozen.
- Don't defrost frozen meat at room temperature, which is warm enough to give germs the chance to grow. Defrost frozen meat or other frozen foods in a fridge. If you don't have a fridge, defrost food in a cool place. Microwave ovens are also good for quick defrosting.

Keep hot foods hot:

- Eat food as soon as possible once it's been cooked. Don't store foods that have cooled down at room temperature.
- Don't keep food at room temperature for more than two hours. After this time period, bacteria start multiplying. Be suspicious of cold cooked food that has been kept at room temperature for longer.
- Refrigerate leftovers. If you don't have a fridge, keep food covered in a cool place.
- Store foods in airtight containers or cling wrap.
- When you eat cooked leftovers, reheat them to a high temperature to kill germs.

Take extra care when travelling:

- you are likely to come into contact with new germs that your body isn't used to.
- Only drink bottled or boiled water, or canned drinks. Avoid ice in drinks, unless you know it has been boiled first.
- Don't eat raw fruits and vegetables unless you have peeled them yourself.
- Make sure that food has been properly cooked.
- Don't eat food sold by street vendors.

Kitchen hygiene

- Wash surfaces like the kitchen table, counter or sink, before and after preparing food there. Keep food storage areas (like shelves and fridges) clean.
- Clean up spills immediately.
- Use separate cleaning cloths for the kitchen and other parts of the house.
- Disinfect kitchen cloths, sponges and scourers with bleach, and dry them in sunlight, which helps kill germs. If you have a microwave, heating cloths and sponges for 60 seconds helps kill bacteria.
- Wash the kitchen floor at least once a week, with cloths that are only used for that purpose.
- Wash dishes, cutlery and cutting boards well – preferably in hot soapy water that you replace when it gets too dirty. Rinse dishes with clean water, if possible.
- Replace cracked or badly scratched utensils. Germs live in cracks in cups and dishes and scratches in plastic containers and cutting boards.
- Use a cutting board for raw foods. Preferably, use one cutting board for meat, poultry and fish, and another for other foods. Or, clean the board well with hot water soapy after cutting each food type. Plastic or stone cutting boards are safest for raw meat.
- Don't reuse utensils after they have touched raw meat, fish or chicken, until you have washed them very thoroughly.

- Keep rubbish in a covered bin that you empty and clean regularly.

Keep the kitchen door and windows open as much as possible to provide good ventilation; this helps prevent the growth of mold and fungus.

Disposal of faeces

Many of the germs responsible for food poisoning are spread through faeces. You should aim to:

- use a latrine and keep it clean and free from flies;
- keep the surroundings clean;

wash clothes, bedding and surfaces that might have been contaminated with.

Cooking and storage of food

Germs multiply more quickly in warm food. Storing food in a refrigerator or cool place slows down this growth. Cooking on a high heat can also kill most germs. Food should be eaten as soon as it is cooked.

- Cover and store food in containers away from insects, rodents and other animals.
- Store fresh food in a cool place or refrigerator where available.
- Cook food thoroughly, but do not overcook vegetables.
- Serve food immediately after cooking. Do not leave the food standing at room temperature before eating, to avoid germs multiplying.
- Do not store raw and cooked food together; use containers to avoid contact between them.
- Avoid storing leftovers unless they can be kept in a refrigerator or a cool place. Do not store them for more than one or two days and always reheat them at a high temperature.

Animal foods

- Cook meat and fish well; meat should have no red juices.
- Wash utensils and surfaces touched by animal products with hot water and soap before preparing other foods.
- Keep meat and fish separate from other foods.
- Eggs should be hard boiled. Do not eat soft-boiled eggs, raw eggs, cracked eggs or any foods containing raw eggs.

However careful one is, food-borne infections may happen. The advice for diarrhoea in Chapter s 11 will help, but when a person has serious food poisoning it is important to see a health worker without delay in order to avoid weight loss and further illness.

Taking care of people living with HIV/AIDS

Nutritional needs must be seen in context with other needs. Nutrition education should be provided alongside other components that contribute to well-being, including health care, economic and social support and, especially, positive living.

Taking care of yourself - advice for the person with HIV/ AIDS

Nutrition education has a place alongside other advice and support directed at promoting well-being and positive living. General recommendations for taking care of yourself are as follows :-

The body needs extra rest. Try to sleep for eight hours every night. Rest whenever you are tired.

- Try not to worry too much. Stress can harm the immune system. Relax more. Relax with people you love, your family, your children and your friends. Do things you enjoy, e.g. listen to music or read a newspaper or a book.
- Be kind to yourself. Try to keep a positive attitude. Feeling good is part of being healthy.
- Take light exercise. Choose a form of exercise that you enjoy.
- Find support and get good advice. Ask for advice from health workers. Many medical problems can be treated.
- Ask for help and accept help when it is offered.
- Stop smoking. It damages the lungs and many other parts of the body and makes it easier for infections to attack your body.
- Alcohol is harmful to the body, especially the liver. It increases vulnerability to infection and destroys vitamins in the body; under the influence of alcohol you may forget to practise safe sex.
- Avoid unnecessary medicines. They often have unwanted side-effects and can interfere with food and nutrition. If you do take medicines, read the instructions carefully.

Caring for a person with HIV/AIDS

The carer looking after a person with HIV/AIDS may be a member of the family or, if the person lives alone, a neighbour, relative or friend. It is not easy to care for a person with HIV/AIDS and whoever grows, prepares, cooks food and serves it to a person with HIV/AIDS needs support. The task involves meeting the needs of the sick person and balancing these with the needs of other members of the family. Too much help may be overprotective and take away the dignity, independence and self-respect of the person with HIV/AIDS while too little help may not provide the support that is needed to ensure that the person eats well and has the strength to resist infection.

Guidelines for carers

- Spend time with the person living with HIV/AIDS. Discuss the foods they need to maintain and gain weight and manage their illness. Get to know what kind of foods they like and do not like. Involve them in planning their meals.
- Keep an eye on their weight. If possible, weigh them regularly and keep a record. Look out for any unexpected weight loss and take action.
- Check the medicines they are taking. Read the instructions to find out when they need to be taken, what foods to be avoided and any side-effects.
- Be encouraging and loving. If people want to have food of their choice at any time of the day, try to get it for them. They may suddenly stop liking a food, refuse what has been prepared and want something different. They are not trying to be difficult. These sudden changes in taste are a result of their illness.
- Be firm about the importance of eating and encourage them to eat frequently, but do not force them to eat. Giving them too much food at one time may cause them to refuse.
- If they are too sick to leave their beds, make sure that they have something to drink and a snack nearby.
- Keep a watchful eye. Look around to see if the house is clean, that there are no hygiene problems and there is enough food.

- If the sick person lives alone, invite them to join your family for a meal. Encourage others in the community to visit them and invite them out.

Carers will have their own concerns and worries, fears for the future, for their families and for their own health. It is important that they take care of themselves, get enough rest and have the appropriate information and support to carry out their difficult task. The important messages given below cannot be emphasized enough.

- HIV/AIDS is not spread by food or water.
- HIV/AIDS cannot be spread by sharing food, dishes or cooking utensils such as cups, plates, knives and forks with a person who is HIV positive.
- HIV/AIDS cannot be spread by touching another person, hugging, shaking hands or holding other people in a normal way. There is no need to avoid body contact with a person living with HIV/AIDS.

Eat and travel safe

When travelling or attending social gatherings, it may be a time you eat foods different from your normal diet. Take precautions to keep yourself safe from illness. Be prepared for delays in travelling and unexpected extended stays.

Tips when attending a party

- Eat a healthy snack before you go to the party. Do this just in case you are not satisfied the food being served has been safely prepared, handled, or stored, or are not your food preferences.
- Eat when the food is first served and make sure the cold foods are cold, and the hot foods hot.
- Avoid foods that you suspect were made with raw eggs such as homemade eggnog or Caesar salad dressing.
- Eat and drink only pasteurized dairy products (milk, cream, cheese) and eggnog and juices.
- Avoid raw fish or foods that contain raw fish.
- Avoid undercooked protein foods, such as chicken that is still pink, meat that is red, or runny eggs.
- Avoid fresh fruit or vegetables served raw unless you know they were washed prior to cutting.

- Wash your hands after having contact with others to avoid spread of germs.

If you experience diarrhoea easily

- Watch out for fried foods, high fat foods, foods that contain lactose, such as most dairy products, spicy foods, caffeinated beverages, popcorn, nuts, or insoluble fiber, such as the skins and seeds of fruits and vegetables. Small amounts may be fine.
- Foods that can help decrease diarrhoea include white rice, bananas, white toast, applesauce, skinless mashed potatoes, yogurt with active cultures, or a dose of Metamucil, Citrucel, Konsyl, psyllium, or other soluble fibre powder taken before the party, daily, or as needed.

Tips to remember while travelling

- Follow the same food safety guidelines above. What is considered "safe" for others may not be safe for you.
- Take medications along for an extra three to ten days. This should allow time for mail to reach you with a new supply if needed.
- Have the names and numbers of medical services and HIV knowledgeable doctors on the way to and at your destination in case of an emergency, or if you have to go to an ER, you can always ask for the ID (infectious disease) doctor on call.
- Travel with your medication in their original prescription containers in your backpack, pockets or in a bag that is with you at all times. Checked bags can be delayed or lost during travel.
- If you don't have your prescription bottles, ask your doctor for a list of your medications to identify them as necessary for a medical condition or ask your pharmacist for a copy of the prescription label for each medication.
- Avoid changes in the medication regimen shortly before travel to ensure that no side effects or complications of a new regimen occur while traveling.
- Take anti-diarrhoeal medicine with you in case you need it.
- Consult your doctor about prescribing Cipro, a broad-spectrum antibiotic, as prophylaxis against pathogens.

- Norvir (ritonavir) and Kaletra (which contains ritonavir) in the soft gel need to be stored below 77 degrees Fahrenheit (25 degrees Celsius.) However the new formulation of Kaletra does not need refrigerated. Carry a small cooler with cold packs to keep medications safe from the heat. Do not leave medications in the car where the temperatures may go over 77 degrees F. Protect Norvir from the light.
- Fuzeon or T20 needs to be stored at 77 degrees Fahreneheit or 25 degrees Celsius. Once mixed with water (reconstituted), it should be stored under refrigeration to 36-46 degrees Fahrenheit or 2-8 degrees Celsius and used within 24 hours. Look for hotels, motels, inns that have small in-room refrigerators. Consider taking a refrigerator thermometer to make sure it does not get too cold and freeze your medication or keep it at sub-optimal temperatures.
- Always travel with safe fluids and snacks. Use ice or ice packs to keep refrigerated foods cold.
- Use safe water. Avoid tap water. Drink only bottled water that has been distilled or that has gone through reverse osmosis or water that has been boiled and cooled properly, or bottled (carbonated) or canned beverages. Make sure the seal on the cap has not been broken. Avoid ice cubes, fountain drinks: anything with tap water.
- Use safe water for brushing your teeth.
- Wash your hands often. Carry moist hand towelettes or waterless hand cleaners for temporary hand washing until you can properly wash your hands.
- Avoid food purchased from street vendors.
- Keep current with necessary vaccines.

Choose Wisely and Eat Safely

- Purchase fresh produce without bruises, soft spots, slime, mold or broken skins.
- Wash ALL fruits and vegetables, including melons, oranges, and bananas, before cutting, slicing and eating. Scrub with a brush under cool running water to remove any dirt, pesticides and unhealthy bacteria.
- Store in the fruit/vegetable drawer in the refrigerator or in a cool place. Once cut or sliced, all fruits and vegetables should

be placed in refrigerator in tightly sealed plastic bags and consumed within 2 to 3 days. Do not let cut fruit and vegetables sit at room temperature.

- Freeze fruits and vegetables that cannot be consumed in two to three days to cut down on waste and spoilage. Note that the consistency will be slightly changed once thawed.

Planning Meals for PLWHAs

It is important to work with households to select foods that are easily available, acceptable, and affordable to prepare. In planning meals, the following elements should be considered:

- The nutrient value and variety of the available foods (e.g., animal foods, legumes, nuts, fruits, vegetables, staples, and fats);
- The nutritional needs of the person(s), including the additional energy requirements due to infections and stage in the life cycle (e.g., pregnancy, lactation, childhood, adolescence);
- The personal food preferences of the PLWHAs;
- The effects of taking drugs, such as ARVs, on diet or drug food interactions
- The time required for food preparation and
- The cost and availability of food.Persons caring for PLWHAs need to plan meals that are adequate and satisfy their physical and emotional needs. Compared to the requirements of healthy, non-HIV-infected people of the same age, sex, and physical activity level, HIV-infected asymptomatic persons need 10 percent more energy and HIV infected symptomatic persons need 20 to 30 percent more energy. Meals should contribute to good health, be visually appealing, and provide aromas and tastes that stimulate the appetite.

In planning a meal for an HIV-infected individual, follow three steps:

1. Begin by assessing the stage in the disease based on the presence or absence of symptoms and opportunistic infections, the medications being taken, the food preferences and dietary practices of the PLWHAs, the quantity of food consumed, the frequency of meals, and the types of foods that are regularly consumed including staple foods.

Tips to help you pick, store, and prepare your fruits and vegetables

Food	*How to pick*	*How to store*	*How to prepare*
Tomatoes	Slightly soft, with rich red color.	Store at room temperature away from direct sunlight then refrigerate when ripe for up to 4 days.	May be eaten raw or cooked or part of another dish.
Sweet corn	Fresh green husks, not dry. Plump kernels with no dents.	Remove husks and silk, put in zip log bag and refrigerate for up to 2 days for optimal freshness.	Boil 3-5 minutes or microwave on high 3 to 4 minutes per ear.
Strawberries	Rich red color and firm.	In the refrigerator, unwashed in airtight container for 2-4 days.	Wash when ready to eat. Handle gently. Eat raw, sliced in cereal or salad.
Cantaloupes	Slightly oval and 5 inches or more in diameter with yellow or golden background color.	At room temperature for 2 to 3 days or store in refrigerator up to 1 week.	Scrub with brush under running water, before cutting and eating. Serve with or without rind.

(Contd.)

(Contd. Table)

Food	How to pick	How to store	How to prepare
Honeydew	Look for a waxy white rind barely tinged with green. The blossom end should give to gentle pressure.	At room temperature for 2 to 3 days or store in refrigerator for up to 1 week.	Scrub with brush under running water, before cutting and eating. Serve with or without rind.
Watermelon	Symmetrical shape, a dull rather than shiny surface, and an underside that's yellowish or beginning to turn cream-colored.	As above, or to hasten ripening, place melon inside loosely closed paper bag, or store in refrigerator for up to one week.	Scrub with brush under running water, before cutting and eating. Serve with or without rind.
Spinach	Pre-washed in plastic bag or in a bunch with deep green healthy looking leaves, not yellow, wilted or slimy.	In the refrigerator for 2 to 3 days, do not wash until ready to use.	Rinse the spinach from the bag once. Bunches should be washed in several changes of water until there is no grit left in bowl. Steam, sauté, or serve raw in salad.

2. Identify and reinforce good dietary practices. Identify the nutrients not adequately covered through food consumption. Analyze the reasons for the inadequacy and opportunities to meet these needs.
3. Based on the assessment, plan a varied diet with the client. Work with households to select foods that are easily available, acceptable, and affordable.

Good Dietary Practices:

Good dietary practices play an important role in maintaining a healthy lifestyle and healthy body. An HIV-infected person already has a weakened immune system. A nutritious diet can help maintain the proper functioning of the immune system and provides needed energy, protein, and micronutrients during all stages of the HIV infection. Programme managers can promote a number of dietary practices that HIV-infected individuals and their families can follow.

The following suggestions are provided as general principles in responding to the nutritional needs of HIV-affected populations. Maintaining adequate nutritional status means consuming a variety and adequate quantity of foods to meet energy, protein, and micronutrients needs. PLWHAs should eat a balanced and diverse diet consisting of starchy staples (e.g., rice, maize, potato, cassava, banana, yam) with cooked legumes (e.g., beans, peas), nuts and nut butters, animal foods, fat and oil, fruits, and vegetables. A balanced diet will ensure that the individual consumes sufficient nutrients to maintain energy, normalize weight, and ensure the body's proper functioning. The main types of food people need to live a healthy life include energy-providing foods (i.e., carbohydrates, fats), body-building foods (i.e., proteins, minerals), and protective foods (i.e., vitamins, minerals). Carbohydrates (i.e., sugars, starches) and fats provide the body with energy.

These foods:

- Provide energy to make bodies work and keep active;
- Are found in various starchy staple foods such as maize, rice, sorghum, millet, and green banana and roots and tubers such as cassava, taro, potato, and sweet potato; and
- Are usually more affordable and available than high-protein foods. HIV-infected people have increased energy requirements

because of HIV disease and coinfections. Consuming a variety of foods from each of the main groups of energy sources on a daily basis is important to maintaining good nutritional status to help fight illness. In addition, good nutritional status may ensure that a person is able to survive an opportunistic infection such as TB or pneumonia without further compromising health and nutritional status. Proteins and minerals are found in bodybuilding foods.

These foods:

- Contain proteins for cell repair and growth nutrients such as iron for blood and calcium and phosphorus for strong bones;
- Help build bones and cells important for growth and development;
- Help fight infection and repair the body during times of illness; and
- Are obtained from legumes (e.g., beans, lentils, cowpeas, pigeon peas, groundnuts, nuts), milk products (e.g., cow or goat milk, yogurt, cheese, human breast milk), animal foods (e.g., fish, eggs, chicken, pork, beef, birds, rodents, other meat products, insects), whole grains and cereals (e.g., wheat, maize, millet, sorghum, rice). Animal products are important sources of nutrients but may not be feasible to consume every day because they are usually more expensive than vegetable protein sources. Daily consumption of a cereal with a protein source such as legumes is recommended. Foods rich in micronutrients (e.g., vitamins A, B, C, D, E) and minerals (e.g., iodine selenium, zinc, iron) are called protective foods. Micronutrient-rich foods:

- Help the body absorb and utilize protein and carbohydrates;
- Help fight infections and digest and absorb other nutrients; and
- Are found in dark green, leafy vegetables (e.g., collard greens, cassava and potato leaves, spinach, callaloo, pumpkin leaves, cabbage) and yellow and orange fruits and vegetables (e.g., mango, papaya or paw paw, sweet potato, pumpkin, carrots, tomato, avocado, oranges, lemons, bananas).

16

Nutrition and HIV/AIDS

Helping families and communities to cope

Although human immunodeficiency virus/acquired immunodeficiency syndrome (HIV/AIDS) is recognized predominantly as a health problem, the epidemic has multiple social and economic dimensions and implications since it affects adults in their most productive years of life. A health approach alone is not sufficient to prevent the spread of the disease or to mitigate its impact on both individuals and society. The spread of HIV/AIDS has become a major constraint to development in affected areas and must, therefore, become a major consideration in the programme planning of governments and agencies. The detrimental impact of the HIV/AIDS epidemic on nutrition and household food security in affected areas requires attention, and strategies to address these problems should be incorporated in programme planning.

The interaction between HIV/AIDS and nutrition can basically be seen from two perspectives:

- the *biological* perspective, which is the association between nutritional status and risk of infection, as well as the relationship of nutritional status and the evolution of the disease;
- the *socio-economic* perspective, which considers the consequences of the disease for the food and nutrition situation of affected households and communities through lack of food, insufficient care and lack of time to ensure hygiene.

HIV/AIDS and nutritional status

Biologically, there are multiple relations between HIV/AIDS and nutritional status. Research shows that the chance of infection with the HIV virus might be reduced in individuals who have good nutritional status, with micronutrients and, especially, vitamin-A playing significant roles. At the same time, the onset of the disease and even death might be delayed in well-nourished HIV-positive individuals.

Because the virus damages the immune system, AIDS patients are vulnerable to multiple infections. A diet rich in protein, energy and micronutrients, especially vitamin-A, contributes to resistance to opportunistic infections in AIDS patients (Friis, 1998). Higher nutrient intakes are required when the patient suffers from a secondary disease. When diarrhoea occurs, extra liquids are required to restore the balance.

In these vulnerable individuals, the prevention of food-borne illnesses is extremely important as these would further increase the patients' needs and, at the same time, reduce their absorption of nutrients. Hygienic food handling and access to safe foods are, therefore, imperative.

Impact of HIV/AIDS on household food security and nutrition

HIV/AIDS has a detrimental impact on household food security and nutrition in endemic areas. Household food security is defined as the ability of the household to secure, either from its own production or through purchases, adequate food to meet the dietary needs of its members so that they can lead a healthy and active life.

In HIV/AIDS-affected households, problems start as soon as the first adult becomes sick. This results in increased spending for health care, decreased ability to carry out work and higher demands on time for care. Children might be forced to discontinue their schooling as the household needs their help and can no longer afford the school expenses. Eventually the AIDS patient dies, additional expenditures are made for the funeral and the productive capacity of the household is permanently reduced. Socio-cultural practices may further aggravate the problems of the household, for example, when the surviving spouse cannot maintain access to the property of the deceased.

In the next stage the patient's partner may become sick, problems increase and accumulate and the downward spiral accelerates. The household may find itself without cash reserves; often it becomes indebted and is forced to sell livestock and other productive resources. Traditional solidarity systems may wear out, and the family may progressively slide into destitution. Eventually, the household is reduced to elderly people and children. Essential skills are lost to the family and the community as active adults die.

Households affected by AIDS are at risk nutritionally: access to food is difficult; demand for care soars, together with time constraints; and it becomes increasingly difficult to preserve health.

The impact of the epidemic on food and agriculture is clearly related to people's livelihoods and will vary according to the different ecological zones, farming systems and stage of the epidemic. It may result in a shift from cash crops to less labour-intensive food crops, to more basic and less varied food production or to a reduction of productivity and cash income with corresponding adverse effects on household food security (FAO, 1995). Research carried out in Uganda showed that food insecurity and malnutrition (rather than medical treatment and drugs) were foremost among the immediate problems faced by female-headed AIDS-affected households (Topouzis and Hemrich, 1996). This further aggravates the situation, as good nutrition is of great importance to the victims of the AIDS epidemic as well as to children and pregnant and lactating women.

Types of Food and Nutrition Supplements

Nutrition and food-based interventions often include the term 'supplement', which refers to any food or nutritional product that is provided to supplement or add to the daily diet.

Three types of supplements should be considered:

1. **Food to manage HIV-related symptoms and secondary infections**; maintain weight and treat mild weight loss; manage the nutrition-related side effects of ART; and address nutritional needs in food insecure areas.

   For PLWHAs, foods that are enriched, easy to prepare and digest, and palatable during illness are preferred. Programmed food is intended to supplement the food that an individual or household has available, except in emergency situations.

2. **Nutrition supplements** for specific HIV positive groups at risk of malnutrition.

   This includes multi-vitamin supplements for HIV-positive children, special fortified foods for non-breastfed children six months and older, and nutritional supplements for pregnant and lactating women, according to WHO or national protocols. Such supplements may include iron-folic acid pills for pregnant women and to treat iron deficiency anemia, and multiple micronutrient (MM) supplements.

3. **Therapeutic foods for rehabilitation of moderate and severe malnutrition** in HIV-positive adults and children.

   This includes nutrient-dense foods that can be used for clinic-based stabilization and home- or community-based care as per WHO or national nutrition rehabilitation protocols. The foods and protocols used to treat severe and moderate malnutrition in the general population may be used for HIV-positive patients, although some adaptations may be required for adults and those experiencing severe symptoms. There are increased daily energy needs (10-30 percent) to maintain or recover weight loss and there is a heightened need to have palatable and easy-to-digest foods for those suffering from anorexia, oral sores, diarrhea, and other symptoms that affect ability to eat. Nutrient dense foods or food-spreads are an excellent way to insure that nutritional needs are being met in people with reduced appetite or ability to eat or absorb nutrients.

   When PLWHAs are questioned about their priority needs, food—not drugs, health services, or relief from stigma—is often the predominant response. The call for food may reflect the physical lack of food in the household, but it often echoes a lack of means or income to acquire food, despite the availability of food in the community or markets. Food aid can play an important role in bridging short-term food gaps, protecting the income and livelihood capacity of households affected by HIV/AIDS and, consequently, supporting both short- and long-term food security.

   Food can be obtained from external donations or locally. While it is recognized that external food aid is not a sustainable resource, the intention is to make the best use of food to ensure that no harm is done and, eventually, communities will be able to respond to food security shocks. In the long term, sustainable strategies should include local ownership, skills development, infrastructure development, income-generating activities, and sustainable agricultural and natural resource development particularly focused on locally available resources and foods. In designing programs using food aid, it is important to do a thorough analysis of vulnerability to food insecurity in the specific communities affected by HIV/AIDS. An analysis should include documentation of all major factors that are contributing to food insecurity, including drought and climactic factors, economic factors, conflict and displacement, and acute or chronic disease, including HIV/AIDS. Livelihood and coping mechanisms and local capacities should also be assessed. Such analyses should be done for programs distributing a general ration, as well as for those targeting PLWHAs and affected individuals, households, and communities. It is important to focus on what communities can do to address the food insecurity impacts of HIV/AIDS and other care issues.

The goals and objectives of nutrition and food interventions for PLWHAs vary according to the disease stage of the individual, and whether or not they are receiving ART and other treatments for secondary infections. Goals and objectives will also vary according to the group being targeted for interventions. Interventions for which an adequate evidence base currently exists and that should be immediately included in program are listed below. Other interventions, including food aid and food security programs, are likely to be effective in certain situations and may be supported on a pilot basis while further evidence is gathered.

Food-based Approach to Support HIV/AIDS-affected Households and Communities

A food based programme can be used to support the HIV/AIDS-affected Households and Communities in the following areas:-

Treatment of PLWHAs, including children

- Food to improve adherence to ART
- Food to improve treatment efficacy
- Food to help manage drug side effects

Prevention of HIV infection

- Food as an income transfer and asset protection
- Food to prevent or reduce high-risk behaviors or reliance on negative coping strategies
- Food as an incentive for voluntary testing and counseling
- Food as an incentive for participation in PMTCT and PMTCT+

For Communities in high prevalence or high risk areas

- Food as incentive to participate in HIV/AIDS awareness and behaviour change programmes
- Food as an incentive for voluntary testing and counseling
- Food as an income transfer and asset protection and to prevent or reduce high-risk behaviours or reliance on negative coping strategies

Care and Support of PLWHAs

- Food to supplement daily nutritional requirements and special dietary needs, such as increased energy requirements
- Food to support nutritional management of symptoms of opportunistic infections (e.g., anorexia, diarrhea, nausea)
- Food for use in hospitals and hospices as a part of palliative care
- Food to provide safety net and income transfer
- Food as an income transfer and asset protection
- Food for training in life skills, life planning, alternative livelihood strategies

For Affected households :

- Food to supplement daily nutritional requirements of affected household members
- Food to provide safety net and income transfer for affected households and guardians
- Food for education as a nutritional supplement, income transfer and guardianship incentive

- Food as an income transfer and asset protection
- Food as an income transfer to encourage school attendance
- Food for training in life skills, life planning, alternative livelihood strategies
- Food as a bridge for adopting new technologies and practices or establishing new

As livelihood strategies in institutions

- Food to supplement daily nutritional requirements
- Food as an income transfer to assist with costs of care, free-up cash resources for provision of other critical services, and facilitate school and training programme attendance for Street children
- Food to supplement daily nutritional requirements
- Food to encourage attendance at skills training or counseling sessions Communities in high prevalence or high risk areas
- Food as an income transfer or to cover opportunity costs to voluntary care providers
- Food for training voluntary care providers
- Food as a bridge for establishing community-based social safety nets (e.g., food banks) and care and support services
- Food as an income transfer and asset protection and to prevent or reduce high risk behaviours or reliance on negative coping strategies

What is the Appropriate Way to Deliver:

Food Aid in a Community? A programme manager should work with the community to determine the most effective and efficient means of distributing the food based on the human, financial, and other resources the community can provide. If food is available, two approaches to distribute food are take-home rations and on-site feeding. The decision is between a more flexible and administratively simpler take-home option and the more controlled on-site feeding option.

Take-home Rations. This is the most common method of food distribution, in which food rations are provided to households to be taken home for storage, preparation, and consumption. Take-home rations are targeted to households with the greatest need or provided generally to a community, as in the case of emergencies or natural disasters.

On-site Feeding. Food is prepared at a center, and participants consume the meal or snack, such as biscuits, on site. Snacks provided at schools can help increase school attendance as well as address children's nutritional needs. Providing a meal to all students—not just to orphans—can forestall the stigma and resentment that can arise in community-based feeding programme. Communities affected by HIV/AIDS have created a variety of institutions to care for and provide services to affected children.. Food aid has been used to help support such self-help efforts, but programmes should be monitored carefully to ensure that they do not undermine community integration or development.

Each method has advantages and disadvantages.

Take-home rations generally require fewer resources to manage and take less time to establish a distribution system. In addition, this approach is less time-consuming for recipients, who do not have to travel long distances to obtain food every day. However, in cases where only certain groups are targeted for food distribution and the programme seeks to prevent dilution to other family members.

On-site feeding may be more advantageous. It may also be more effective where firewood and cooking utensils are in short supply and households are unable to prepare meals or where the security situation is poor and beneficiaries are at risk when carrying food home.

It is recommended that in each community, an existing group be identified to help manage the food programme. This group should already be actively engaged in assisting vulnerable persons in the community, preferably drawing mostly or entirely on locally available resources. If no such group exists, a committee can be organized by the external agency or a partner. If a programme wants to provide take-home rations to households with PLWHAs or orphans, a team should be employed to be responsible for the logistics. This includes advance planning and ordering of food, receiving and storing the food from the donor, delivering food to the recipient households, and establishing a simple monitoring system to keep track of the food provided to each household. In an on-site feeding programme, the committee selects community members to be responsible for preparing and serving the meals. An exit strategy that defines more sustainable food interventions should be developed, since food donations will not continue indefinitely. As part of the exit strategy, the committee should also define criteria for deciding when a household should stop receiving donated foods and become involved in other interventions that promote livelihood security.

Who are the Beneficiaries and What are their Energy Needs? Once the approach for food distribution is decided, it is important to determine who the beneficiaries will be and the appropriate eligibility criteria. A programme working with community leaders may want to review whether it will be providing food for all households in a community or targeting specific groups such as households with PLWHAs or orphans or, more specifically, orphans under the age of five.

Priority Nutrition and Food-based Actions The goals and objectives of nutrition and food interventions for PLWHAs vary according to the disease stage of the individual, and whether or not they are receiving ART and other treatments for secondary infections. Goals and objectives will also vary according to the group being targeted for interventions.

Impact on services and institutions

The epidemic takes a heavy toll on national development staff. The health, education and agriculture extension services usually provided to the population will be disrupted as the staff operating these activities become ill and die. Provision of care to sick family members, attendance at funerals and observation of mourning times further reduce the staff's productive time. This disruption in services further aggravates the local situation and undermines households' capacity to cope with the illness.

HIV/AIDS issues in nutrition and agricultural development strategies

The HIV/AIDS epidemic and strategies for mitigating its impact are often not given specific attention by rural development workers and/or agriculture project staff. This frequently leads to further marginalization and destitution of affected households.

With an estimated 16 000 new infections per day, worldwide, and the rapid decreases in life expectancy in the most affected countries, the AIDS epidemic should be a primary focus of development assistance in affected countries . For organizations working in agriculture, the natural entry point to mitigate the impact of the epidemic is through improving household food security. Knowledge of the local dynamics among HIV/AIDS, food insecurity and malnutrition, including households' coping strategies (to offset labour shortages, decline in income, etc.) will allow projects to identify and design activities according to existing needs and constraints and help to mitigate the impact of the epidemic.

Targeting affected households

Projects operating in HIV/AIDS endemic areas do not always reach the households struck by the epidemic. In such areas, HIV/AIDS-affected households should systematically be included in the target groups of household food security and nutrition projects. These projects need to be able to identify where the most affected communities are located and which households are living with HIV/AIDS. Project activities should not obstruct the provision of care to the sick, infants and young children, including orphans, and special activities might need to be developed to support these. Training and support for youth will be essential to the survival of the household as a whole.

Raising awareness of field staff

In many countries, HIV/AIDS is not openly discussed. Raising awareness among field staff about the disease and prevention methods is the first step to be taken. Before HIV/AIDS considerations can be addressed, staff need to be trained to understand the impact of HIV/AIDS on food security and the specific constraints suffered by affected households. Field staff from all technical and institutional backgrounds need to be trained on how to identify affected households and help them to find solutions to the constraints they face.

To use food effectively as a means of providing care and support to HIV-affected households and mitigate the impact of HIV/AIDS, programme managers should pursue a four-step process:

1. Facilitate a community-led assessment of local food sources and care practices to determine effective uses of all food;
2. to design and implement a food strategy in collaboration with the community stakeholders, based on decisions about the purpose of the food, how food will be delivered and stored, and who is eligible to participate, including an exit or transition strategy phasing down the reliance on food aid;
3. Decide and calculate ration composition and size and frequency of schedule for distribution; and
4. Link communities to other services, including health, hygiene, water, sanitation, growth promotion, and other food security interventions.

Facilitating a Community-led Situation Assessment

In designing a programme to address a particular dimension of food insecurity, especially the additional burden of HIV/AIDS, it is necessary to work backwards from the immediate manifestations of food insecurity to the root causes of the problem. Understanding the causes of food insecurity requires a significant amount of information gathering. Normally, quantitative information will be available to begin this analysis from data collected routinely by the host government agriculture, health, or planning ministries, national survey data sets . In addition, it is also typically necessary to conduct field studies using a combination of qualitative and quantitative methods to ensure an understanding of local conditions in the intended programme area. It is advisable to work with the community to ensure that the community conducts its own assessment of the situation and then devises an appropriate action plan based on the findings. In most cases, a series of simple and related questions can provide a very general structure to guide the information-gathering process. While the questions themselves are simple, obtaining their answers may be quite complex, requiring expertise from a variety of relevant technical disciplines.

The questions to begin the information gathering process include:

- Where do households get their food?
- What factors limit the ability of households to obtain food from each of these sources?
- How do households obtain their cash income, and what factors limit the ability of households to obtain income from each of these sources?
- What factors limit how well households use their food to meet the dietary needs of the individuals within them?
- Who are the most food insecure or vulnerable population groups? Involving community leaders, health workers, educators, household members and PLWHAs in both the gathering and analysis of the information is useful for obtaining accurate information and designing an intervention that will be beneficial to all members of the community.

Issues that may need to be included are:

- What traditional community feeding and care practices promote good health and nutrition for adults and adolescents and which practices promote appropriate breastfeeding and complementary feeding practices for infants and young children?
- What traditional feeding and care practices exist for special needs groups such as PLWHAs, pregnant and lactating women ,and orphans and vulnerable children?
- What locally available foods are used for household consumption or sold or traded, and what is their availability throughout the seasons? This should include all items consumed by the family, including insects, herbs, fruits, vegetables, legumes, nuts, and other plant and animal products that are purchased, bartered, grown, or gathered by households.
- What food preparation and storage techniques are commonly used?

- What are the market services, including where people buy food and medicines, micronutrients, or herbal supplements for promoting good health, including traditional medicines?
- What are the links to health services and other government and nongovernmental assistance?
- What are the available sources and types of food aid provided in safety net and other programmes? Programme managers may be able to obtain existing information from governmental and nongovernmental reports, household surveys, and food consumption surveys. Rapid food security assessments and qualitative data using techniques such as key informant interviews, focus group discussions, and observational studies are some of the methods that can be used to gather and complement this information. This phase is also important for identifying the beneficial and harmful practices that support or undermine good health; knowing these is useful for designing programmes and developing messages for good nutrition.

Designing and Implementing a Food Programme : The initial assessment should provide an understanding of food security conditions and constraints in a given area. Programme managers should continue to work with the community to develop a set of programme goals and objectives where the probability of a successful intervention is highest while addressing constraints. A clear and measurable set of goals and objectives is the first step towards developing performance indicators and establishing an effective monitoring and evaluation system. Once the goals and objectives have been established, it is necessary to agree on how the objectives will be met, including developing a strategy for delivering food and other services. In many instances, it is preferable to work with existing organizations and committees in a community rather than creating entirely new structures. Experience has shown that mobilizing groups for the sole purpose of receiving and distributing external aid often results in weak short-lived structures that are less able and willing to mobilize their own local resources in the long term.

What is the Purpose of Introducing a Food Programme to the Community?

Food aid can have multiple uses Food-based programmes should be integrated with HIV/AIDS activities where appropriate and that the objectives of food-based programmes must be clearly stated. Any food based programme should meet the following broad programme objectives :-

- Nutritional care and support;
- Incentive for participation in HIV/AIDS related activities; and
- Income transfers to people infected with or affected by HIV/AIDS.

The broad objectives of food aid programming in the context of HIV/AIDS include:

- Prevent malnutrition and mortality among the *general population* due to deteriorating food security where HIV is one of a number of critical determinants of vulnerability through provision of a general food ration integrated with complementary inputs;
- Prevent nutritional deterioration among *individual PLWHAs* by providing general food rations and specialized foods with specific nutrient profiles and acceptability to improving treatment adherence by helping patients manage gastrointestinal side effects of ARVs;
- Provide incentives as a form of income-in- kind to increase participation in the prevention of mother-to-child transmission (PMTCT), PMTCT+, and other prevention, treatment, or palliative care programs, as well as partial payment for care and increasing enrollment in schools for orphans and vulnerable children; and
- Protect livelihoods through supporting safety net programmes, asset protection and food-for-work or training programmes such as skill enhancement targeting *communities and households affected by HIV/AIDS.* In some programmes, food serves multiple purposes. For example, in maternal and child health programmes, food plays a preventative nutritional role and is an incentive for mothers to participate in key health services such as immunization and counselling. The use of the food will determine its type and quantity, who is eligible,

and the likely result. It is important to understand and agree on the use of the food. The use can change over time and in response to a community emergency such as a flood or drought. In programmes to assist HIV-affected households, food is sometimes focused on helping household members maintain their nutritional status. This is because most households seriously affected by HIV/AIDS experience chronic food shortages that affect all members. There are examples of specialized foods being promoted to be used by PLWHAs.

Linking Communities with Other Services

Providing food can play an important role in providing nutritional support to HIV-infected individuals, including management of drug related side effects of ARV therapies; assisting HIV-affected households to cope with a member who is living with AIDS; providing extra food to overburdened households caring for children orphaned by the disease; and assisting households that have suffered the recent loss of a member to allocate resources to cover other expenses associated with an illness or loss. If food aid is provided, it should be part of an overall intervention strategy that builds the capacity of AIDS-affected households and communities to sustain them over the long term. Programmes that use food to provide nutritional support to households are most efficient when combined or linked to other services such as:

- Prevention of HIV transmission, including the prevention of MTCT during pregnancy, delivery, and infant care; Treatment of HIV infection with HAART;
- Nutrition education and counseling to ensure proper utilization, preparation, and storage of foods;
- Growth promotion, breastfeeding, and basic child health services to promote the health of young children;
- Health services to manage and treat infections, especially diarrhea, TB, and Malaria, which can worsen malnutrition;
- Reproductive health services, particularly pre- and post-natal care to assist pregnant and lactating women;
- Psychosocial support for PLWHAs and family members to cope with the illness and plan for the future; and

- Other types of economic and social support, including microfinance, agricultural training, vocational training, and school feeding programmes, and programmes that help HIV-affected households maintain their income, savings, and overall livelihood security. The actual increases in consumption required by individual HIV-positive beneficiaries will depend on their age, sex, and symptoms.

Institution-based Feeding Programmes Institutions, such as orphanages, community groups, hospitals, hospices, and health clinics provide on-site and take-home rations for specific groups, including HIV/AIDS-affected people. These programmes are usually targeted to people who are living with AIDS who come for medical treatment and care, children who have lost a parent to HIV/AIDS, or street children. Designing a complete diet for participants fed at institutions requires careful consideration of how to meet nutritional needs and ensure that food is appealing, culturally acceptable, and easy to prepare, serve and consume and that resources are available to ensure needs can be met over time. The role of food aid should be to complement locally available foods, especially fruits and vegetables.

Institutional and Home-based Care for Severely Malnourished Individuals In some cases, people suffering from AIDS or children orphaned by the death of a parent may become severely malnourished and need therapeutic foods and medical care to reduce the risk of death or excessive morbidity. Severe acute malnutrition occurs once AIDS has developed, but these children are often underweight and stunted even before AIDS symptoms are evident. More significant, however, is that the indirect impact of HIV on nutrition by the underlying poverty, which also results in acute malnutrition events. HIV-positive children do respond to treatment for severe acute malnutrition using special foods. The nature of the HIV results in bouts of infection and weight loss and is therefore difficult to treat. The approach to using specialized foods for HIV positive people should combine both supplementary feeding approaches with therapeutic feeding. In therapeutic feeding, a person receives both medical and nutritional care until he/she gains sufficient weight. The timeframe for rehabilitating a severely malnourished child without HIV infection is generally four to six weeks and can be longer. For HIV-infected adults and children, however, weight gain may not be sufficient or relapse, and programmes will need to assess with households whether nutritional care or more intensive medical treatment is needed. In addition to center-based therapeutic care, home-based or Community Therapeutic Care (CTC) can be used to deal with rehabilitation of severely malnourished adults and children. Often, critical to home based or CTC is the availability of ready-to-use therapeutic food (RUTF) and includes vitamins and minerals, and consists of locally produced foods like peanut, butter, oil, full cream milk, and sugar.

Developing strategies with the communities

The participatory nutrition approach promoted by the Food and Agriculture Organisation's (FAO) Food and Nutrition Division includes the joint development of local household food and nutrition strategies by the different stakeholders. In HIV/AIDS-affected areas, organizing local planning and training workshops to discuss local food security and nutrition problems among various local groups and institutions would help identify possible interventions that could mitigate the negative impact of the epidemic.

Participatory appraisal of the impact of HIV/AIDS on food security in a given community can help identify affected households and clarify local dynamics among HIV/AIDS, food insecurity and malnutrition, including households' coping strategies.

Strategies to improve the coping mechanisms of affected households might include activities aimed at:

- reorienting food production to facilitate access to a nutritious diet;
- seeking alternative income-generating opportunities;
- decreasing people's workload through labour-saving technologies and improving access to labour and resources through gender sensitization and the promotion of more gender-balanced extension approaches;
- improving community organization for the exchange of labour;
- developing community-based care strategies for patients and small children, including orphans;
- encouraging HIV-positive and sick patients to teach their skills and knowledge to others and assisting households to plan for the future;

- developing appropriate communication strategies to prevent the marginalization of affected households and helping the community to deal with the epidemic.

Nutrition education

All field staff, in particular agricultural extension workers, should be informed of the beneficial impact of good nutritional status, both on the prevention of HIV infection and on the course of the disease, so that they can provide advice to families and reorient their own activities accordingly. Nutrition education and communication strategies in the affected areas should include appropriate dietary recommendations for individuals suffering from the disease, taking into account local food sources and production systems. Collaboration with local male and female leaders (e.g. traditional and religious leaders) needs to be sought.

Transfer of knowledge and skills

The training of staff and community members and the timely transfer of essential skills are needed to mitigate the destructive impact on households and institutions. If required, and where possible, individuals who already suffer from the disease should be involved in this process.

Since nutrition requires an integrated approach to household food security, health and care, it forms a logical entry point for assisting affected communities in coping with the epidemic.

Several key points should be considered:

- Appropriate nutrition education is required as well as the transfer of knowledge and skills to prevent their loss to the household and the wider community.
- Participatory techniques are fundamental in the development of a comprehensive understanding of the specific constraints that HIV/AIDS-affected communities are facing, as well as in the design of adequate responses.
- Since behavioural change is needed for effective prevention and mitigation of the epidemic, and since HIV/AIDS issues are highly sensitive, the development of appropriate communication strategies is crucial.

- The inclusion of HIV/AIDS considerations into agricultural and nutrition strategies is a relatively new field. Cross-sectoral and inter-institutional collaboration is required to develop appropriate strategies through operation research and documentation and the evaluation of experiences.

17

Frequently Asked Questions about HIV/AIDS and Nutrition

1. **What is Good Nutrition**

   Good nutrition means eating foods each day that will give you the vitamins, minerals, and other things you need to keep your body strong. It means eating foods that give you enough calories to have a healthy body weight. It means getting enough protein to keep your body built up and repair any damage it may have.

2. **Why is nutrition important for people living with HIV/AIDS ?**

   Nutritional care and support promote well-being, self-esteem and a positive attitude to life for people and their families living with HIV/AIDS. Healthy and balanced nutrition should be one of the goals of counselling and care for people at all stages of HIV infection. An effective programme of nutritional care and support will improve the quality of life of people living with HIV/AIDS, by:

   - maintaining body weight and strength;
   - replacing lost vitamins and minerals;
   - improving the function of the immune system and the body's ability to fight infection;

- extending the period from infection to the development of the AIDS disease;
- improving response to treatment; reducing time and money spent on health care;
- keeping HIV-infected people active, allowing them to take care of themselves, their family and children; and
- keeping HIV-infected people productive, able to work, grow food and contribute to the income of their families.

3. What is the role of vitamins and mineral intake in HIV/AIDS ?

Vitamins and minerals are essential to keep healthy. They protect against opportunistic infection by ensuring that the lining of skin, lungs and gut remain healthy and that the immune system functions properly. Of special importance are vitamin A, vitamin C, vitamin E, certain B-group vitamins and minerals such as selenium, zinc and iron. A mixed diet should provide enough of these vitamins and minerals.

4. What is the role of micronutrient supplementation in HIV/AIDS ?

When food intake is low, multivitamin and mineral supplements - often in the form of pills - can help to meet increased requirements.

If supplements are considered necessary, the following guidelines should be adhered to:

- Discuss your intake of vitamin and mineral supplements with your health worker or nutritionist.
- Always take vitamin pills on a full stomach. Be consistent and take them regularly.
- It is probably cheaper to take a combined product with minerals rather than several pills containing different vitamins and minerals. However, iron may be a problem for people with HIV/AIDS as it can increase the activity of some bacteria. Supplements that do not contain iron are therefore better.
- Take any vitamin or mineral supplementation according to the advice on the label. More is not better. Taking

high doses can cause nausea, vomiting, decreased appetite and liver and kidney problems as well as interfere with the immune system. This is particularly true for vitamin A, vitamin E, zinc and iron.

Micronutrient supplements can be useful but cannot replace eating a balanced and healthy diet.

5. Why do people living with HIV/AIDS have special nutritional needs ?

A person who is infected with HIV/AIDS and is not showing signs of illness does not need a specific diet. However, those infected with HIV should make every effort to adopt healthy and balanced nutrition patterns in order to meet their increased protein and energy requirements and maintain their nutritional status.

Once people with HIV/AIDS become ill they will have special needs

5.1 Why do People living with HIV/AIDS have increased nutrient needs?

When infected with the HIV virus the body's defence system - the immune system - works harder to fight infection. This increases energy and nutrient requirements. Further infection and fever also increase the body's demand for food. Once people are infected with HIV they have to eat more to meet these extra energy and nutrient needs. Such needs will increase even further as the HIV/AIDS symptoms develop.

5.2 Why don't people with HIV/AIDS eat enough?

People with HIV/AIDS often do not eat enough because:

- the illness and the medicines taken for it may reduce the appetite, modify the taste of food and prevent the body from absorbing it;
- symptoms such as a sore mouth, nausea and vomiting make it difficult to eat;
- tiredness, isolation and depression reduce the appetite and the willingness to make an effort to prepare food and eat regularly;

- there is not enough money to buy food.

5.3. Why do HIV/AIDS reduces the absorption of food?

- Food, once eaten, is broken down by digestion into nutrients. These nutrients pass through the gut walls into the bloodstream and are transported to the organs and tissues in the body where they are needed. One of the consequences of HIV and other infections is that since the gut wall is damaged, food does not pass through properly and is consequently not absorbed.
- Diarrhoea is a common occurrence in people with HIV/AIDS. When a person has diarrhoea the food passes through the gut so quickly that it is not properly digested and fewer nutrients are absorbed.
- Reduced food intake and absorption lead to weight loss and malnutrition.

6. How can I Prevent weight loss during and after illness?

Infection increases the body's requirements for nutrients. Illness also reduces the appetite and the ill person will eat less food, causing weight loss. Firs you have to treat the underlying cause of weight loss like loss of appetite, diarrhoea, vomiting, sore mouth and nausea etc. Early treatment of infection is important to maintain body weight. If infection persists and cannot be cured by nutritional management within a couple of days, advice and treatment should be sought from a doctor, nutritionist, nurse or local health worker. Once the infection is over and the person is feeling better, he or she should start eating normally again. It is important to regain the weight lost as soon as possible and to restore the body's nutritional reserves.

7. How can I gain weight ?

HIV/AIDS affects weight. When a person does not eat enough food, or the food eaten is poorly absorbed, the body draws on its reserve stores of energy from body fat and protein from muscle. As a result, the person loses weight because body weight and muscles are lost. The weight loss may be so gradual that it is not obvious. There are two basic ways to discover whether weight is being lost.

- Weigh the person on the same day once a week and keep a record of the weight and date. For an average adult, serious weight loss is indicated by a 10 percent loss of body weight or 6-7 kg in one month. If a person does not have scales at home it might be possible to make an arrangement with a chemist, clinic or local health unit to weigh him or her.
- When clothes become loose and no longer fit properly.
- If a person loses weight he or she needs to take action to increase weight to the normal level.

Weight is gained by eating more food, either by eating larger portions and/or eating meals more frequently, using a variety of foods.

Here are some suggestions for gaining weight:

- Eat more staple foods such as rice, maize, millet, sorghum, wheat, bread, potatoes, sweet potatoes, yams and bananas.
- Increase intake of beans, soy products, lentils, peas, groundnuts, peanut butter and seeds, such as sunflower and sesame.
- Include all forms of meat, poultry, fish and eggs as often as possible. Minced meat, chicken and fish are easier to digest. Offal (such as kidney and liver) can be the least expensive source.
- Eat snacks regularly between meals. Good snacks are nuts, seeds, fruit, yoghurt, carrots, cassava crisps, crab crisps and peanut butter sandwiches.
- Slowly increase the fat content of the food by using more fats and oils, as well as eating fatty foods - oilseeds such as groundnuts, soy and sesame, avocados and fatty meat. If problems with a high fat intake are experienced (especially diarrhoea), reduce the fat intake until the symptoms are over and then gradually increase it to a level that the body can tolerate.
- Introduce more dairy products such as full-cream milk, sour milk, buttermilk, yoghurt and cheese into the diet.

- Add dry milk powder to foods such as porridge, cereals, sauces and mashed potatoes. However, do not use coffee and tea whiteners, which do not have the same nutritional benefits as milk. Note that some people may find milk difficult to digest. It should be avoided if it causes cramps, a feeling of being full or skin rashes.
- Add sugar, honey, jam, syrup and other sweet products to the food.

Make meals as attractive as possible.

8. What About Junk Food?

Sometimes is very tempting to eat junk food instead of healthy food. A bag of chips, a cola and a candy bar seem so much easier to eat, and taste good too. Some facts about junk food can help you make your own decisions about whether or not to eat it.

First of all, some things that people call "junk food" are really good for you. Pizza, hamburger, tacos, sandwiches, and ice cream are all very nutritious. You can feel good about eating them. Some other "junk foods" are not as nutritious. Candy, chips, and soft drinks are mostly made of fat and sugar. They have very little protein, vitamins and minerals. If you eat too much of them, you may find you are not hungry for foods in the basic food groups which give you what your body needs. Junk food usually has a lot of calories. Eating foods with a lot of calories can make people gain weight. When you are infected with HIV, you may find yourself losing more weight than is good for you. Candy, cookies, and soft drinks may help you gain weight at these times. You can enjoy them along with foods from the basic food groups for extra calories and good nutrition too!

9. What problems could make it hard for me to eat a healthy diet?

You might have trouble eating if you have sores in your mouth, diarrhoea, nausea or just a poor appetite. If you have trouble eating or exercising, talk to your doctor.

10. What are some good tips for eating right?

A few simple steps can help you make sure your food is healthy and safe:

- Wash your hands with soap and water before you eat so you won't get an infection from germs on your hands.
- Wash fruits and vegetables before you eat them or cook them.
- Wash your hands with soap and water after you touch raw fish, chicken or meat so you won't get an infection.
- Be sure that meat, eggs and fish are well cooked before you eat them.

Here are some ways to put good nutrition into your diet:

- Have high-calorie protein drinks or shakes. Adding powdered milk can increase the nutrition in other drinks.
- Drink 8 to 10 glasses of filtered water each day.
- Keep nutritious snacks on hand.
- Eat high-calorie foods if you're losing weight.
- Call your doctor if you lose 5 pounds or more when you didn't want to.
- Talk to your doctor about taking a multivitamin every day. Take your multivitamin with a meal so your stomach won't get upset.

11. What can I do if I'm having trouble eating?

- If you don't have an appetite—Try to eat your favourite foods. Instead of eating 3 big meals each day, eat 6 to 8 small meals. Drink high-calorie protein shakes with your meals or between meals.
- If you have diarrhoea—Don't eat fried foods and other high-fat foods like potato chips. Don't eat high-fibre foods. Instead, eat bland foods like bread, rice and applesauce. Ask your doctor about taking nutritional supplements, such as Ensure.
- If you have mouth sores—Avoid citrus fruits like oranges and grapefruit. Avoid very hot or cold foods. Don't eat spicy foods. Try not to eat hard foods like chips and pretzels. Use a straw to drink liquids.

- If you have nausea and vomiting—Avoid drinking any liquid with your meals. Eat 6 to 8 small meals each day instead of 3 large meals. Eat foods with a mild flavour. Eat foods at a medium temperature, not hot or cold. Drink nutritional supplements and sports drinks. Sit and relax for 30 minutes after you eat.

12. What is the role of Traditional medical treatments in HIV/AIDS ?

Traditional treatments differ greatly from region to region and are often very specific to a location. Therefore, locally known and available treatments and their advantages and disadvantages discussed. People with HIV/AIDS often become frustrated with management of the disease. Many are willing to try anything in the hope of staying healthy and living longer. HIV/AIDS is not a traditional illness and so far there is no hard evidence to believe that traditional medicines can treat HIV and cure AIDS. However, certain traditional medicines may help to treat many of the symptoms of opportunistic infections that are part of AIDS. While some of these medicines may be undoubtedly helpful, others may be dangerous because they may do more harm than good, they are expensive and therefore reduce money available for buying food, and they may require avoidance of certain foods. It is therefore recommended always to discuss treatments with a health worker or nutritionist and avoid any treatment or practice, such as fasting, that could possibly reduce food intake and cause weight loss.

Herbs and spices

Herbs and spices can improve digestion, stimulate appetite and preserve foods. A list of herbs and the beneficial effects claimed by people living with HIV/AIDS are given in the following table opposite. The effects may not be the same for all people. People can try these herbs and decide for themselves whether they are helpful. They may also know of other remedies used in their country that they want to add.

Herb	*Benefits found by some people living with HIV/AIDS*	*How to use*
Aloe	Helps to relieve constipation	Use as extract; boil and drink the concentrated water. To be used in limited amounts; stop immediately if it causes cramps or diarrhoea
Basil	Helps to relieve nausea and aid digestion; has an antiseptic function for mouth sores	Add to food to treat nausea and digestive problems. Use as gargle for mouth sores
Calendula	Flower heads have antiseptic, anti-inflammatory and healing function. Helps with infections of the upper digestive tract	Use as a compress to treat infected wounds. Prepare as tea to help digestion
Cardamom	Helps with digestive problems, pain, diarrhoea, nausea, vomiting and loss of appetite	Add to food during cooking or prepare as tea
Cayenne	Stimulates appetite, helps fight infection, heals ulcers and intestina inflammation	Add a pinch to cooked or raw foods. For an energizing drink add to fruit juice or water

(Contd.)

(Contd Table.)

Herb	*Benefits found by some people living with HIV/AIDS*	*How to use*
Camomile	Helps digestion and provides relief for nausea	Prepare tea from the leaves and flowers and drink several cups throughout the day
Cinnamon	Good for colds and for weakness after colds or flu. Also used when feeling cold, for diarrhoea and nausea. Stimulates appetite. Gently stimulates digestive juices, encouraging bowel movements	Either add to meals or in tea, particularly ginger cinnamon tea for chesty colds or tuberculosis (see recipe in Annex 1)
Cloves	Stimulate appetite, help weak digestion, diarrhoea, nausea and vomiting	Use in soups, stews, warmed fruit juice and tea
Coriander	Helps to increase appetite and reduce flatulence. Controls bacteria and fungi	Add herb to meals
Eucalyptus	Has an antibacterial function, particularly for lungs and during bronchitis. Eucalyptus oil from leaves increases the blood flow and reduces the symptoms of inflammation	Prepare tea from the leaves or extract (see recipe in Annex 1)

(Contd.)

(Contd Table.)

Herb	*Benefits found by some people living with HIV/AIDS*	*How to use*
Fennel	Helps to increase appetite, combat flatulence and expel gas	Add as spice to foods or prepare tea from the seeds. Use in limited amounts
Garlic	Has antibacterial, antiviral and antifungal function, particularly in the gut, intestines, lungs and vagina. Helps digestion and feeling of weakness. Also good for thrush, throat infections, herpes and diarrhoea	Prepare tea or energy drink (see recipe in Annex 1), or use in food
Ginger	Improves digestion, energizes, relieves diarrhoea and stimulates appetite. Used for treating common colds, flu and nausea	Use either as a spice in meals or prepare a ginger tea (see recipe in Annex 1)
Lemon	Is antibacterial and helps digestion	Add lemon juice to food or drinks
Lemon grass	Has a calming effect as well as soothing digestion and alleviating stress	Use as tea
Mint	Has an anti-inflammatory effect and helps digestion	Use as tea or gargle for mouth sores. Chew mint leaves to aid digestion

(Contd.)

(Contd Table.)

Herb	*Benefits found by some people living with HIV/AIDS*	*How to use*
Neem	Brings down fever	Cut a fresh twig, remove the leaves and boil the bark in water; drink as tea. The bark can also be chewed
Parsley	Reduces intestinal colic. Stimulates stomach secretions and activities and produces a feeling of hunger. The seed is used to remove excess water from the body	Add raw or cooked to food
Peppermint	May help nausea. Reduces colic (abdominal pain and cramps), helps to control diarrhoea and stop vomiting. Used for relieving tension and sleeplessness	Prepare as tea, by boiling the leaves for about ten minutes. Add to food. (Peppermint can easily be grown in the garden and or in a pot near the house)

(Contd.)

(Contd Table.)

Herb	*Benefits found by some people living with HIV/AIDS*	*How to use*
Thyme	Has antiseptic and antifungal function. Relaxes nervous coughing and increases mucosal secretions. (particularly effective in the gut) Stimulates digestion and the growth of the good intestinal flora in the gut	Use as gargle or mouthwash, as a vaginal douche or as tea
Turmeric/ yellow root	Digestive aid, antiseptic and antioxidant	Use powdered in rice, cereals, etc.

Remember that all herbs and spices should be used in moderate amounts. Exceeding these amounts may cause problems and have a toxic effect; moreover, the function of the herbs and spices will not be increased. They cannot replace healthy eating and should not be used in place of a healthy and balanced diet.

Herbal treatments and remedies

The advice presented here is based on knowledge gained from people living with HIV/AIDS about useful herbal treatments and remedies. It does not claim that all herbs and remedies have the same effect on all people.

Many communities have their own knowledge of health and nutrition, based on local traditions and culture. It is important to understand and be sensitive to these traditional beliefs and the many kinds of traditional care available. They represent alternatives to formal general medicine and for many people will be the only options they have. Any external medical recommendations that people receive will be compared with their cultural practices and the recommendations of their traditional healers. People will only take action if the recommendations they receive appear to make sense and provide some benefit.

Some traditional beliefs and food practices may not be useful. It will be important to find out about local practices and explain both to people with HIV/AIDS and to traditional healers whenever and why such practices should not be followed. However, beneficial traditional practices that provide readily accessible, effective and low-cost remedies should be identified and promoted.

13. What To do if I am invited to be Involved In a Drug Trial Or Research Project

Drug trials provide the opportunity to start on new or unapproved drugs well before they are available to the general public. Remember: trials are developed and designed to evaluate the effectiveness of a particular treatment and its potential toxicity. Before deciding to take part in a trial special consideration to the possible pro's and con's of each trial should be considered.

In most trials, one arm (group of people who receive identical treatment) includes the unapproved drug and the other arm is a drug or drugs previously shown to have some benefit. Trials may contain several arms which study drugs at different dosage levels. This allows the researchers to compare the results of the new treatment to treatments which have already been approved for use by the Food and Drug Administration (FDA). Currently, many trials compare combinations that include protease inhibitors to combinations of non-protease inhibiting drugs that have already been shown to inhibit HIV replication. People have to decide if they are willing to risk being assigned to an arm that may contain drugs that are not as effective as the ones currently available through their health care provider.

Many health care plans have been slow to offer the viral HIV RNA test. These tests are generally agreed to be the most important test to track the progression of HIV. One way to get a free viral load test is to join a drug trial. Most trials will run these tests because they are the best tool to evaluate the efficacy of the new drugs. Before joining a trial, find out if the researchers will release viral RNA results to clients; also see if the tests will be released in a timely manner, or whether they wait until the end of the trial to release the HIV RNA results. If trials don't provide access to a viral load test, or if the trial is not going to release the results frequently, it may be better not to join the trial.

Some trials may ask participants to stop taking particular medication or may ask them not to start taking other medication. Always find out before starting a trial what restrictions will be place on participants. People who are even slightly uncomfortable with the requirements of the trial, should consult their health care provider before joining. Once in a trial, people should try to be as compliant with trial protocols as possible. If severe side effects appear, the investigators should be notified, and the option to withdraw from the trial should be considered. Trials can provide excellent opportunities for people to access drugs and tests that they would not otherwise have access to. Careful examination of the trial protocols and consultation with a health care provider are crucial when considering new drug trails.

14. What methods are available to measure the body lean mass ?

Weights and Measurements

Body weight alone is not the best indicator of body composition. Various other metrics can give a better sense of relative proportions of lean body mass and fat. Each method has its pros and cons; ask your healthcare provider which are most appropriate given your individual situation.

Body mass index (BMI): an equation that relates weight to height (weight in kilograms divided by height in meters squared). BMI below 18.5 indicates that a person is underweight; 18.5-24.9 is normal weight; 25.0-29.9 is overweight; and 30.0 or above is obese.

Waist-to-Hip Ratio: waist measurement (at the narrowest point) divided by hip measurement (at the widest point). Weight carried around the waist (an "apple" shape) is associated with greater cardiovascular risk than weight distributed around the hips and thighs (a "pear" shape). A healthy waist-to-hip ratio is below 0.9 for men or 0.8 for women. This measure may not be appropriate for HIV positive individuals with lipodystrophy.

Bioelectrical impedance analysis (BIA): a technique for determining body composition using a mild electrical current that travels more easily through muscle than fat.

Skinfold thickness: a technique that uses calipers to assess the amount of subcutaneous fat under the skin at multiple sites.

Hydrostatic weighing: a technique for assessing body density in which a person's weight measured when dry is compared to his or her underwater weight, accounting for residual air in the lungs and gastrointestinal tract.

Magnetic resonance imaging (MRI): a noninvasive method for viewing soft tissues of the body using a magnetic field.

Dual-energy X-ray absorptiometry (DEXA): an X-ray technique used to measure body composition, including proportion of fat and bone mineral density.

Computerized tomography (CT or CAT scans): a method of visualizing tissues of the body using X-rays.

15. What are the cardio vascular risks of people with HIV/ AIDS ?

Traditional cardiovascular risk factors — advancing age, male sex, cigarette smoking, high LDL cholesterol and triglyceride levels, insulin resistance, elevated blood pressure, and being overweight — are as important for HIV positive people as for anyone else . Obesity, and in particular visceral abdominal fat, has been linked to increased risk of cardiovascular disease. Lifestyle changes, including diet modification, weight loss (if needed), exercise, and smoking cessation, are the first line of defense against cardiovascular disease. In order to lose weight, HIV positive people must follow the same rules as everyone else: burn more calories than one takes in. But reducing the amount of fat and cholesterol in the diet is not always enough to reverse fat accumulation or bring blood lipids within a healthy range, and exercise may not have much effect on visceral fat. When this is the case, lipid-lowering medications (including the statin and fibrate classes) are often used. Altering one's antiretroviral regimen to include drugs less linked to high blood fat — such as substituting atazanavir (Reyataz) for another PI — is often effective.

16. What is the role of physical exercise in HIV/AIDS ?

Regular exercise makes a person feel more alert, helps to relieve stress and stimulates the appetite. Exercise is the only way to strengthen and build up muscles. The body uses muscles to store energy and protein that the immune system can draw upon when required. Exercise is therefore especially important for maintaining the health of people with HIV/AIDS.

It may be that everyday activities such as cleaning, working in the field and collecting firewood and water provide enough exercise. If a person's work does not involve much exercise, an enjoyable exercise programme should be found that can be part of his or her daily life. Exercise should not be tiring or stressful; gentle muscle-building exercise is recommended.

Walking, running, swimming or dancing are all suitable. People living with HIV/AIDS need to make an effort to find the exercise that they enjoy and that suits their situation.

17. How can I increase my strength?

An aerobic exercise like walking will help make you stronger. It's good to begin exercising slowly. Little by little, increase the amount of exercise. For example, you might start walking for 20 minutes 3 times a week. Then, after you get a little stronger, you can increase the walking time to 30 minutes 4 times a week. Talk with your doctor before you start.

Weight lifting is also a good way to increase your strength. The pictures below show several basic exercises. Start by trying to do a weight lifting exercise with a weight light enough that you can lift it 10 times. Lifting it once is called a "repetition." More than one repetition is called a "set." Try to do 2 sets of 10 repetitions. Rest for 90 seconds between each set.

You don't need to have fancy exercise equipment to do weight lifting. You can use soup or juice cans, books and other objects you have in the house. Start by lifting a weight that's comfortable for you and doesn't cause too much strain.

In the first week, do 1 or 2 different weight lifting exercises for each body part once or twice in the week. Start with a small weight in each hand, like 10 to 15 ounces (a can of soup or a can of beans), depending on the exercise. Each week increase the number of exercises you do and the number of times you exercise. Rest for 1 to 2 days between exercise sessions. When you're feeling sick, either exercise less or stop for a while.

Dumbbell bench press (for your chest, shoulders and the back of your arms)

Lie on a bench on your back. Hold a dumbbell in each hand, with your hands lined up with your shoulders. Have the palms of your hands facing down (toward your toes). Lower the dumbbells until your elbows are below the bench (left picture). Don't relax your arms at the bottom of this movement. As soon as your elbows are as low as they can go, move your arms up again to the starting position. Don't "lock" your elbows at the top of the movement (right picture). (This means, don't make your arms be exactly straight—leave a tiny little bend in your elbows.)

Remember: You can use cans of soup instead of dumbbells in these exercises.

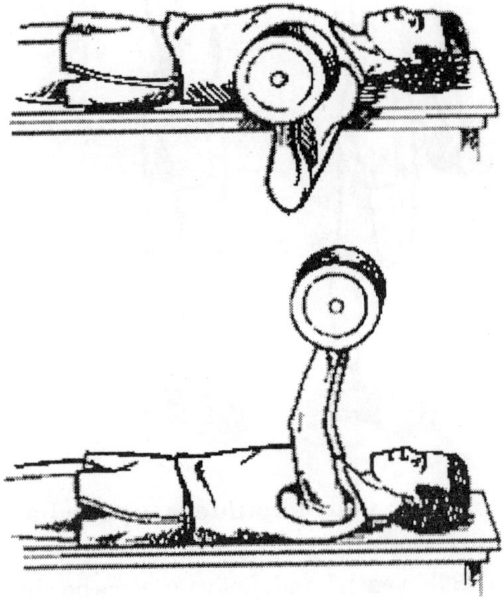

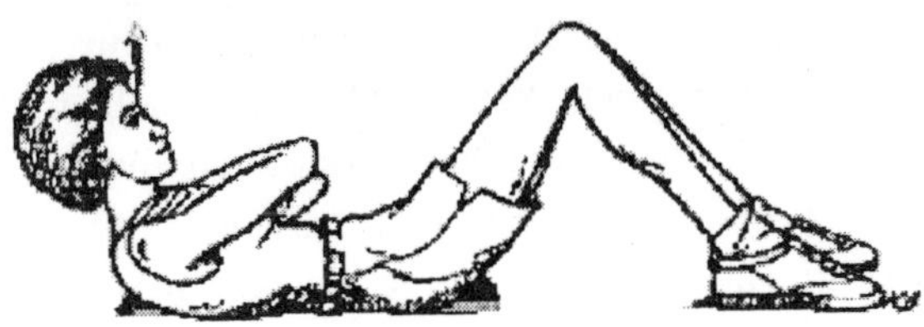

Crunches (for your abdomen)

Lie on your back on the floor. Keep your feet on the floor and your knees bent. Fold your arms across your chest. Now raise just your head and shoulders from the floor. This is a small and slow movement, like a curl. Your back stays on the floor. Slowly lower your head and shoulders back to the floor. When you are curling your head up, keep your chin up and your eyes looking at the ceiling. You can add resistance to this exercise by holding a weight on your chest.

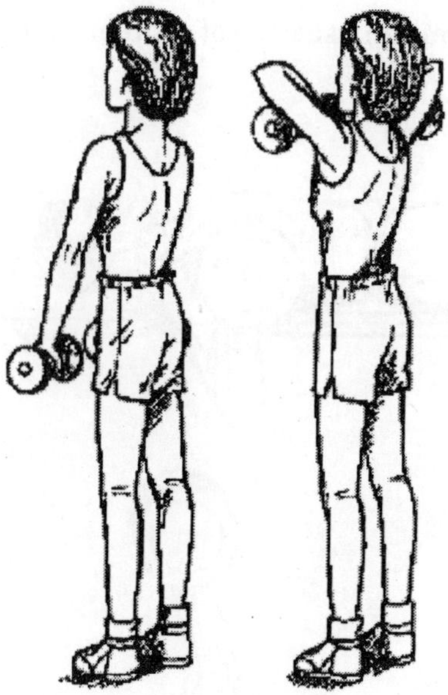

Upright row (for your shoulders, upper back and the front of your arms)

Hold a dumbbell in each hand. Let your arms be almost straight and resting on the front of your thighs. Your palms should face toward your legs. Now pull the dumbbells up to the level of your shoulders. Your elbows should go up first. When your elbows are about even with your ears, lower the dumbbells to your thighs again. Keep your knees bent just a tiny bit. Don't let yourself lean backwards.

Lunge (for the front and back of your legs and your buttocks)

Hold a dumbbell in each hand. Keep your arms down at your sides. Your palms should face your legs. Your feet should be even with your shoulders. Take a large step forward with your left leg. Lower your right knee until it's 1 inch above the floor. Now straighten your left leg and step back to the starting position. Repeat on the other leg. Remember that the movement is up and down, not really forward. Keep your back straight and your head up. Don't let yourself lean forward.

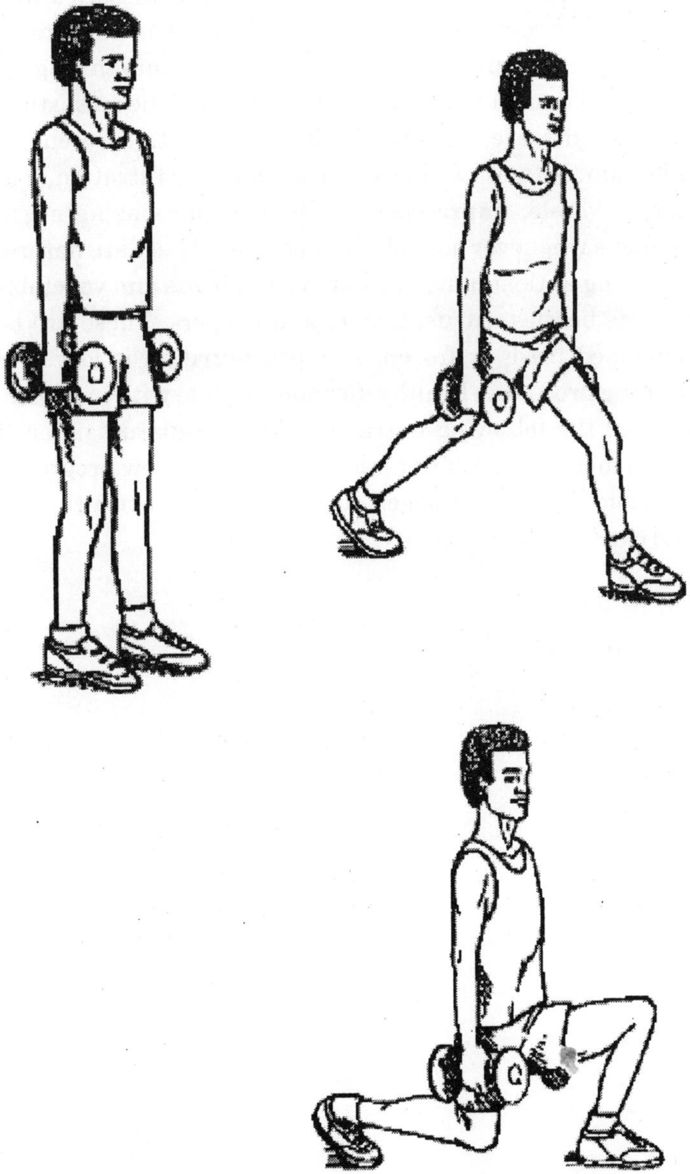

18. How can I protect myself against Free-Radical damage?

Fortunately, our bodies have a defence system to protect our cells from oxidative damage. Antioxidants, which are manufactured within our body or extracted from the food we eat, help neutralize the free radicals in our bodies. In order to protect and repair the cells in your body, it is important to make sure you are getting enough antioxidants through the food you eat and/or nutritional supplements. The most studied antioxidants are vitamin C, vitamin E, beta-carotene and selenium. Vitamin C. For this reason water filtration, a diet rich in whole, unprocessed foods, and purchasing organic products whenever possible is important . There are naturally occurring antioxidants present in fresh fruits and vegetables, such as berries, citrus, tomato and peppers. These are best consumed fresh or frozen, as much nutrition is lost in the canning process. A healthy diet and lifestyle with inclusion of some of the following nutrients will help guard against the inevitable damage of free-radicals and may slow progression of tissue damage. Dosages depend on patient health status and existing conditions.

Glossary

Adherence: Compliance with a drug regimen, as in taking medications correctly and on time. It encompasses the patient's active participation in his or her own healthcare, seeking medical advice, keeping appointments, following recommendations concerning lifestyle, as well as following medical regimens.

Anaemia: A lower than normal number of red blood cells.

Anorexia: The lack or loss of appetite that leads to significant decline in weight.

Antibody: A protein that is manufactured by lymphocytes (a type of white blood cell) to neutralize an antigen or foreign protein. Bacteria, viruses, and other microorganisms commonly contain many antigens.

Atherosclerosis: an inflammatory disease resulting in the accumulation of cholesterol-laden plaque in artery walls. Rupture of atherosclerotic plaque results in clot formation, which may result in myocardial infarction or ischemic stroke.

Bacteria : Single-celled organisms that can exist independently, symbiotically (in cooperation with another organism) or parasitically (dependent upon another organism, sometimes to the detriment of the other organism). Examples of bacteria include acidophilus (found in yogurt), streptococcus the cause of strep throat, and E. coli (a normal intestinal bacteria, as well as a disease-causing agent).

Blood sugar: Fuel source for the body, also known as glucose. Normal values are 70-120 mg/dl.

Body mass index (bmi): A measure of body fat based on height and weight that applies to both adult men and women.

Bone marrow: Soft tissue located in the cavities of the bones where blood cells such as erythrocytes, leukocytes, and platelets are formed.

Bone marrow suppression: A side effect of many anticancer and antiviral drugs, including AZT. Leads to a decrease in white blood cells, red blood cells, and platelets. Such reductions in turn result in anemia, bacterial infections, and spontaneous or excess bleeding.

Candidiasis: An infection with a yeast-like fungus of the Candida family, generally Candida albicans. Candidiasis of the esophagus, trachea, bronchi, or lungs is an indicator disease for AIDS. Oral or recurrent vaginal candida infection is an early sign of immune system deterioration.

Carnitine a compound that is required to transport long chain fatty acids across the inner membrane of the mitochondria, in the form of acyl-carnitine, where they can be metabolized for energy.

CD4 (T4) or CD4+ CELLS: A type of T cell involved in protecting against viral, fungal, and protozoal infections. These cells normally orchestrate the immune response, signaling other cells in the immune system to perform their special functions. Also known as T helper cells. HIV's preferred targets are cells that have a docking molecule called "cluster designation 4" (CD4) on their surfaces. Cells with this molecule are known as CD4- positive (or CD4+) cells. Destruction of CD4+ lymphocytes is the major cause of the immune deficiency observed in AIDS, and decreasing CD4+ lymphocyte levels appear to be the best indicator for developing opportunistic infections. Although CD4 counts fall, the total T cell level remains fairly constant through the course of HIV disease, due to a concomitant increase in the CD8+ cells. The ratio of CD4+ to CD8+ cells is therefore an important measure of disease progression.

Combination therapy: Two or more drugs or treatments used together to achieve optimum results against HIV infection and/or AIDS. Combination drug therapy has proven more effective in decreasing viral load than monotherapy (single-drug therapy). An example of combination therapy would be the use of two nucleoside analog drugs plus either a protease inhibitor or a non-nucleoside reverse transcription inhibitor.

Congestive heart failure (CHF) : a condition, in which the heart loses the ability to pump blood efficiently enough to meet the demands of the body. Symptoms may include edema (swelling), shortness of breath, weakness and exercise intolerance.

Crohn's disease : an inflammatory bowel disease that usually affects the lower part of the small intestine or upper part of the colon, but may affect any part of the gastrointestinal tract.

Cryptosporidiosis: A diarrheal disease caused by the protozoa Cryptosporidium which grows in the intestines. Symptoms include abdominal cramps and severe chronic diarrhea. It is considered an AIDS defining opportunistic infection in persons with HIV infection. Cryptosporidiosis usually occurs late in the course of HIV disease as immunological deterioration progresses.

Dementia : significant impairment of intellectual abilities such as attention, orientation, memory, judgment or language. By definition, dementia is not due to major depression or psychosis. Alzheimer's disease is the most common cause of dementia in older adults.

Dental caries : cavities or holes in the outer two layers of a tooth—the enamel and the dentin. Dental caries are caused by bacteria which metabolize carbohydrates (sugars).to form organic acids which dissolve tooth enamel.

Dermatitis : inflammation of the skin. This term is often used to describe a skin rash.

DEXA : dual energy X-ray absorptiometry. A precise instrument that uses the energy from very small doses of X-rays to determine bone mineral density (BMD) and to diagnose and follow the treatment of osteoporosis.

Diabetes mellitus : a chronic metabolic disease, characterized by abnormally high blood glucose (sugar) levels, resulting from the inability of the body to produce or respond to insulin. Type 1 diabetes mellitus, formerly known as insulin-dependent or juvenile-onset diabetes, is usually the result of autoimmune destruction of the insulin secreting beta-cells of the pancreas. The most common form of diabetes is type 2 diabetes mellitus, formerly known as noninsulin-dependent or adult onset diabetes, which develops when the tissues of the body become less sensitive to insulin secreted by the pancreas. Condition that occurs when there is (1) a fasting blood sugar level greater than or equal to 126 mg/dl on two separate occasions or (2) if diabetes symptoms exist and a blood sugar taken at any time is greater than or equal to 200, and a second test shows the same results.

Diabetic ketoacidosis : a potentially life-threatening condition characterized by ketosis (elevated levels of ketone bodies in the blood) and acidosis (increased acidity of the blood). Ketoacidosis occurs when diabetes is not adequately controlled.

Dialysis : a medical procedure to filter waste products from the blood. Dialysis is needed to perform the work of the kidneys if they can no longer function effectively. Two types of dialysis are hemodialysis and peritoneal dialysis.

Diuretic : an agent that increases the formation of urine by the kidneys, resulting in water loss from the individual using the diuretic.

DNA : deoxyribonucleic acid; a double-stranded nucleic acid composed of many nucleotides. The nucleotides in DNA are each composed of a nitrogen containing base (adenine, guanine, cytosine or thymine), a 5-carbon sugar (deoxyribose), and a phosphate group. The sequence of bases in DNA encodes the genetic information required to synthesize proteins.

DRUG-DRUG interaction: A modification of the effect of a drug when administered with another drug. The effect may be an increase or a decrease in the action of either substance, or it may be an adverse effect that is not normally associated with either drug.

Dyspnoea: Difficult or labored breathing.

Electrolytes : ionized (dissociated into positive and negative ions) salts in the body fluids. Major electrolytes in the body include sodium, potassium, magnesium, calcium, chloride, bicarbonate, phosphate.

Emphysema : a chronic obstructive pulmonary (lung) disease, characterized by damage to the small air sacs (alveoli) and difficulty breathing. Damage to the alveoli decreases their elasticity and results in hyperinflation of the lungs, which impairs gas exchange. Smoking is the most common cause of emphysema.

Enzyme : a biological catalyst. That is, a substance that increases the speed of a chemical reaction without being changed in the overall process. Enzymes are vitally important to the regulation of the chemistry of cells and organisms.

Erythema: Redness or inflammation of the skin or mucous membranes.

Fasting blood sugar: Test taken when you have not eaten eight to 12 hours before the blood draw to measure sugar in the blood .

Fatty acid : an organic acid molecule consisting of a chain of carbon molecules and a carboxylic acid (COOH) group. Fatty acids are found in fats, oils, and as components of a number of essential lipids, such as phospholipids and triglycerides. Fatty acids can be burned by the body for energy

Fortification : the addition of nutrients to foods to prevent or correct a nutritional deficiency, to balance the total nutrient profile of food, or to restore nutrients lost in processing. referring to or affecting the digestive tract, which includes the mouth, phyarynx (throat), esophagus, stomach and intestines.

Food-drug interaction: When food affects the ingredients in a medication, preventing the medicine from working the way it should. Some nutrients can affect the way certain drugs metabolize by binding with drug ingredients, thus reducing their absorption or speeding their elimination. Taking medicationsat the same time as eating may interfere with the stomach and intestines' absorption of medications.

Food security: When all people at all times have both physical and economic access to sufficient food to meet their dietary needs for a productive and healthy life. To be food secure, households and individuals need to have available food, access to food and the ability to fully utilize it once it is consumed.

Fortified foods: The addition of nutrients to foods for the purpose of ensuring the nutritional equivalence of substitute foods.

Gene : a region of DNA that controls a specific hereditary characteristic, usually corresponding to a single protein.

Gestation : the period of time between fertilization and birth. In humans, normal gestation is usually about 40 weeks.

Glucose : a 6-carbcn sugar which plays a major role in the generation of energy for living organisms. Major fuel source of the body, also known as blood sugar.

Glucose tolerance : the ability of the body to maintain normal glucose levels when challenged with a carbohydrate load (see impaired glucose tolerance

Glutathione : a tripeptide consisting of glutamate, cysteine and glyceine. Glutathione is an endogenous intracellular antioxidant, and is also required for some phase II biotransformation reactions.

Glycogen : a large polymer (repeating units) of glucose molecules, used to store energy in cells, especially muscle and liver cells.

Glycoside : a compound containing a sugar molecule that can be cleaved by hydrolysis to a sugar and a nonsugar component (aglycone).

Gout : a condition characterized by abnormally high blood levels of uric acid (urate). Urate crystals may form in joints, resulting in inflammation and pain. Urate crystals may also form in the kidney and urinary tract, resulting in kidney stones. The tendency to develop elevated blood uric acid levels and gout is often inherited.

HDL : high density lipoproteins. HDL transport cholesterol from the tissues to the liver where it can be eliminated in bile. HDL-cholesterol is considered good cholesterol, because higher blood levels of HDL-cholesterol are associated with lower risk of heart disease.

Heme : compounds of iron complexed in a characteristic ring structure known as a porphyrin ring.

Hemodialysis : the process of removing blood from an artery, removing waste products from the blood through dialysis, and returning it to the body through a vein. Hemodialysis is used to treat end stage renal failure.

Hemoglobin : the oxygen-carrying pigment in red blood cells.

Hemolysis : rupture of red blood cells.

Hemorrhage : excessive or uncontrolled bleeding.

Hepatitis : literally, inflammation of the liver. Hepatitis caused by a virus is known as viral hepatitis. Other causes of hepatitis include toxic chemicals and alcohol abuse.

Highly active antiretroviral therapy (HAART): The name given to treatment regimens recommended by leading HIV experts to aggressively suppress viral replication and progress of HIV disease. The usual HAART regimen combines three or more different drugs, such as two nucleoside reverse transcriptase inhibitors (NRTIs) and a protease inhibitor, two NRTIs and a non-nucleoside reverse transcriptase inhibitor (NNRTI), or other combinations. These treatment regimens have been shown to reduce the amount of virus so that it becomes undetectable in a patient's blood.

Hormone : a chemical, released by a gland or a tissue, which affects or regulates the activity of specific cells or organs. Complex bodily functions, such as growth and sexual development, are regulated by hormones.

Human papilloma virus (HPV) : a group of viruses that may cause papillomas (growths or warts) on the skin or other parts of the body, including the genitals and the larynx (voice box). Infection with particular strains of HPV is associated with increased risk of cervical cancer.

Hydrolysis : cleavage of a chemical bond by the addition of water. In hydrolysis reactions, a large compound may be broken down into smaller compounds when a molecule of water is added.

Hyperparathyroidism : excess secretion of parathyroid hormone by the parathyroid glands resulting in the disturbance of calcium metabolism. Symptoms may include increased blood levels of calcium (hypercalcemia), decreased blood levels of phosphorus, loss of calcium from bone, and kidney stone formation.

Hypertension : high blood pressure. Hypertension is defined by the Joint National Committee on Prevention, Detection, Evaluation and Treatment of High Blood Pressure as a systolic blood pressure of 140 mm Hg or higher and/or a diastolic blood pressure of 90 mm Hg or higher.

Hyperthyroidism : an excess of thyroid hormone which may result from an overactive thyroid gland or nodule, or from taking too much thyroid hormone.

Hypoglycemia : an abnormally low blood glucose concentration. Symptoms may include nausea, sweating, weakness, faintness, confusion hallucinations, headache, loss of consciousness, convulsions, or coma.

Hypoparathyroidism : a deficiency of parathyroid hormone, which may be characterized by low blood calcium levels (hypocalcemia).

Hypothalamus : An area at the base of the brain that regulates bodily functions, such as body temperature, hunger, and thirst.

Hypothyroidism : a deficiency of thyroid hormone which is normally made by the thyroid gland, located in the front of the neck.

Incontinence : inablility to control the evacuation of urine or feces.

Inflammation : a response to injury or infection, characterized by redness, heat, swelling, and pain. Physiologically, the inflammatory response involves a complex series of events, leading to the migration of white blood cells to the inflamed area.

Insulin: Hormone released into the blood by the pancreas. Insulin removes glucose and other nutrients from the blood and into cells where they are used or stored.

Insulin resistance: diminished responsiveness to insulin. - Term for when the normal amount of insulin is not enough to maintain normal blood glucose levels, causing the pancreas to release even more insulin.

Jaundice : a yellowish staining of the skin and whites of the eyes due to increased bilirubin (a bile pigment) levels in the blood. Jaundice can be an indicator of red blood cells rupturing (hemolysis), or disease of the liver or gallbladder.

Ketone bodies : any of three acidic chemicals (acetate, acetoacetate, and beta-hydroxybutyrate). Ketone bodies may accumulate in the blood (ketosis) when the body has inadequate glucose to use for energy, and must increase the use of fat for fuel. Ketone bodies are acidic, and very high levels in the blood are toxic and may result in ketoacidosis.

Kidney stones : solid masses resulting from the crystallization of minerals and other compounds found in urine. Common types of kidney stones include those composed of calcium oxalate, calcium phosphate and urate. Kidney stones may form in the kidney, ureters or urinary bladder.

LDL : low density lipoprotein. LDLs transport cholesterol from the liver to the tissues of the body. Elevated serum LDL-cholesterol is associated with increased cardiovascular disease risk.

Legumes : members of the large family of plants known as leguminosae. In this context the term refers to the fruits or seeds of leguminous plants (e.g., peas and beans) that are used for food.

Lens : the transparent structure inside the eye that focuses light rays onto the retina (the nerve cells at the back of the eye).

Leukemia : an acute or chronic form of cancer that involves the blood-forming organs. Leukemia is characterized by an abnormal increase in the number of white blood cells in the tissues of the body with or without a corresponding increase of those in the circulating blood, and is classified according to the type of white blood cell most prominently involved.

Leukocytes : white blood cells. Leukocytes are part of the immune system. Monocytes, lymphocytes, neutrophils, basophils and eosinophils are different types of leukocytes.

Lipids : a chemical term for fats. Lipids found in the human body include fatty acids, phospholipids, triglycerides and cholesterol.

Lipoproteins : particles composed of lipids and protein that allow for the transport of lipids through the bloodstream. A lipoprotein particle is composed of an outer layer of phospholipids, which renders it soluble in water, and a hydrophobic core that contains triglycerides and cholesterol esters. Different types of lipoproteins are distinguished by their surface proteins (apoproteins), their size and the types and amounts of lipids they contain.

Malabsorption syndrome: Decreased intestinal absorption resulting in loss of appetite, muscle pain, and weight loss.

Mastitis: An infection of the breast. It usually only occurs in women who are breastfeeding their babies. In the process, unaccustomed to the vigorous pull and tug of the infant's suck, the nipples may become sore, cracked, or slightly abraded. This creates a tiny opening in the breast, through which bacteria can enter. The presence of milk, with high sugar content, gives the bacteria an excellent source of nutrition. Under these conditions, the bacteria are able to multiply, until they are plentiful enough to cause an infection within the breast. Mastitis usually begins more than two to four weeks after delivery of the baby. Mastitis may increase the chances of HIV transmission from infected mother to child during breastfeeding.

Metabolism: The chemical changes in living cells by which energy is provided for vital processes and activities and new material is assimilated.

Methionine : a sulfur containing amino acid, required for protein synthesis and other vital metabolic processes. It can be obtained through the diet in protein or synthesized from homocysteine.

Micronutrient : a nutrient required by the body in small amounts, such as a vitamin or a mineral.

Migraine headache : a type of headache thought to be related to abnormal sensitivity of blood vessels (arteries) in the brain to various triggers resulting in rapid changes in the artery size due to spasm (constriction). Other arteries in the brain and scalp then open (dilate), and throbbing pain is perceived in the head. The tendency toward migraine appears to involve serotonin, a neurotransmitter that can trigger the release of vasoactive substances in the blood vessels.

Mitochondria : energy-producing structures within cells. Mitochondria possess two sets of membranes, a smooth continuous outer membrane, and an inner membrane arranged in folds. Among other critical functions, mitochondria convert nutrients into energy via the electron transport chain.

Morbidity: The condition of being diseased or sick; also the incidence of disease or rate of sickness.

Myocardial infarction (MI) : death (necrosis) of heart muscle tissue due to an interruption in its blood supply. Commonly known as a heart attack, an MI usually results from the obstruction of a coronary artery by a clot in people who have coronary atherosclerosis (heart disease).

Myopathy : any disease of muscle.

Nausea: A stomach distress with distaste for food and an urge to vomit.

Necrosis : unprogrammed cell death, in which cells break open and release their contents, promoting inflammation. Necrotic cell death may be the result of injury, infection or infarction.

Nephropathy : kidney damage or disease.

Neuropathy : nerve damage or disease.

Neurotoxic : toxic or damaging to nervous tissue (brain and peripheral nerves).

Neurotransmitter : a chemical that is released from a nerve cell and results in the transmission of an impulse to another nerve cell or organ (e.g., a muscle). Acetylcholine, dopamine, norepinephrine and serotonin are neurotransmitters.

Oedema : swelling; accumulation of excessive fluid in subcutaneous tissues (beneath the skin).

Osteoblasts : bone cells that are responsible for the formation of new bone mineral in the bone remodeling process.

Osteoclasts : bone cells that are responsible for the breakdown or resorption of bone in the bone remodeling process.

Osteomalacia : a disease of adults that is characterized by softening of the bones due to loss of bone mineral. Osteomalacia is characteristic of vitamin D deficiency in adults, while children with vitamin D deficiency suffer from rickets.

Osteoporosis : a condition of increased bone fragility and susceptibility to bone fracture due to a loss of bone mineral density (BMD)

Oxidation : a chemical reaction that removes electrons from an atom or molecule.

Oxidative stress : a condition, in which the effects of pro-oxidants (e.g. free radicals, reactive oxygen and reactive nitrogen species) exceed the ability of antioxidant systems to neutralize them.

Peripheral neuropathy : a disease or degenerative state affecting the nerves of the extremities (arms and legs). Symptoms may include numbness, pain, and muscle weakness.

Phosphorylation : the creation of a phosphate derivative of an organic molecule. This is usually achieved by transferring a phosphate group ($-PO_4$) from ATP to another molecule.

Placebo : an inert treatment that is given to a control group while the experimental group is given the active treatment. Placebo-controlled studies are conducted to make sure that the results are due to the experimental treatment, rather than another factor associated with participating in the study.

Pneumonia : a disease of the lungs, characterized by inflammation and accumulation of fluid in the lungs. Pneumonia may be caused by infectious agents (e.g., viruses or bacteria) or by inhalation of certain irritants.

Pneumonia (pneumocystis carinii pneumonia): An infection of the lungs caused by Pneumocystis carinii, which is thought to be a protozoa but may be more closely related to a fungus. P. carinii grows rapidly in the lungs of persons with AIDS and is a frequent AIDS-related cause of death. P. carinii infection sometimes may occur elsewhere in the body (skin, eye, spleen, liver, or heart).

Polymerase chain reaction (PCR): A laboratory process that selects a DNA segment from a mixture of DNA chains and rapidly replicates it to create a large, readily analyzed sample of a piece of DNA. As related to HIV: a sensitive laboratory technique that can detect and quantify HIV in a person's blood or lymph nodes (also called RT-PCR). It is an FDA-approved test to measure viral load.

RDA : recommended dietary allowance. Established by the Food and Nutrition Board of the Institute of Medicine, the RDA is the average daily dietary intake level of a nutrient sufficient to meet the requirements of nearly all healthy individuals in a specific life stage and gender group.

Retrovirus: A type of virus that, when not infecting a cell, stores its genetic nformation on a single-stranded RNA molecule instead of the more usual double-stranded DNA. HIV is an example of a retrovirus. After a retrovirus penetrates a cell, it constructs a DNA version of its genes using a special enzyme called reverse transcriptase. This DNA then becomes part of the cell's genetic material.

RNA : ribonuceic acid; a single-stranded nucleic acid composed of many nucleotides. The nucleotides in RNA are composed of a nitrogen containing base (adenine, guanine, cytosine or uracil), a 5-carbon sugar (ribose) and a phosphate group. RNA functions in the translation of the genetic information encoded in DNA to proteins.

Saturated fatty acid : a fatty acid with no double bonds between carbon atoms.

Sexually transmitted disease (STDs): Also called venereal disease (VD) (an older public health term) or sexually transmitted infections (STIs). Sexually transmitted diseases are infections spread by the transfer of organisms from person to person during sexual contact. In addition to the "traditional" STDs (syphilis and gonorrhea), the spectrum of STDs now includes HIV infection, which causes AIDS; Chlamydia trachomatis infections; human papilloma virus (HPV) infection; genital herpes; chancroid; genital mycoplasmas; hepatitis B; trichomoniasis; enteric infections; and ectoparasitic diseases (i.e., diseases caused by organisms that live on the outside of the host's body). The complexity and scope of STDs have increased dramatically since the 1980s; more than 20 micro-organisms and syndromes are now recognized as belonging in this category.

Syndrome : a combination of symptoms that occur together and is indicative of a specific condition or disease.

vasoconstriction : narrowing of a blood vessel.

Vasodilation : relaxation or opening of a blood vessel.

Virus a microorganism, which cannot grow or reproduce apart from a living cell. Viruses invade living cells and use the synthetic processes of infected cells to survive and replicate.

Vitamin : an organic (carbon-containing) compound necessary for normal physiological function that cannot be synthesized in adequate amounts, and must therefore be obtained in the diet.

Viral load test: In relation to HIV: Test that measures the quantity of HIV RNA in the blood. Results are expressed as the number of copies per milliliter of blood plasma.

Research indicates that viral load is a better predictor of the risk of HIV disease rogression than the CD4 count. The lower the viral load, the longer the time to AIDS diagnosis and the longer the survival time. Viral load testing for HIV infection is being used to determine when to initiate and/or change therapy.

Viral replication: There are generally six steps that take place in viral replication. Adsorption (attachment to the host cell), penetration, uncoating, genome replication (viral synthesis), maturation, and release.

Xenograft : a transplant of tissue from a donor of one species to a recipient of another species.

Zollinger-Ellison syndrome : a rare disorder caused by a tumor called a gastrinoma, most often occurring in the pancreas. The tumor secretes the hormone gastrin, which causes increased production of gastric acid leading to severe recurrent ulcers of the esophagus, stomach, and the upper portions of the small intestine.

Bibliography

A Bendich, "Antioxidant Nutrients and Immune Functions - Introduction", pp 1-12 *Antioxidant Nutrients and Immune Function*, ed A Bendich, M Phillips, RP Tengerdy, Plenum Press (Advances in Experimental Medicine and Biology, v 262, 1990).

Agatston AS. The end of the diet debates? All fats and carbohydrates are not created equal. *Cleve Clin J Med*. 72(10):946-50, 2005.

American Diabetes Association. Nutrition recommendations and principles for people with diabetes mellitus. Diabetes Care **2000**; 23(Suppl 1):S43-6

Amorosa, V. and others. A tale of two epidemics: the intersection between obesity and HIV infection in Philadelphia. *JAIDS*. 39(5): 557-561. August 15, 2005.

Ashbrook, D. W., "Carnitine Supplementation in Human Carnitine Deficiency", pp 120-134 in *Clinical Aspects of Human Carnitine Deficiency*, ed. P. R. Borum, Pergamon Press, 1986.

AM Tang, NMH Graham, AJ Kirby, D McCall, WC Willett, AJ Saah, "Dietary Micronutrient Intake and Risk of Progression to Acquired Immunodeficiency Syndrome (AIDS) in Human Immunodeficiency Virus Type 1 (HIV-1)-infected Homosexual Men", *Amer J Epidemiology 138*:1993:937-951.

Association of Nutrition Services Agencies. Nutrition guidelines for agencies providing food to people living with HIV disease, 2nd ed. Washington, DC: ANSA; **2002**. Available at: http://www.aidsnutrition.org/Guidelines.aspx.

Agarwal KN, Tripathi AM, Sen S, Kaliyar GP. (1974). Physical growth and adolescence. *Ind. Paediatr.*, **11:** 93-97.

Baum, M.K. and others. High risk of HIV-related mortality is associated with selenium deficiency. *JAIDS*. 15(5): 370-374, August 15, 1997.

Baum MK and others, "Micronutrients and HIV-1 disease progression", *AIDS* 9:1995:1051-1056.

Baum MK, Shor Posner G, Zhang G, et al. HIV-1 infection in women is associated with severe nutritional deficiencies. J Acquir Immune Defic Syndr Hum Retrovirol **1997**; 16:2728

Baum MK, Cure N, Shor-Posner G, "The B-Complex Vitamins, Immune Regulation, Cognitive Function, and HIV-1 Infection", Chapter 7 in *Nutrition and AIDS*, ed. RR Watson, CRC Press, Boca Raton, 1994.

Bendich A, "A Role for Carotenoids in Immune Function", *Clinical Nutrition* 7:1988:113-117.

Bendich A, "Antioxidant Nutrients and Immune Functions - Introduction", in *Antioxidant Nutrients and Immune Functions*, ed. A Bendich, M Phillips, RP Tengerdy, Series Advances in Experimental Medicine and Biology, Plenum Press, 1990.

Bendich A, "Antioxidant Vitamins and their Functions in Immune Responses", in *Antioxidant Nutrients and Immune Functions*, ed. A Bendich, M Phillips, RP Tengerdy, Series Advances in Experimental Medicine and Biology, Plenum Press, 1990b.

Brown P, Crane L. Avascular necrosis of bone in patients with human immunodeficiency virus infection: report of 6 cases and review of the literature. Clin Infect Dis **2001**; 32:12216.

Buhl, R., Jaffe, H. A., Holroyd, K. J., Wells, F. B., Mastrangeli, A., Saltini, C., Cantin, A. M., Crystal, R. G., "Systematic Glutathione Deficiency in Symptom-free HIV-seropositive Individuals", Lancet *2*(1989)1294-1298.

Babat, R. and others. Safety and efficacy of zinc supplementation for children with HIV-1 infection in South Africa: a randomised double-blind placebo-controlled trial. *The Lancet* 366(9500): 1862-1867. November 26, 2005.

B de Quay, R Malinverni, BH Lauterberg, "Glutathione depletion in HIV-infected patients: role of cysteine deficiency and effect of oral N-acetylcysteine", *AIDS* 6:1992:815-819

Boomgarden, ZT Definitions of the Insulin Resistance Syndrome, The 1st World Congress on the Insulin Resistance Syndrome. *Diabetes Care*. 27:3,824-830, 2004.

Braverman, E. R., Pfeiffer, C. C., *The Healing Nutrients Within*, Keats Publishing, Inc., 1987.

Campa, A. and others. HIV-related wasting in HIV-infected drug users in the era of highly active antiretroviral therapy. *CID* 41(8): 1179-1185. October 15, 2005.

Campell, T.C. and Haynes, J.R. Role of Nutrition in the Drug - metabolizing Enzyme System. 1974 Pharmacological Reviews, 26 (3): 171-197.

Carr A, Cooper DA. Adverse effects of antiretroviral therapy. Lancet **2000**; 356:142330.

Chandra RK, "Excessive Intake of Zinc Impairs Immune Responses", *JAMA* 252:1984:1443-1446.

Chandra, R. K., "Micronutrients and Immune Functions - An Overview", in *Micronutrients and Immune Functions: Cytokines and Metabolism*, Ann. N. Y. Acad. Sci. *587*(1990)9-16.

Chlebowski RT, Grosvenor MB, Bernhard NH, et al. Nutritional status, gastrointestinal dysfunction, and survival in patients with AIDS. Am J Gastroenterol **1989**; 4:128892

C. H. Halsted, R. B. Rucke; *Nutrition and the Origins of Disease*, ed. r, Academic Press, 1989. *Nutrition & HIV*, Proceedings of the 1992 International Symposium on Nutrition and HIV/AIDS including the Nutrition Algorithm and Nutrition Initiative of the Physicians Association for AIDS Care.

Clark, TD, and RD Semba. 2001. Iron supplementation during human immunodeficiency virus infection: A double-edged sword? *Med Hypotheses* 57(4):476-79.

Coodley and others, "ß-Carotene in HIV Infection", *J Acquir Immun Deficien Syndr* 6:1993:272-276.

Coodley GO, "Vitamins in HIV Infection", Chapter 7 in *Nutrition and AIDS*, ed. RR Watson, CRC Press, Boca Raton, 1994.

Currier, J. S. Metabolic Complications of antiretroviral therapy and HIV infection. *Medscape HIV/AIDS Annual Update* 2001.

DJ Reed, "Interaction of Vitamin E, Ascorbic Acid, and Glutathione in Protection Against Oxidative Damage", pp 269-281 *Vitamin E in Health and Disease* (Chapter 21), ed L Packer, J Fuchs, Marcel Dekker, 1993.

D GerardMonnier, J Chaudiere, "Metabolism and antioxidant function of glutathione", *Pathologie Biologie* 44:1996:75-85.

D. P. Kotler, Gastrointestinal and Nutritional Manifestations of the Acquired Immunodeficiency Syndrome, ed., Raven Press, 1991. Journal of . Nutrition 122(1992) - Symposium: History of Nutritional Immunology.

DP Stites, AI Terr, *Basic and Clinical Immunology*, Appleton & Lange, 1991.

de Quay, B., Malinverni, R., Lauterburg, B. H., "Glutathione Depletion in HIV-Infected Patients: Role of Cysteine Deficiency and Effect of Oral N-acetylcysteine", AIDS *6*(1992)815-819.

Expert Group of ICMR. (1981). *Recommended Dietary Intakes for Indians.* New Delhi: Indian Council of Medical Research.

Expert Group of ICMR. (1990). *Nutrient Requirements and Recommended Dietary Allowances for Indians.* New Delhi: Indian Council of Medical Research.

FASEB Life Sciences Research Office, FDA Contract No. 223-88-2124, 1990.

Nutrition and HIV Infection: A Review and Evaluation of the Extant Knowledge of the Relationship between Nutrition and HIV Infection,

Galvin TAG, "Micronutrients: Implications in human immunodeficiency virus disease", *Top Clin Nutr* 7:1992:63-73.

GE Kaugars, S Silverman, JGL Lovas, RB Brandt, JS Thompson, "A Review of the Use of Antioxidant Supplements in the Treatment of Human Oral Leukoplakia", *J Cell Biochem 17F*:1993:S292-S298.

GL Gilliland, "Glutathione proteins", *Current Opinion in Structural Biology* 3:1993:875-884.

Gorbach SL, Knox TA, Roubenoff R. Interaction between nutrition and infection with human immunodeficiency virus. Nutr Rev **1993**; 51:22634.

G Pantaleo, C Graziosi, AC Fauci, "The Immunopathogenesis of Human Immunodeficiency Virus Infection", *N Engl J Med 328*:1993:327-335.

Granberry MC, Fonseca VA. Cardiovascular risk factors associated with insulin resistance: effects of oral antidiabetic agents. *Am J Cardiovasc Drugs*. 5(3):201-9, 2005.

Grunfeld, C., "Metabolic Disturbances, Anorexia, and Wasting in HIV/AIDS", Proc. of the 1992 International Symposium on

Nutrition and HIV/AIDS including the Nutrition Algorithm and Nutrition Initiative of the Physicians Association for AIDS Care, Nutrition & HIV/AIDS, 1(1992)9-15.

Guengerich, F.P. Effects of Nutritive Factors on Metabolic Process Involving Bioactivation and Detoxification of Chemicals. 1984 Annual Review Nutrition, 4:207-231.

GT Keusch, DM Thea, "Malnutrition in AIDS", *Med Clin N.A.* 77:1993:795-814.

Guenter P, Muurahainen N, Simons G, et al. Relationships among nutritional status disease progression, and survival in HIV infection. J Acquir Immune Defic Syndr **1993**; 6:11308

Gopalan C, Ramashastry BY, Balasubramaniam Sc. Table of Food Composition: Nutritive Value of Indian Foods. National Institute of Nutrition, Indian Council of Medical Re-search, Hyderabad, 1993.

Gopalan C, Ramasastry BV, Balasubramanyam SC, Narasinga Rao BS, Deosthale YG, Pant KC. (1990). *Nutritive Value of Indian Foods.* Hyderabad: National Institute Of Nutrition.

Hart, A.M. and others. Acetyl-l-carnitine: a pathogenesis based treatment for HIV-associated antiretroviral toxic neuropathy. *AIDS* 18(11): 1549-1560. July 23, 2004.

Hadigan C, Rabe J, Grinspoon S. Sustained benefits of metformin therapy on markers of cardiovascular risk in human immunodeficiency virus-infected patients with fat redistribution and insulin resistance. *J Clin Endocrinol Metab*. 87(10):4611-5, 2002.

Heredia, A. and others. In vitro suppression of latent HIV-1 activation by vitamin E: potential clinical implications. *AIDS* 19(8): 836-837. May 20, 2005.

Hellerstein, M. K., "Pathophysiology of Lean Body Wasting and Nutrient Unresponsiveness in HIV/AIDS: Therapeutic Implications", Proc. 1992 Internat. Symp. on Nutrition and HIV/AIDS, including the Nutrition Algorithm and Nutrition Initiative of the Physicians Association for AIDS Care, Nutrition and HIV/AIDS *1*(1992)17-25.

Hunt, S. M., Groff, J. L., *Advanced Nutrition and Human Metabolism*, West Publishing Co., 1990.

Hamill PVV, Drizd TA, Johnson CL, Reed RB, Roche AF, Moore WM. (1979). Physical growth: National Centre for Health Statistics percentiles. *Am. J. Clin. Nutr.,* **32:** 607-629. MEDLINE

J Arnaud, P Chappuis, MC Jaudon, J Bellanger, "Biological Indices Used for the Assessment of Zinc, Copper and Selenium Status in Huamns", *Annales de Biol Clinique* 51:1993:589-604.

J Jensen, MBA, MPH, RD, monographs "Modern Food Safety", "Anyone for Another Dozen Pills?", "Diarrhea", "Diarrhea and What you Can do About It", "Mouth Care", "What About Dairy?", "Body Weight Basics", "Your Weight-Gain Program".

JE Kinsella, B Lokesh, S Broughton, J Whelan, "Dietary Polyunsaturated Fatty Acids and Eicosanoids: Potential Effects on the Modulation of Inflammatory and Immune Cells: An Overview", Nutrition *6*(1990)S24-S44.

JT La Brooy, "Enteropathy in HIV Infection", *J acquir immun defic syndr 6*:1993:S16-S19.

JM Jacobson, JS Greenspan, J Spritzler, N Ketter, JL Fahey, JB Jackson, L Fox, M Chermoff, AW Wu, LA MacPhail, GJ Vasquez, DA Wohl, "Thalidomide for the treatment of oral aphthous ulcers in patients with human immunodeficiency virus infection", *N Engl J Med 336*:1997:1487-1493.

Jelliffee DB. (1966). *Assessment of the nutritional status of the community.* WHO Monograph Series no. 53. Geneva: WHO.

Krishnaswamy K, Vijayaraghavan K, Shastry JG. Twenty Five Years of National Nutrition. Monitoring Bureau: National Institute of Nutrition, Indian Council of Medical Research, Hyderabad,1997.

Kelley DS and others, "Effects of low-copper diets on human immune response", *Am J Clin Nutr* 62:1995:412-416.

Knowler WC, Barrett-Connor E, Fowler SE, Hamman RF, Lachin JM, Walker EA, Nathan DM; Diabetes Prevention Program Research Group. Reduction in the incidence of type 2 diabetes with lifestyle intervention or metformin. *N Engl J Med.* 7;346(6):393-403, 2002.

Kotler, D. P., "Causes and Consequences of Malnutrition in HIV/AIDS", Proc. of the 1992 International Symposium on Nutrition and HIV/AIDS including the Nutrition Algorithm and Nutrition Initiative of the Physicians Association for AIDS Care, Nutrition & HIV/AIDS, 1(1992)5-8.

Layman DK, Evans E, Baum JI, Seyler J, Erickson DJ, Boileau RA. Dietary protein and exercise have additive effects on body composition during weight loss in adult women. *J Nutr.* 135(8):1903-10, 2005.

LA Herzenberg, SC De Rosa, JG Dubs, M Roederer, MT Anderson, SW Ela, SC Deresinski, LA Herzenberg, "Glutathione deficiency is associated with impaired survival in HIV disease", *Proc Natl Acad Sci USA* 94:1997:1967-1972.

L Badgley, *Healing AIDS Naturally*, Human Energy Press, 1986.

JD Bogden, H Baker, O Frank, G Perez, F Kemp, K Bruening, D Louria, "Micronutrient Status and Immunodeficiency Virus (HIV) Infection", Micronutrients and Immune Functions: Cytokines and Metabolism, *Ann N.Y. Acad Sci* 587:1990:189-195.

Jaeckel E, Cornberg M, Wedemeyer H, Santantonio T, Mayer J, Zankel M, Pastore G, Dietrich M, Trautwein C, Manns MP (Nov 2001). "Treatment of acute hepatitis C with interferon alfa-2b". New England Journal of Medicine ***345*** *(20): 1452-1457.* PMID 11794193.

Lohninger, A., Kaiser, E., Legenstein, E., Staniek, H., "Carnitine, Metabolism and Function", pp 1-25 in *Carnitine -It s Role in Lung and Heart Disorders*, ed. E. Kaiser, A. Lohninger, Karger, 1987.

Los Angeles County Commission on HIV Health Services. Guidelines for implementing HIV/AIDS Medical Nutrition Therapy protocols. Los Angeles, CA: Los Angeles County Commission on HIV Health Services, **1999**

McGovern B, Wurcel A, Kim A, Schulze zur Wiesch J, Bica I, Zaman M, Timm J, Walker B, Lauer G (2006). "Acute hepatitis C virus infection in incarcerated injection drug users.". Clin Infect Dis ***42*** *(12): 1663-70.* PMID 16705568.

McComsey, G. and others. Effect of antioxidants on glucose metabolism and plasma lipids in HIV-infected subjects with lipoatrophy. *JAIDS* 33(5): 605-607. August 15, 2003.

Mangili, A. Metabolic Syndrome and Markers of Early Atherosclerosis in a Cohort of HIV-infected Subjects from Nutrition for Health Living (Abstract 861). Abstract presented at the 12th Conference on Retroviruses and Opportunistic Infections, Boston, USA. February, 2005.

Miller, E. and other. Meta-analysis: high-dosage vitamin E supplementation may increase all-cause mortality. *Annals of Internal Medicine* 142(1): 37-46. January 4, 2005.

MK Baum, L Cassetti, P Bonvehi, G Shor-posner, Y Lu, H Sauberlich, "Inadequate Dietary Intake and Altered Nutrition Status in Early HIV-1 Infection", *Nutrition 10*:1994:16-20;

Monier P, McKown K, Bronze MS. Osteonecrosis complicating highly active antiretroviral therapy in patients infected with human immunodeficiency virus. Clin Infect Dis **2000**; 31:148892

Mori TA, Bao DQ, Burke V, Puddey IB, Watts GF, Beilin LJ. Dietary fish as a major component of a weight-loss diet: effect on serum lipids, glucose, and insulin metabolism in overweight hypertensive subjects. *Am J Clin Nutr*. 70(5):817-25, 1999.

M Ott, B Lembcke, H Fischer, R Jäger, H Polat, H Geier, M Rech, S Staszeswki, EB Helm, WF Caspary, "Early Changes of Body Composition in Human Immunodeficiency Virus-infected Patients: Tetrapolar Body Impedance Analysis Indicates Significant Malnutrition", *Am J Clin Nutr* 57:1993:15-19.

NIH Consensus Development Panel on Osteoporosis, Prevention, Diagnosis, and Therapy. Osteoporosis prevention, diagnosis, and therapy. JAMA **2001**; 285:78595

Negredo E, Gel S, Arisa ER, et al. Bone mineral density (BMD) in HIV-1infected patients [abstract 626]. In: Program and abstracts of the 8th Conference on Retroviruses and Opportunistic Infections (Chicago). Washington, DC: Foundation for Retroviruses and Human Health, **2001**; 232.

National Family Health Survey-Bihar. Mumbai, International Institute for Population Sciences, 1995.

National Nutrition Monitoring Bureau. (1999). *Report of Second Repeat Survey¾Rural (1996-1997).* Hyderabad: NIN.

Nutrition Foundation of India. (1989). *Growth of affluent Indian girls during adolescence.* Scientific Report no. 10, pp 41-48, New Delhi: Nutritional Foundation of India.

Office of Special Health Issues and Division of Antiviral Drug Products. Nucleoside reverse transcriptase inhibitor (NRTI) and non-nucleoside reverse transcriptase inhibitor (NNRTI) drug interactions. Washington, DC: US Food and Drug Administration, **2001**

Pan XR, Li GW, Hu YH, Wang JX, Yang WY, An ZX, Hu ZX, Lin J, Xiao JZ, Cao HB, Liu PA, Jiang XG, Jiang YY, Wang JP, Zheng H, Zhang H, Bennett PH, Howard BV. Effects of diet and exercise in preventing NIDDM in people with impaired glucose tolerance. The Da Qing IGT and Diabetes Study. *Diabetes Care* 1997;20:537-44.

Periquet BA and others, "Micronutrient levels in HIV-1 infected children", *AIDS* 9:1995:887-893.

P. Singer, D. P. Katz, L. Dillon, O. Kirvelä, T. Lazarus, J. Askanazi, Amer. J. Gastroent*; Nutritional Aspects of the Acquired Immunodeficiency Syndrome,. 87*(1992)265-273.

Reaven GM. The insulin resistance syndrome: definition and dietary approaches to treatment. *Annu Rev Nutr*. 25:391-406, 2005.

RS Rivlin, "The Clinical Significance of Micronutrients in Relation to Immune Functions", in *Micronutrients and Immune Functions: Cytokines and Metabolism, Ann NY Acad Sci 587*:1990:55-58.

Recommended Dietary Allowances(RDA), 10th edition, National Academy Press, 1989.

R Ullrich, M Zeitz, W Heise, M L'age, G Hö ken, EO Riecken, "Small Intestinal Structure and Function in Patients Infected with Human Immunodeficiency Virus (HIV): Evidence for HIV-Induced Enteropathy", *Ann Intern Med 111*:1989:15-21.

Sabin, C. Changes Over Time in the Use of Antiretroviral Therapy and Risk Factors for Cardiovascular Disease in the D:A:D Study (Abstract 866). 12th Conference on Retroviruses and Opportunistic Infections, Boston, USA. February 2005.

S Baruchel, G Bounous, P Gold, "Place for an antioxidant therapy in human immunodeficiency virus (HIV) infection", in *Oxidative Stress, Cell Activation and Viral Infection*, ed. C Pasquier et al, Birkhäuser Verlag, Basel, 1994.

SM Hunt, JL Groff, *Advanced Nutrition and Human Metabolism*, West Publishing Co., 1990.

Shevitz, A. and Knox, T. Nutrition in the era of highly active antiretroviral therapy. *CID* 32(12): 1769-75. June 15, 2001.

Sabin, C. Deaths in the Era of HAART: Contributions of Abnormal Lipid and Liver Function Markers (Abstract 957). 12th Conference on Retroviruses and Opportunistic Infections, Boston, USA, February 2005.

S Cunningham-Rundles, "Nutritional Factors in Immune Response", pp 233-244, *Malnutrition: Determinants and Consequences*, ed., PL White, N Selvey, AR Liss, 1984.

Shevitz, A. and Knox, T. Nutrition in the era of highly active antiretroviral therapy. *CID* 32(12): 1769-75. June 15, 2001.

Singer P, Katz DP, Dillon L, Kirvelä O, Lazarus T, Askanazi J, "Nutritional Aspects of the Acquired Immunodeficiency Syndrome", 87:1992:265-273.

Singer, P., Katz, D. P., Dillon, L., Kirvelä, O., Lazarus, T., Askanazi, J., "Nutritional Aspects of the Acquired Immunodeficiency Syndrome", *The American Journal of Gastroenterology,. 87*(1992)265-273.

Sirtori CR, Paoletti R, Mancini M, Crepaldi G, Manzato E, Rivellese A, Pamparana F, Stragliotto E. N-3 fatty acids do not lead to an increased diabetic risk in patients with hyperlipidemia and abnormal glucose tolerance. Italian Fish Oil Multicenter Study. *Am J Clin Nutr*. 65(6):1874-81, 1997.

SM Finegold, WL George, editors, *Anaerobic Infections in Humans*, Academic Press, 1989.

S. M. Hunt, J. L. Groff,, *Advanced Nutrition and Human Metabolism*, West Publishing Co., 1990. *Annals of the New York Academy of Sciences*, vol. 585 (about vitamin B_6), 1990.

Storlien LH. KANWU Study. Substituting dietary saturated for monounsaturated fat impairs insulin sensitivity in healthy men and women: The KANWU Study. *Diabetologia*. 44(3):312-9, 2001.

Sutinen, J. and others. Uridine supplementation increases subcutaneous fat in patients with HAART-associated lipodystrophy: a randomised placebo-controlled trial. 7th International Workshop on Adverse Drug Reactions and Lipodystrophy in HIV. Abstract 7.

Siegel S. **(1956).** ***Non-parametric Statistics for the Behavioural Services.*** **New York: McGraw-Hill.**

TA Galvin, "Micronutrients: Implications in Human Immunodeficiency Virus Disease", *Top Clin Nutr* 7:1992:63-73.

Tang, A.M. and others. Increasing risk of 5% or greater unintentional weight loss in a cohort of HIV-infected patients, 1995-2003. *JAIDS* 40(1): 70-76. September 1, 2005.

Tang, A.M. and others. Micronutrients: current issues for HIV care providers. *AIDS* 19(9): 847-861. June 10, 2005.

Tang A and others, "The Effect of Micronutrient Intake on Survival in HIV-1 Infection", presentation by N Graham, Toronto, 1995.

Tuomilehto J, Lindstrom J, Eriksson JG, Valle TT, Hamalainen H, Ilanne-Parikka P, Keinanen-Kiukaanniemi S, Laakso M, Louheranta A, Rastas M, Salminen V, Uusitupa M; Finnish Diabetes Prevention Study Group. Prevention of type 2 diabetes mellitus by changes in lifestyle among subjects with impaired glucose tolerance. *N Engl J Med* 2001;344:1343-50.

Tershakovec AM, Frank I, Rader D. HIV-related lipodystrophy and related factors. *Atherosclerosis*. 174(1):1-10, 2004.

Tomazic J, Karner P, Vidmar L, Maticic M, Sharma PM, Janez A . Effect of metformin and rosiglitazone on lipid metabolism in HIV infected patients receiving protease inhibitor containing HAART. *Acta Dermatovenerol Alp Panonica Adriat.* 14(3):99-105, 2005.

Ullrich R, "HIV Enteropathy", International Conference Nutrition and HIV Infection, Cannes, 1995.

Ullrich and others, "Serum Carotene Deficiency in HIV-Infected Patients", *AIDS* 8:1994:661-665.

Van de Laar FA, Lucassen PL, Akkermans RP, Van de Lisdonk EH, Rutten GE, Van Weel C. Alpha-glucosidase inhibitors for type 2 diabetes mellitus. *Cochrane Database Syst.* Apr 18;(2):CD003639, 2005.

Vessby B, Unsitupa M, Hermansen K, Riccardi G, Rivellese AA, Tapsell LC, Nalsen C, Berglund L, Louheranta A, Rasmussen BM, Calvert GD, Maffetone A, Pedersen E Gustafsson IB, Wohl, D.A. and others. Randomized study of the safety and efficacy of fish oil (omega-3 fatty acid) supplementation with dietary and exercise counseling for the treatment of antiretroviral therapy-associated hypertriglyceridemia. *CID* 41(10): 1498-1504. November 15, 2005.

Vijayaraghavan K, Singh D, Swaminathan MC. (1971). Heights and weights of well nourished Indian School Ghildren. *Ind. J. Med. Res.,* **59:** 648-654.

WR Beisel, "Trace Elements in Infectious Processes", *Med Clin N. A.* 60:1976:831-849.

WR Beisel, "Single Nutrients and Immunity", *Am J Clin Nutr 35*:1982:S417-S468.

WHO. (1995). *Physical status: the use and interpretation of anthropometry*. WHO Technical Report Series no. 854. Geneva: WHO.

Yarasheski KE, Tebas P, Stanerson B, et al. Resistance exercise training reduces hypertriglyceridemia in HIV-infected men treated with antiviral therapy. J Appl Physiol **2001**; 90:1338.

Zazzo JF and others, "Effect of Zinc on the Immune Status of Zinc-depleted AIDS Related Complex Patients", *Clin Nutr* 8:1989:259-261.

Index

D

E

F

I

J

K

L

M

W

Y

Z